CW01669120

DIABETES & YOU

The essential guide

NEW EDITION

FORMERLY DIABETES & YOU

AN OWNER'S MANUAL

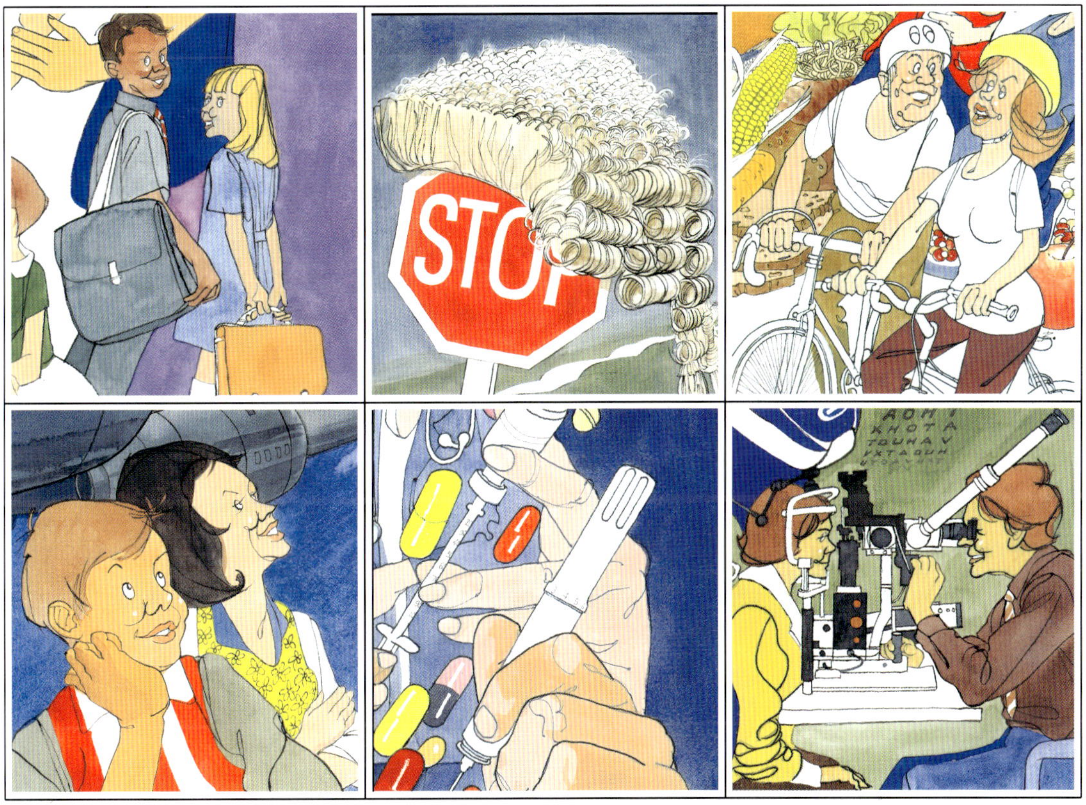

The official reference
for people with diabetes

DIABETES AUSTRALIA

- First published 1991
  Under the title
  Diabetes & You – An owner's manual
  by Diabetes Australia
- Reprinted June, 1993
- Second edition May, 1994

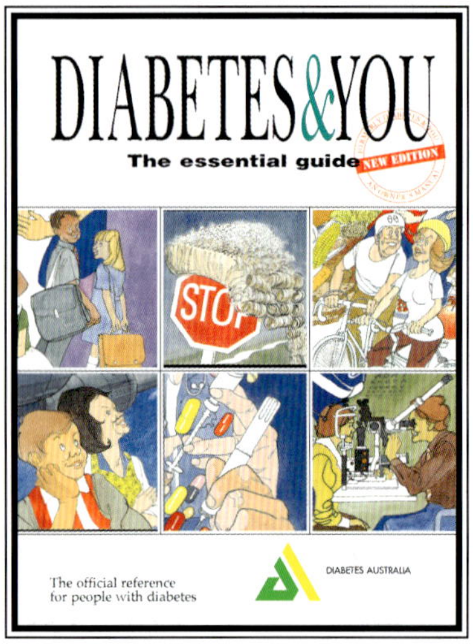

Publishers: Diabetes Australia
Editor-in-Chief: Dr Pat Phillips
Editors: Lynette Brown, Trisha Dunning, Bernie Ayers
Design and Production: Stephen Dennis
News Management, Pyrmont, NSW
Editorial Coordinator: Joanne Sainsbury
Writer: Susie Foster
Illustrator: Earl Budden
Printers: Phoenix Offset
Typesetting: Graphic Type, Mudgeeraba, Qld.
Sponsor: Aza Research Pty Ltd
ISBN: 1-875690-14-X

© Diabetes Australia, 1999

This work is copyright. Reproduction for educational use is encouraged. Reproduction for commercial usage or sale requires written permission from Diabetes Australia, Canberra.

DIABETES AUSTRALIA
A.C.N. 008 528 461

An Australian Company supporting Australian Research

Contents

INTRODUCTION

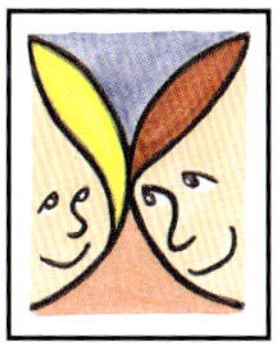

1. Living with someone with type 1 diabetes 1
2. Living with diabetes 3
3. Diabetes – what goes wrong? 5

MANAGEMENT AND LIFESTYLE

4. Diabetes and Lifestyle 8
5. Healthy Eating and Diabetes 10
6. The Use of Tablets 14
7. Diabetes and Exercise 16

INSULIN AND MONITORING

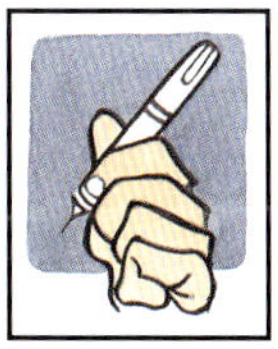

8. Insulin and its Role 21
9. Injections and Injectors 25
10. Self-monitoring of Blood Glucose 31
11. Testing Urine 36
12. Hypoglycaemia and Hyperglycaemia 39
13. Diabetes and Other Medications 43
14. Sick Days – Feeling Unwell? 47

COMPLICATIONS

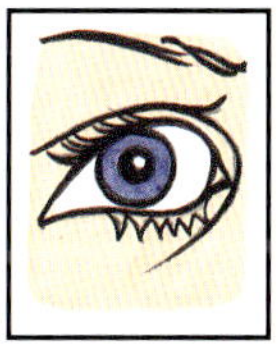

15. Long Term Complications of Diabetes 51
16. Diabetes and Eyes 56
17. Foot Care and Foot Wear 59
18. Diabetes and Oral Health 62
19. Sexual Problems in Men 64
20. Diabetes and Women's Health 66
   – Diabetes and Pregnancy 68
   – Diabetes, Menopause and Hormone Replacement Therapy (HRT) 72

SPECIAL GROUPS

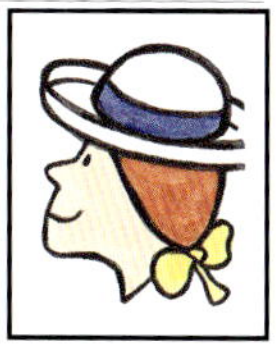

21. The School Child with Diabetes 76
22. Diabetes and Teenagers 80
23. Diabetes in the Elderly 82
24. Diabetes in Aboriginal People 86
25. Diabetes – A Problem in Any Language 89

SOCIAL ISSUES

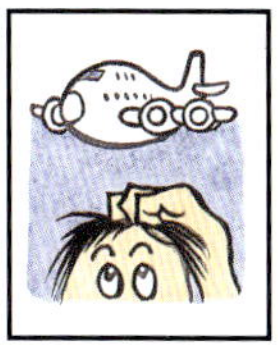

26. How to Work with Your Health Care Team 93
27. Rights and Responsibilities 96
28. Diabetes in General Practice 99
29. Travelling with Diabetes 101
30. Diabetes and Discrimination 107
31. Insurance and Diabetes 110
32. Further Resources 113

SPECIAL ISSUES

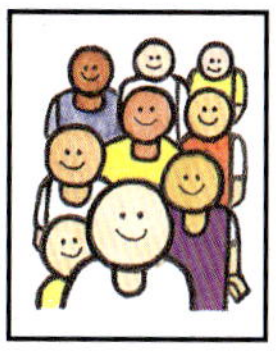

33. The Genetics of Diabetes 117
34. Around the World with Diabetes 120
35. The Impact of Diabetes 123
36. National Diabetes Strategy 126
37. Diabetes: Back to the Future 128

Quick Read **132**

Glossary **138**

Abbreviations and measures **142**

Index **143**

Your information ally

THE key to successfully living with diabetes is information. *Diabetes & You – The essential guide* contains the most comprehensive and up to date information available on diabetes management.

Based on *Diabetes & You – An owner's manual*, which sold over 20,000 copies, the essential guide contains more chapters from Australia's leading experts in diabetes education and care and is the official reference guide of Diabetes Australia.

My sincere thanks must go to the authors who without their contributions this book would not have happened, and to the editorial and production teams who did a marvellous job in bringing all the contributions together into an easy to read and professional publication.

Special mention must also be made of the generosity of Aza Research for sponsoring *the essential guide* and the two other books in the *Diabetes & You* series – *Living with Insulin* and *All About Type 2 Diabetes*.

If you have diabetes *the essential guide* will provide you with the knowledge needed to fight diabetes and to take charge of your life. If you care for someone with diabetes or have a person with diabetes in your family, or you are a health professional, this book will be an invaluable guide.

LAWRENCE BURR
National President
Diabetes Australia

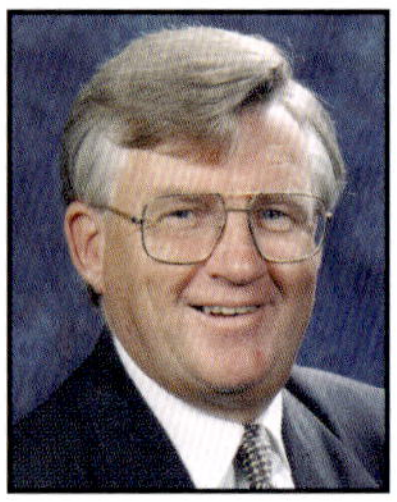

Acknowledgments

Diabetes Australia is grateful to the following experts in diabetes education and care for contributing their time to ensure the continuing success of this book.

Bernie Ayers
Health Promotion and Research
Diabetes Australia
Braddon, ACT

Jeannette Baldwin
National Diabetes Strategy
Diabetes Australia
Braddon, ACT

Karen Barfoot
Chief Executive Officer
Juvenile Diabetes Foundation Australia
St Leonards, NSW

Dr Kerry Bowen
Diabetes Education Centre
Royal Newcastle Hospital
Newcastle, NSW

Lynette Brown
Department of Nutrition
Canberra Hospital
Woden, ACT

Associate Professor Lesley Campbell
Diabetes Centre
St Vincent's Hospital
Darlinghurst, NSW

Dr John Carter
Department of Endocrinology
Hornsby and Ku-ring-gai Hospital, and Concord Hospital
Concord, NSW

Professor Don Chisholm
Metabolic Research Program
Garvan Institute of Medical Research
Darlinghurst, NSW

Dr Thomas Cromer
Potency Enhancement Clinic
Concord Repatriation General Hospital
Concord, NSW

Diabetes Education Service
The Queen Elizabeth Hospital
Woodville, SA

Tony Diment
Diabetes Centre
Royal North Shore Hospital
St Leonards, NSW

Trisha Dunning
Diabetes Education
St Vincent's Hospital
Fitzroy, VIC

Angela Evans
Podiatrist
Oaklands Park, SA

Gillian Harris
Diabetes Centre
Royal North Shore Hospital
St Leonards, NSW

Professor Leonard Harrison
The Walter and Eliza Hall Institute of Medical Research
Royal Melbourne Hospital
Parkville, VIC

Dr Chris Holmwood
General Practitioner
Tusmore, SA

Joy Horton
Research Scientist
Abbotsford, VIC

Dr Warren Kidson
Department of Endocrinology
Prince of Wales, Hornsby and Sydney Children's Hospitals
Parramatta, NSW

Bernadette Lowther
Educational Services
Diabetes Australia-NSW
Glebe, NSW

Dr Daniel McCarty
Epidemiology
International Diabetes Institute
Caulfield, VIC

Dr Aidan McElduff
Department of Endocrinology
Royal North Shore Hospital
St Leonards, NSW

Ian McEwen AM
Past National President
Diabetes Australia
Essendon, VIC

Margaret McGill
Diabetes Centre
Royal Prince Alfred Hospital
Camperdown, NSW

Patricia Marshall
Eastern Perth Public and Community Health Unit
Perth, WA

Melba Mensch
Diabetes Education Centre
Royal Newcastle Hospital
Newcastle, NSW

Associate Professor Paul Mitchell
Department of Ophthalmology
University of Sydney
Westmead Hospital
Westmead, NSW

Clinical Associate Professor Paul Moffitt AM
Faculty of Medicine and Health Sciences
University of Newcastle
Newcastle, NSW

Shirley Murray
President of Diabetes Australia - Tasmania
Hobart, TAS

Dr Alison Nankervis
Department of Diabetes and Endocrinology
Royal Melbourne Hospital
Parkville, VIC

Professor Kerin O'Dea
Nutrition and Preventative Medicine Unit, Department of Epidemiology and Preventative Medicine, Monash University
Clayton, VIC

Dr David O'Neal
Department of Endocrinology and Diabetes, St Vincent's Hospital
Fitzroy, VIC

Dr Mary Parkin
Endocrinologist
East Melbourne, VIC

Dr Pat Phillips
Endocrine and Diabetes Service
The Queen Elizabeth Hospital
Woodville, SA

Dr Phil Popplewell
Department of Medicine
Flinders Medical Centre
Bedford Park, SA

Professor Susan Serjeantson
John Curtin School of Medical Research, Australian National University, Canberra, ACT

Clinical Professor Gillian Shenfield
Department of Clinical Pharmacology
Royal North Shore Hospital
St Leonards, NSW

Professor Martin Silink
Ray Williams Institute of Paediatric Endocrinology, Diabetes and Metabolism
New Children's Hospital
Parramatta, NSW

Dr Alan E Stocks AM
Brisbane Clinic
Brisbane, QLD

Maureen Unsworth
Eastern Perth Public and Community Health Unit
Perth, WA

Dr Timothy Welborn
Department of Endocrinology and Diabetes
Sir Charles Gardiner Hospital
Nedlands, WA

Professor Paul Zimmet
Diabetology
International Diabetes Institute
Caulfield, VIC

How to use this book

EARLIER editions of this book, *Diabetes & You – An owner's manual,* were popular, with more than 20,000 copies sold to people with diabetes throughout Australia. Readers gave us considerable feedback about what was useful and not so useful in past editions.

This time we decided to include a short section on the different ways of using this book. Although you will develop your own style of referring to the information, we have built in some additional aids that may also be of use.

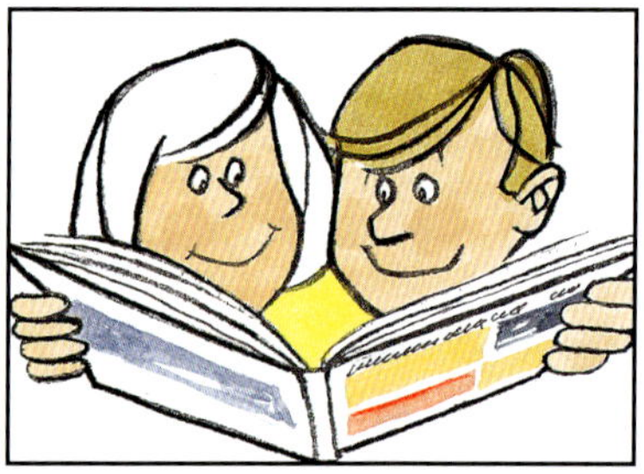

Colour codes

We have grouped chapters into the most logical sections, for example, Management and Lifestyle.

Look at the contents page under each of these sections for the subject you seek. You'll find a colour code representing each subject area is also shown.

Key points

At the start of each chapter there is an At a Glance list of key points. We hope these will be a useful reminder of what the chapter covers and the order in which points are discussed.

Quick Read

At the back of the book we have produced a Quick Read. This is a compilation of all the key points from all the chapters. When you become familiar with the book, you may only need to consult the Quick Read as a ready reference.

Little extras

To make reference even easier, we have included some little extras such as:

The comprehensive glossary
The index – a quick way to look up information
Abbreviations & measures
Important phone numbers

We hope you enjoy this book and adopt it as your main reference to help you achieve better management of your diabetes.

BERNIE AYERS

Editorial advisory board:

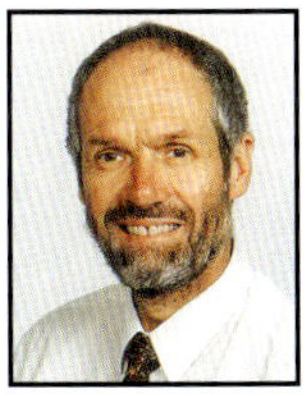

❑ **DR PAT PHILLIPS MB, BS, MA (OXON) FRACP, MRACMA**

Pat Phillips is the Senior Director of Endocrinology at the North Western Adelaide Health Service. He has been actively involved in Diabetes Australia, the Australian Diabetes Society and the Australian Diabetes Educators' Association since he became involved with diabetes care in 1987. In South Australia he has contributed to the development of the South Australian Diabetes Strategy and oversees the unit's two Diabetes Centres and the State Diabetes Outreach Program. Pat lives in Adelaide with a tribe of children, dogs and Burmese cats and enjoys reading, writing, cycling and barbeques.

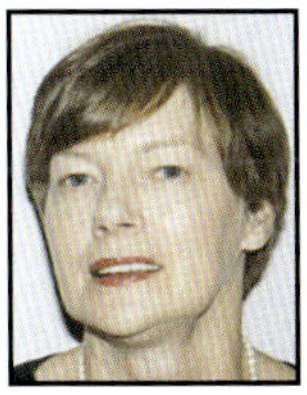

❑ **LYNETTE BROWN Dip Nut & Diet. MDAA**

Lynette Brown is a dietitian and Director of the Nutrition and Dietetics Department, The Canberra Hospital. She is also a member of the Dietitians Association of Australia, the Australian Diabetes Educators' Association and is a life member of Diabetes Australia–ACT. She contributes to diabetes management and education and is a keen advocate for empowerment of the individual over ones own health. She was the editor of the Dietitians Association, professional guidelines for diabetes care.

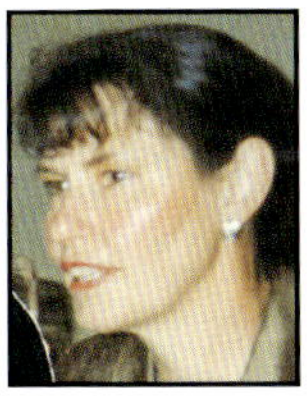

❑ **TRISHA DUNNING RN RN M.Ed FRCNA**

Trisha Dunning is a Clinical Nurse Consultant with the Department of Endocrinology and Diabetes at St Vincent's Hospital in Melbourne. She is a Past National President of the Australian Diabetes Educators' Association, the current Chair of the International Diabetes Federation Consultative Section on Diabetes Education and a member of the Victorian Ministerial Diabetes Taskforce. Trisha lives in Melbourne with her husband, three adult children and a tribe of dogs and horses. She is also a qualified aromatherapist.

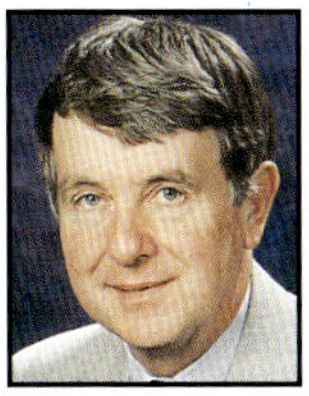

❑ **BERNIE AYERS B Ec**

Bernie Ayers is the Manager, Health Promotion and Research with the National Office of Diabetes Australia. He previously spent five years as National Director, Health Promotion for the Federal Department of Health, Housing and Community Services in Canberra. Bernie has also worked in Denmark as a consultant to the World Health Organisation on health promotion. He is Secretary to the Medical, Education and Scientific Council and the Research Council, of Diabetes Australia. Bernie holds a real estate certificate and enjoys cycling and, more especially, tennis.

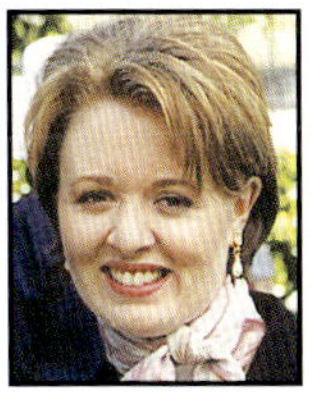

❑ **JOANNE SAINSBURY B Com**

Joanne Sainsbury is Health Promotion and Research Officer with the National Office of Diabetes Australia. Joanne is Editorial Coordinator for *Conquest*, Diabetes Australia's national magazine, and coordinates the production of all national education materials. She has a Bachelor of Commerce in marketing from the University of Newcastle and is member of the Public Relations Institute of Australia. Originally from Newcastle, Joanne currently lives in Canberra with her husband.

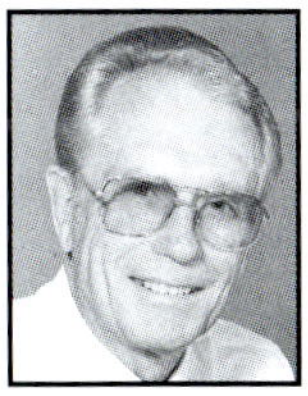

❑ **ASSOC PROF PAUL MOFFITT**

Special Thanks

A special note of thanks must go to Dr Paul Moffitt whose idea to develop a comprehensive manual for people with diabetes was the basis for this book. Dr Moffitt also conceived and instituted Australia's first Diabetes Education and Stabilisation Centre at Royal Newcastle Hospital.

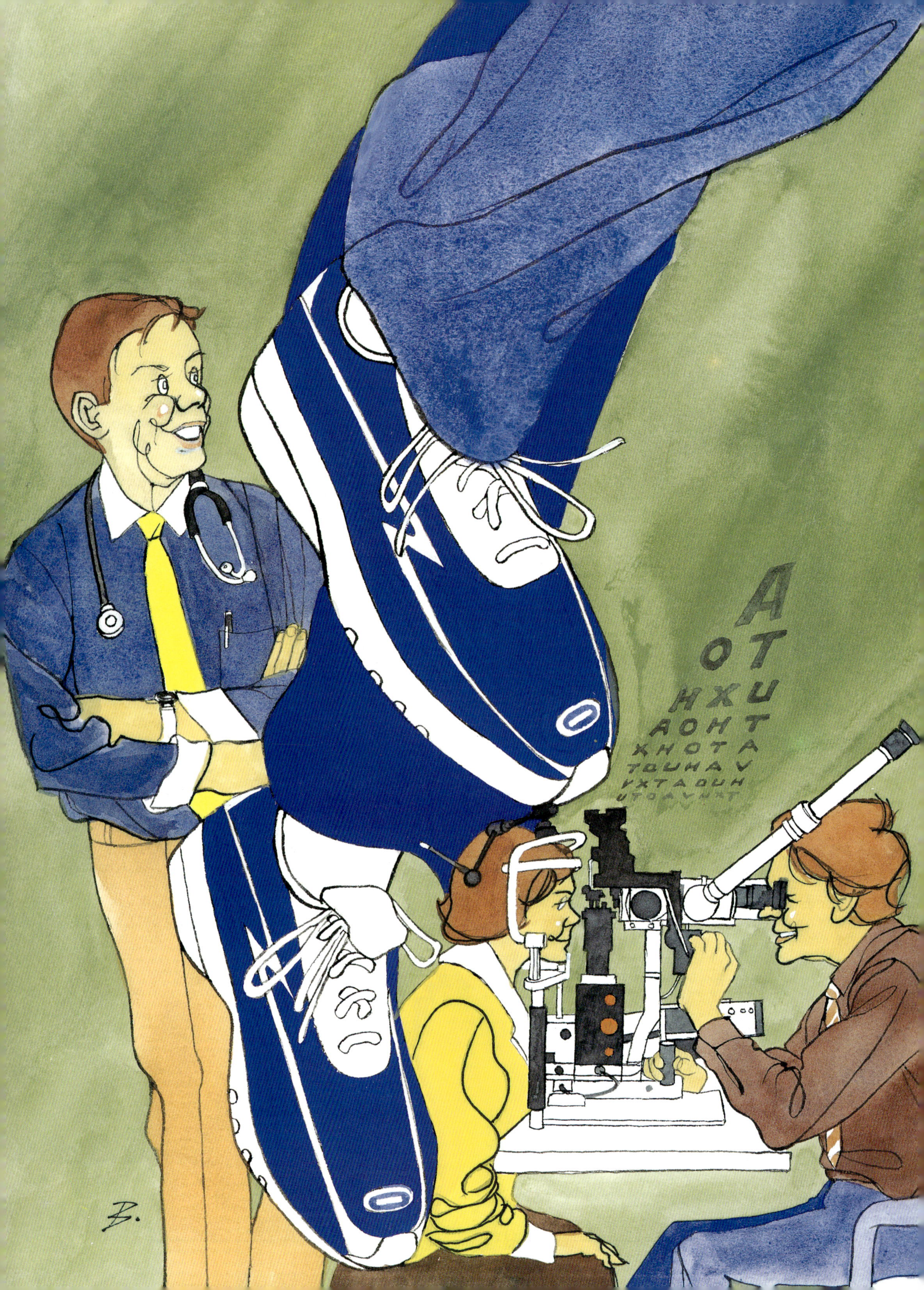
A
O T
H X U
A O H T

Chapter 1

Living with someone with type 1 diabetes

◆ By Joy Horton ◆

WHAT does it mean to live with someone who has type 1 diabetes?

The answer is as varied as the number of people who have the disorder and will change as time passes.

Although we have important guidelines about meal plans, insulin intake, exercise and so on, they must always be balanced against the first-hand knowledge you both accumulate from living with diabetes.

Stress, anger, passion – all emotions count in the equation and are just as important as the length of time with diabetes and the complications encountered.

The question to ask yourself at the start is: What sort of personal consideration should I give to diabetes in this relationship?

There are a number of ways to help yourself to information. You can read books like this, talk to various medical professionals – with or separately from your partner with diabetes – and perhaps attend an education seminar. But no amount of education will ever fully prepare you for the impact diabetes makes.

I can only tell you my own experiences. From these you may gain at least some comfort, knowing someone else is experiencing something similar to you.

Probably your partner has established or is establishing a routine to control diabetes that covers an insulin schedule, exercise of some sort and a list of foods for different circumstances. It is important to discuss these issues early in the relationship as spontaneity can be ruined by an unnerving bout of hypoglycaemia or a high blood glucose level causing nausea.

In the early days of our relationship and on more than one occasion, my flatmate caught my partner scoffing ice-cream straight from the freezer in the middle of the night. Later we learnt that this apparently unusual behaviour was to compensate for a high level of exercise earlier in the day.

Nowadays we both automatically count carbohydrates when we eat together and compare notes last thing at night before the all-important (in his case anyway) night-time insulin. This keeps me in touch and also reassures me that my sleep won't be disturbed by his nocturnal bouts of hypoglycaemia or the tortured dreams and mutterings that accompany his high blood glucose levels.

Nothing replaces experience. It arms you with methods for handling the complexities of diabetes management and teaches you to watch for subtle changes in the way symptoms manifest.

Take heart, for in most cases the person with diabetes has experiences that exceed your own. And be assured, no one gets it right all the time. However, of all the crises to deal with, hypoglycaemia is the worst; the most frightening and challenging, because you cannot ignore it.

Hypoglycaemia tests commitment. Some lucky partners of people with diabetes rarely have to deal with it. Others (myself included) often do.

Hypoglycaemia comes in many guises. The person, who a moment ago you knew and loved, is now different, not responding to you in any way you understood before.

AT A GLANCE

- **Use whatever experiences you can glean from doctors, friends, your partner and literature.**
- **Build trust but not dependence.**
- **Know your personal limits and have a plan in place to hand over to others when it is needed.**
- **Know that no one can understand diabetes better than those who live with it every day.**
- **Above all, remember as a partner of a person with diabetes, you are the second most important person in the health care team.**

Hypoglycaemia episodes can reflect the mood of the moment; sometimes pensive, sometimes wildly laughing, angry, funny and dangerous. Messages can be scrambled. I have known my partner to struggle with a stranger for possession of their ice-cream when he needed sugar; seriously photographing hub caps on the freeway; or he has talked with me on the phone hoping I can tell him where he is.

So how does one cope? First, learn to recognise the symptoms and act fast. Read about the technical details in chapter 12, Hypoglycaemia and Hyperglycaemia.

Every incident adds to your experience and confidence. It is normal for friends and colleagues to freeze, immobilised by ignorance of what to do; or to explain away the episodes as over-exuberance. But let's not beat about the bush, in company, hypoglycaemia can not only be embarrassing, it may be life-threatening.

My partner and I have established hypoglycaemia ground rules. Because they work so well, we share them here:

- Never negotiate during a bout of hypoglycaemia and establish these rules in a quiet moment together.
- Establish confidence that you can identify hypoglycaemia even if they can't. As time passes, people with diabetes may lose the ability to see their own symptoms.
- Communicate effectively. Remember that the capacity of understanding is impaired in the person

with hypoglycaemia. You've got to convince them remedial action is required. Read the symptoms back. 'You are sweating, your feet are dancing, your eyes are glazed, you are slurring...' If necessary, prove your theory with a quick discreet test. Establish trust that 'you *can* pick 'em'. Another method may be to ask a complicated question – sometimes 'what day is it?' suffices! Don't ever ask a question that requires a simple 'yes' answer.

- Get agreement that below a certain blood glucose level, or if the symptoms are accepted, something should be done. Establish agreement on what that remedy will be. (I can remember my partner bravely spitting out apricot nectar with a blood glucose reading of 0.9mmol/L – he hates it! And honey will never pass his lips while he is conscious.)

Be aware that you are fostering trust, not dependence.

I saw this clearly demonstrated when my partner had hypoglycaemia in a swimming pool. While alone, he kept himself above the water, fiercely independent. The moment his trusted partner arrived he slipped under, feeling safe because she was there.

Even with these simple rules, it can still take all your wits to turn a situation around.

After hypoglycaemia, what next? Talk it over with your partner. What went wrong? What can we do to avoid this next time? Who is responsible to make sure the fix happens? Let's keep that blood glucose under control.

Finally, look after yourself. You may have time to join a carers' group where you can learn about diabetes and, more importantly, relieve yourself of your experiences.

Contact Diabetes Australia for information. However, if these more formal groups are not available or are inappropriate, a friend or fellow traveller is essential for that unburdening.

Be aware that the medical community can give the mistaken impression that if you follow their prescribed schedule nothing will go wrong.

Carers and people with diabetes alike may feel they are blamed for non-compliance and feel guilty. Yes, control is extremely important but is frequently not perfect because of the wild cards of emotion, circumstance and freedom to move.

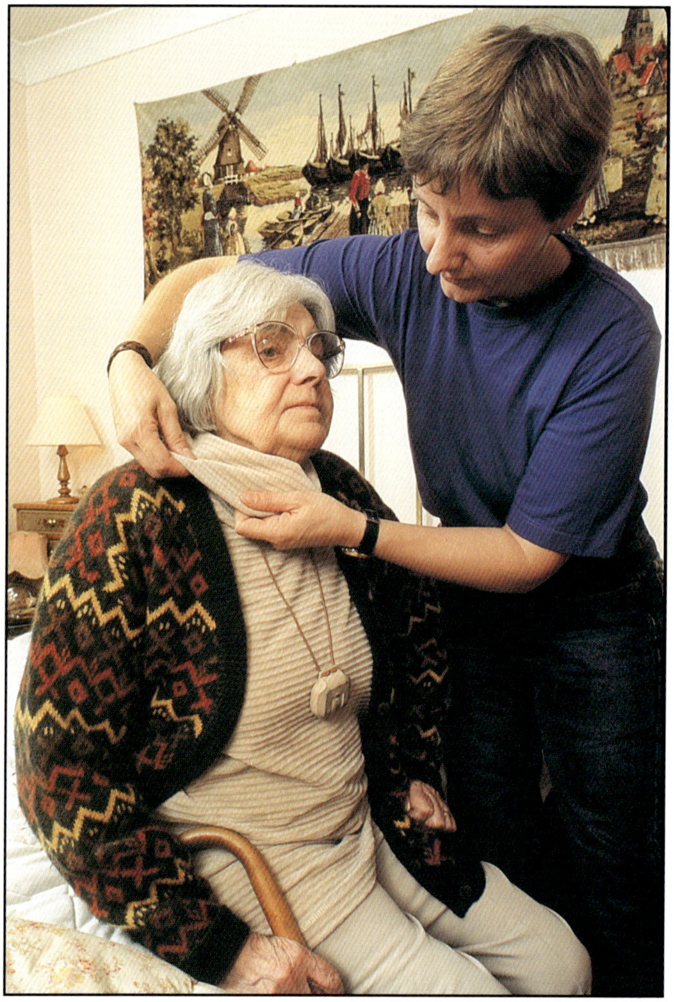

Chapter 2

Living with diabetes

◆ By Ian McEwen AM ◆

SUCCEEDING in life with diabetes is like winning the Cox Plate – Australia's thoroughbred racing championship.

To win the Cox Plate you need absolute team effort from trainer, jockey and horse.

To make a success of life with diabetes you need that same team effort from you, the doctor, the allied health professionals and a fourth element, your family.

My 48 years with diabetes has been a team effort.

I go back to 1951 when the diabetes specialist of the day at New Zealand's Wellington Hospital told me on discharge from two week's stabilisation:

'You're young, you appear intelligent and now we have your diabetes under control, study this book – Dr Lawrence's *The Diabetic Life*. Learn to treat yourself, keep in touch with your doctor and look after your body.'

That advice is as good today as it was then. It remains the best possible advice I can pass on to any person with diabetes, young or old.

Understanding your diabetes is a matter of learning and reading all the literature you can from Diabetes Australia or any other source. But remember, any information you obtain must be authoritative (written by experts in diabetes), not just gained from listening to or reading about other people's experiences. Ask questions and seek answers from your diabetes health care team.

There is enough information about diabetes today to give you a very wide choice and this manual provides an excellent starting point – whether you control your diabetes with insulin, tablets or an eating plan.

For example, not only must you learn about your daily food intake, but also about care of your feet, skin and eyes. It is important that you recognise any change in body functions or appearance. That is where the doctor and health professionals come into your life.

Care of the feet is particularly important. My podiatrist tells me my feet are healthier than many of his patients who do not have diabetes. I achieve this by daily washing, daily application of cream, six-weekly visits to the podiatrist and wearing comfortable shoes and socks.

Food and eating can often be a problem. Often I hear friends with diabetes say: 'I can't eat this or that.'

Sure you can't, but a negative attitude does not help you learn to live with diabetes. If you want a piece of cake, one small piece really won't hurt you as long as you remember at your next meal that you ate it. One small piece is not the whole cake.

And after a hard day's work in the garden, a refreshing glass of beer will quench your thirst, not ruin your eating plan!

This leads to complete understanding of your daily intake of food – knowing precisely what your eating plan is, what it contains and what effect it has on you.

In the old days *substitutes* were common. Today we understand what we are substituting for what.

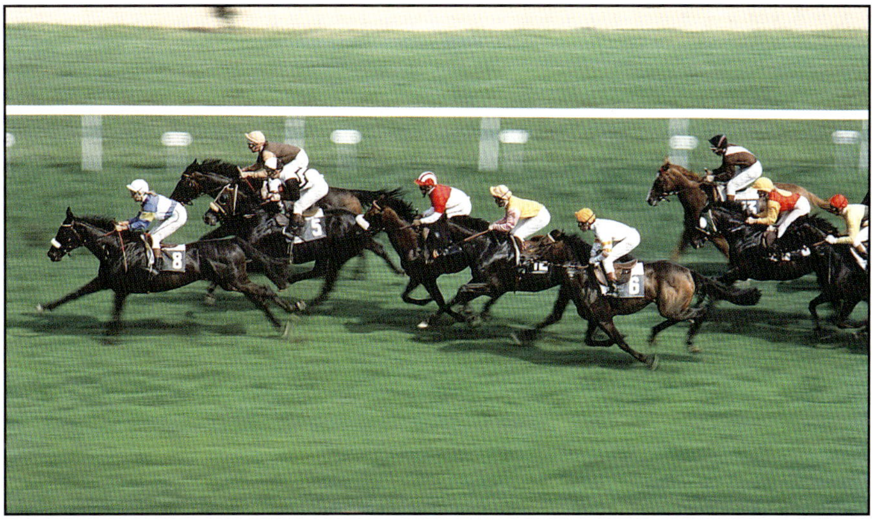

AT A GLANCE

- **Maintain a positive attitude.**
- **Learn to manage your diabetes.**
- **Be diligent with care of your body.**
- **Thoroughly understand your eating plan.**
- **Ask questions of your health care team.**
- **Don't forget to enjoy life.**

In my days at Moonee Valley Racing Club where I was chief executive for 21 years, I worked extended hours, enjoyed extensive social activities and an expanded lifestyle. However, I always coped with blending the requirements of diabetes with my job. I did not see myself as an exception but never hesitated to tell anyone I had diabetes. My four daily injections meant my insulin pen was as common at the dining room table as the knife and fork.

Development of the four-times-a-day injection schedule was accomplished in collaboration with my specialist, who I have consulted at least every six months throughout my 27 years in Australia.

An injection with every meal gives me comfortable control. It was not always like that but refinements in insulin manufacture have improved things. It doesn't

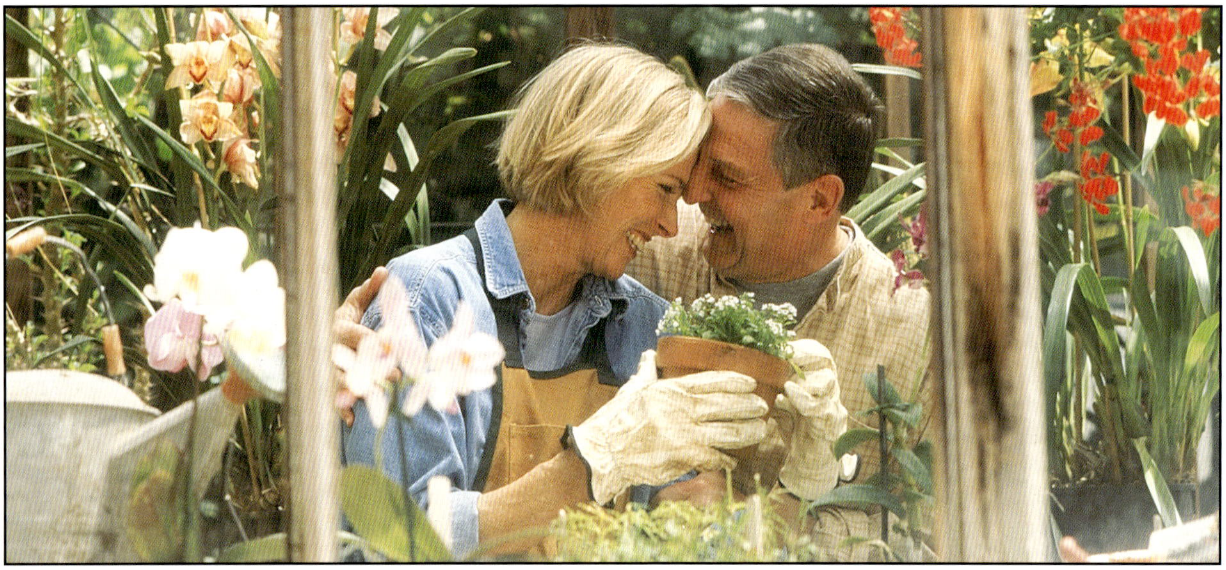

mean it is the ideal schedule for everyone, but it highlights the fact that taking insulin can be varied to suit your needs.

Diabetes should never be your master.

I retired from Moonee Valley in July, 1991, and since then spend half my time tending Angus cows at our farm at Seymour, Victoria.

Retirement has brought no changes to my diet or daily life other than removal of the pressure of a high-powered position.

I survived triple bypass surgery in 1994 and a carotid artery clean out. I also received two lens implants in 1996. Throughout these episodes I was faithful to my life-long schedules of keeping in close contact with my various doctors and looking after my body.

I have seen many changes in treating diabetes during the past 48 years.

In the early 1950s almost every ounce of food was weighed before consumption. Insulin was taken once a day by glass syringe, with needles that were seldom sharp. Urine testing was by boiling up Benedict's solution, which often exploded from a test tube. Meal times were rigid – 8am, 12 noon and 5pm!

How different it is today.

We have come a long way in making the life of the person with diabetes more comfortable. Blood glucose meters, human insulin, single-use syringes, a more lenient approach to a huge variety of foods, plus sugar-free foods.

However, none of this replaces the primary objective – the theme for our first National Diabetes Week of the 1990s – eat well, play well, stay well.

With sensible eating to a healthy meal plan plus adequate exercise, you are much more likely to stay well.

Chapter 3

Diabetes – what goes wrong?

◆ By Dr Pat Phillips ◆

DIABETES was known in ancient times. In fact, the name diabetes comes from the Greek: dia = through, betes = a passing.

This refers to the passing through the body of large volumes of fluid. The full name, *Diabetes mellitus*, refers to sweetness (mellitus = honey). The sweetness of the urine and the body fluids is because of too much sugar. This is the basic problem in diabetes.

Your body needs a special sugar, glucose. Your body makes glucose from starchy foods (carbohydrates like bread, potatoes) and other sugars (like sucrose – table sugar, fructose – fruit sugar). The glucose is carried around the body in the blood and the level is called glycaemia (glyc = glucose; aemia = in the blood).

AT A GLANCE

- **Maintaining your blood glucose at a level just right for you is the essence of managing diabetes.**
- **Understanding the mechanics of diabetes enables you to take control and balance blood glucose within your normal range.**

A question of balance

Your glucose level must be neither too high nor too low ... but just right.

A high level – *hyperglycaemia* – affects the body's machinery:

- Things don't work as well. You feel tired and sleepy.
- The body fluids are concentrated and the lens in your eye changes shape.
- You get blurry vision.
- The kidneys filtering the blood collect more glucose than usual. This glucose must be carried out of the body. You pass a lot of urine (polyuria: poly = lots, uria = urine). You need more water, get thirsty and drink a lot (polydipsia: dipsia = drink).
- Your body is losing glucose from food products. You lose weight, feel hungry and eat more (polyphagia: phagia = to eat).

A low level – *hypoglycaemia* – also affects the body, especially the brain, which relies on glucose. Your brain doesn't like being starved of glucose. It sends urgent signals to the body:

- You feel hungry.
- Your brain doesn't work properly.
- You don't think straight.
- You get trembly.

Controlling diabetes is keeping the balance *just right.*

Where does glucose come from?

The meals you eat have:

- Protein – for body growth and repair.
- Fat – lots of concentrated calories.
- Carbohydrate – starchy foods and sugars. Each is made up of simple units. Starch has hundreds of smaller units joined together. It's a complex carbohydrate. The small units in starch are sugars (like glucose, fructose). They are simple carbohydrates.

Your food is broken down by digestive juices. Starch is digested into sugars which the liver makes into glucose.

Diagram 1

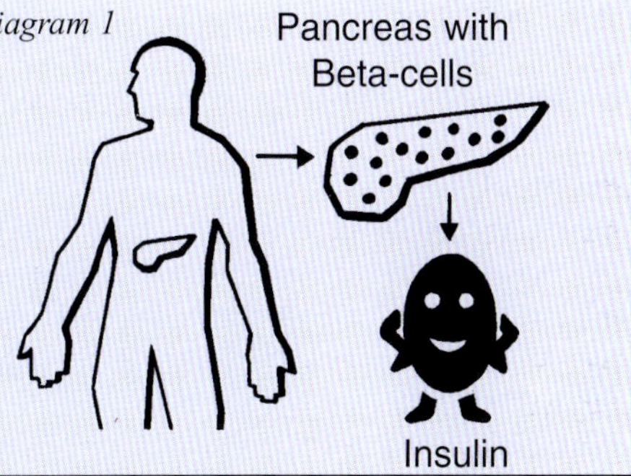

Diagram 2

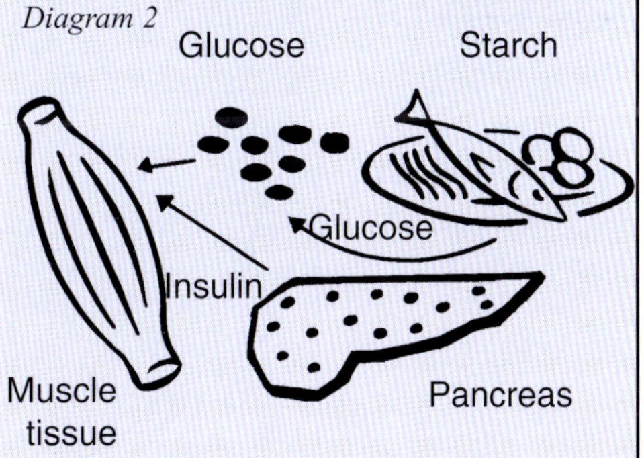

Your body can't change straw into gold (remember the fairytale of Rumple-stiltskin) but it can change bread into glucose!

Insulin enters the story

Now you have changed starch into glucose racing around in the blood stream. But the glucose has to get out of the blood and into the body tissues. The cells in the body tissues actually do the work. Brain cells – so you can think; heart cells – so you can pump blood; muscle cells – so you can walk.

Insulin opens the doors (the glucose channels) that let glucose go from the blood to the body cells.

Insulin comes from the pancreas, a gland sitting just below the stomach – halfway between your belly button and the imaginary line joining your nipples. Most of the cells of the pancreas make digestive juices, but some cells (the beta cells) make insulin which travels in the blood and tells the food products where to go (Diagrams 1 & 2).

Maintaining the balance

Your body is very clever. A high blood glucose level

HYPERGLYCAEMIA	=	high blood glucose levels
HYPOGLYCAEMIA	=	low blood glucose levels
POLYURIA	=	passing lots of urine
POLYDIPSIA	=	drinking lots of fluid
POLYPHAGIA	=	eating lots of food

makes the pancreas put out more insulin. Insulin opens the glucose channels and glucose goes from the blood into the cells. The glucose level falls. The body gets back into balance.

At rest, the cells don't need much glucose.

The glucose channels are difficult to open and there is not much insulin (Diagram 3).

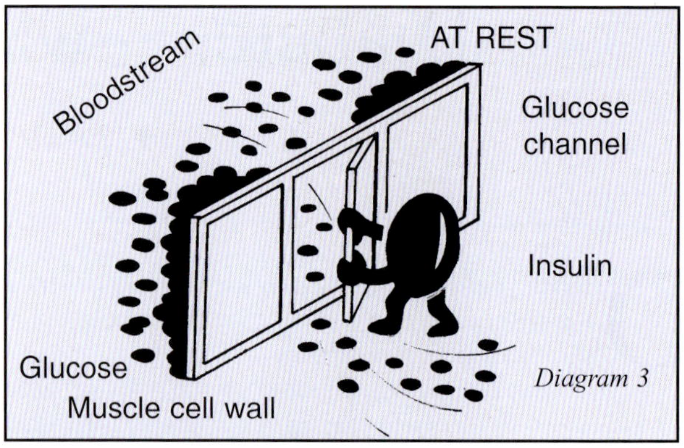

Diagram 3

After a meal containing starch, blood glucose increases. The pancreas releases insulin. Insulin opens glucose channels and the cells use the glucose (Diagram 4).

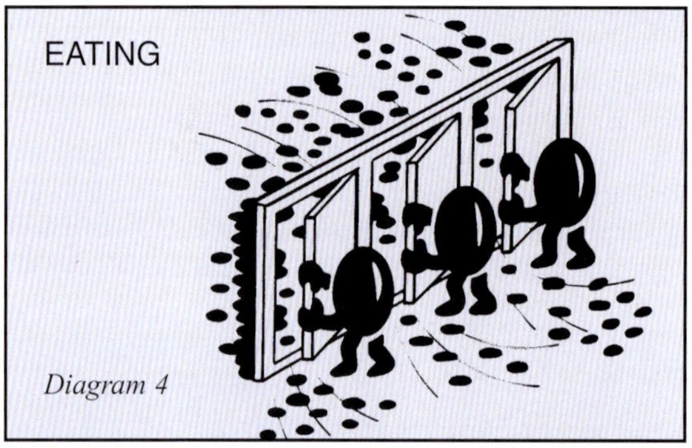

Diagram 4

With exercise, muscle cells need glucose. There is not much insulin, but glucose channels become easy to open and allow enough glucose through (Diagram 5).

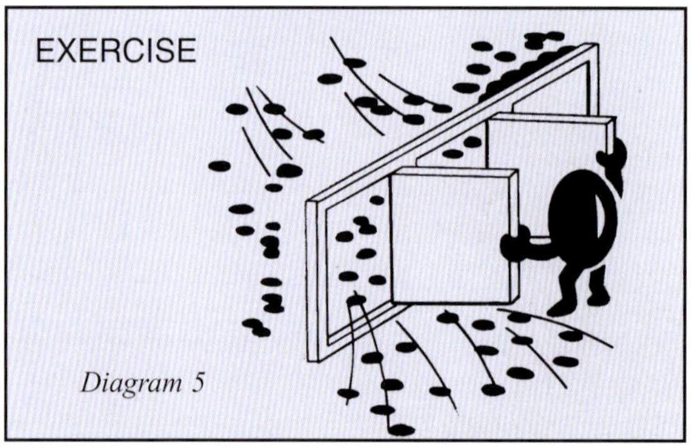

Diagram 5

In diabetes, the insulin levels are decreased or insulin does not work properly. Glucose channels are shut. Glucose builds up in the blood and causes problems.

The balancing act

The aim of diabetes treatment is to keep the blood glucose balanced in the normal range. In diabetes, this is no longer done automatically by the body. People with diabetes must organise and juggle food and stress, insulin/tablets and exercise. They balance:

- the things that raise blood glucose – food and stress.
- the things that lower blood glucose – exercise and insulin/tablets.

If this balancing act is successful, blood glucose doesn't go too high (hyperglycaemia), or too low (hypoglycaemia), but stays in the healthy range (Diagram 6).

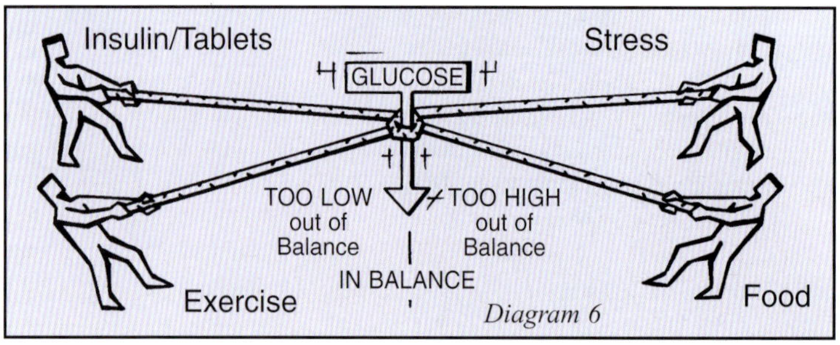

Diagram 6

Highs and lows

Glucose levels go up and down through the day.

Low blood glucose occurs before meals, after exercise, and sometimes in the middle of the night when there is a long gap between meals.

High blood glucose occurs about two hours after meals and when you are under stress.

Blood glucose is measured in millimoles of glucose per litre of blood (mmol/L).

A normal blood glucose level is 5 mmol/L and is equivalent to about one-sixth of a teaspoon of glucose per litre of blood.

What are you aiming for?

The basic problem with diabetes is that the blood glucose level rises. This abnormal chemistry can damage the body. It is important to control blood glucose to avoid problems.

Everyone is different. You and your health care team will work out your own personal goals. In a perfect world, we would aim at the levels which occur in people without diabetes because we believe that this minimises long-term problems. Often though, it is impossible to get this ideal control, and trying too hard causes blood glucose to swing from high to low. It is a question of finding the balance which suits you best.

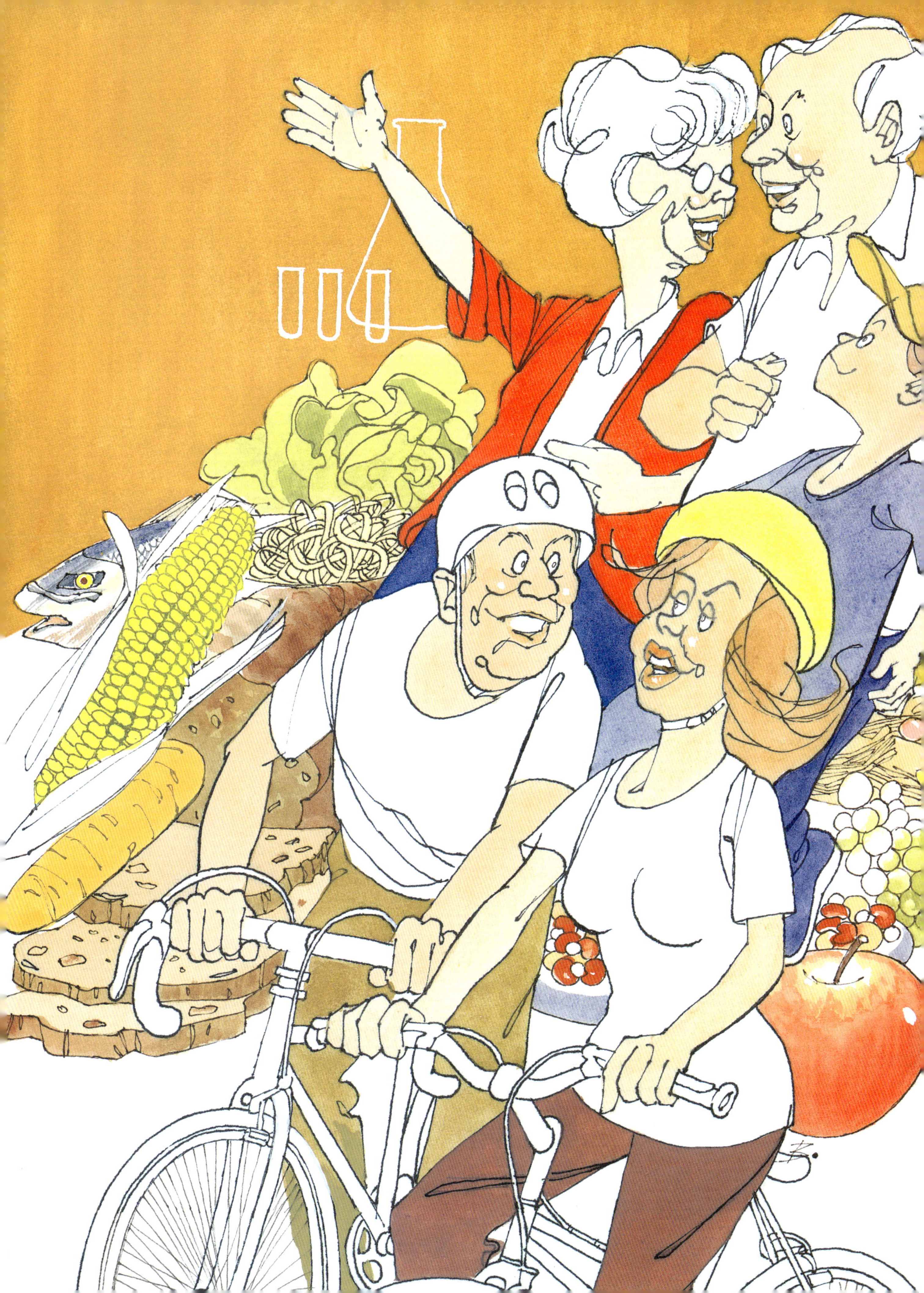

Diabetes and Lifestyle

◆ By Lynette Brown and Dr Pat Phillips ◆

NOT only do you need to maintain a healthy lifestyle to manage diabetes, but also to reduce the risk of it developing.

The most common type of diabetes, type 2, is often called a lifestyle disease. Simply changing your lifestyle may be the main focus of treatment, with attention to exercise and eating habits.

Why is lifestyle so important in diabetes?

The short answer is that our bodies were designed as hunter-gatherers, but during subsequent centuries our lifestyle has changed. We are built to hunt wild animals and fish for their lean meat; to collect fresh fruit, nuts and vegetables and to gather and cook grains.

Our ancestors' bodies adapted to the high activity levels of hunting and gathering plus the low-fat, low-sugar food which were the products of that lifestyle.

However, we have come a long way since the Stone Age. We now live in the Lucky Country, an affluent society where few go hungry.

The down side of this richness is that the way we live does not suit the way our bodies have evolved. We have become fatter and less fit. Our lifestyle has changed but our bodies have not. Cars, buses and bicycles mean less activity. Processed bread, meats and fried and sweet foods mean more fat and sugar.

This applies to all Australians and it applies especially if you have diabetes.

Whether you have type 1 or type 2 diabetes, it is important to follow some rules. These are known as the *Eight Golden Guidelines for Lifestyle*. They are:

1. Don't get fat

Stay trim, taut and terrific. The less extra fat your body has, the better it will respond to insulin.

Check your weight regularly and aim for the healthy weight range for your height. (See chapter 26, How to Work with Your Health Care Team).

2. Eat less fat

Fat and fatty foods contain lots of energy you probably don't need. Fat may block your blood vessels.

3. Eat complex carbohydrate

Fruit, vegetables and cereals all have starch (complex carbohydrate) and only small amounts of the sugars which increase blood glucose levels.

4. Spread your complex carbohydrate

Spreading food throughout the day spreads the load and gives a smooth, steady supply of glucose.

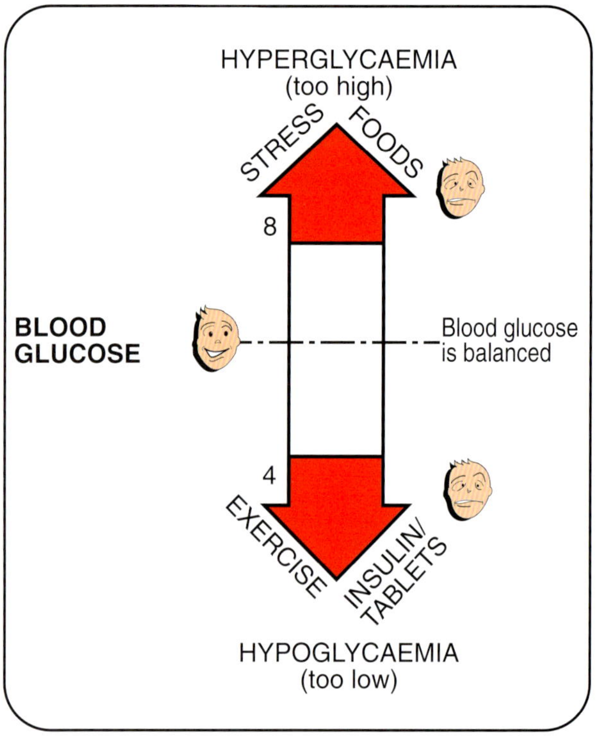

To balance blood glucose you must balance stress, food, exercise and insulin/tablets.

AT A GLANCE

- **Don't get fat.**
- **Eat less fat.**
- **Eat complex carbohydrate.**
- **Spread your meals.**
- **Take 30.**
- **Take time out.**
- **Quit for life.**
- **Drink wise.**

5. Take 30

Thirty minutes of moderate activity each day helps insulin work and helps your blood vessels stay healthy. Consider simple ways to enjoy your activity routines.

6. Take time out – Reduce stress, take time out for yourself

Stress is a problem for everyone, but particularly for people with diabetes. Once again, we can look back at our bodies' design for hunting and gathering. Stress affects our bodies the same way as danger affected our early forebears. When danger threatens we can either fight or take flight. Our bodies get ready, our breathing deepens giving us more oxygen, our heart speeds up providing more blood to the muscles, our glucose stores are released to provide energy, and our muscles tense ready to fight or run.

This is fine for Stone Age folk, but bad news for the modern person with diabetes. The last thing you want is for your glucose stores to be released – your body has enough problems keeping glucose stored in the right place without stress pushing it out again.

Deal with your stress in a healthy way

You may not be able to avoid stress but you can help your body deal with it. Regular activity is one way, plus it helps keep your weight and blood vessels healthy as well.

Because you are an important person, you need to look after yourself, and there are lots of other ways to help your body cope with stress.

Find out more about relaxation

Look in your local newspaper for courses or in your library for books. Ask your doctor or diabetes nurse educator.

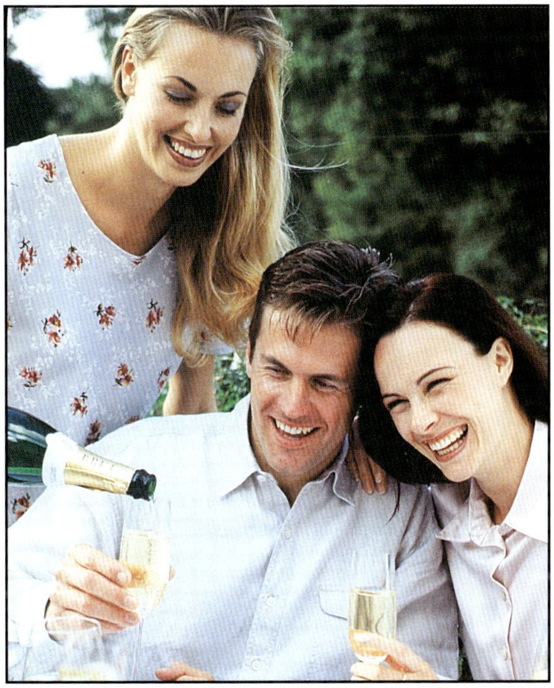

7. Quit for life

The labels on cigarette packets are right – smoking really does damage your health. This is true for everyone, but especially for people with diabetes. Cigarette smoke is a mixture of stimulants like nicotine which affect the brain and give a 'buzz'. Unfortunately, these same stimulants affect blood vessels in both the short term by closing up the walls, and the long term by blocking off the vessels. Also, cigarette smoke has carbon monoxide which stops your blood carrying oxygen.

Add this to the fact that diabetes also damages blood vessels and it is easy to see that smokers with diabetes have 'double trouble' – and that's not even counting other ill effects of cigarettes on lungs, skin, breath, eyes, kidneys and, last but not least, your pocket.

If you do not smoke you have lots of reasons not to smoke. If you do smoke you have lots of reasons to give up – the best one being that you will feel so much better for it. Set a date and quit now!

8. Drink wise – four men and women two

This little slogan refers to standard drinks which contain 10 grams of alcohol – 300 ml of beer, 100 ml of wine. In moderation, that is, four drinks for men and two for women, alcohol is pleasant, sociable and safe.

However, it can cause three special problems for people with diabetes:

1. Overweight – alcohol has lots of energy you may not need if you are trying to control your weight.
2. Loss of judgment – alcohol can impair your ability to make rational decisions concerning food and medication and this can prove costly.
3. Low blood glucose – just as stress releases glucose stores, alcohol can block the release and cause low blood glucose.

Generally, alcohol should be taken with food. Most drinks are suitable or can be made suitable but some have lots of sugar and are best avoided.

So there you have the Eight Golden Guidelines – your challenge is putting them into practice.

Healthy Eating and Diabetes

◆ By Melba Mensch and Dianne van Netten ◆
Revised by Lynette Brown and Patricia Marshall

REGULAR exercise and healthy eating not only help control your weight, but also your blood glucose levels.

If you're overweight, make weight loss your top priority. It will help improve blood glucose control.

At different times in your life you need different quantities of food.

For example, when you retire you may be less active and because you won't burn so much energy you'll need less food.

Children, adolescents, pregnant women and sports people have different energy needs. If you're not sure about how much energy you need, consult a dietitian.

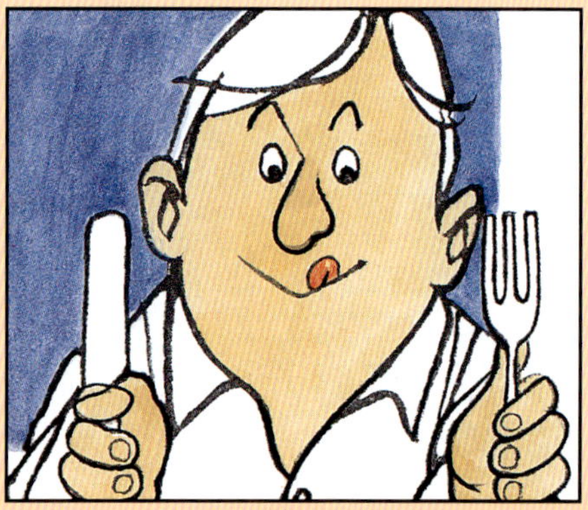

AT A GLANCE

- **Learn basic nutritional facts so you know which foods contain carbohydrates, proteins and fats.**
- **Know the energy values of foods so that wherever you are you can make wise meal choices.**
- **Ask your dietitian to help you review your nutrition needs and to explain aids such as the good-better-best and carbohydrate exchange systems which will assist in your diabetes control.**
- **Limit your fat and oil intake.**
- **Learn to differentiate between good fats and bad fats.**
- **Learn to correctly interpret the nutrition panels on food products.**

What to eat?

Choose:

- Mainly carbohydrates (for example, breads, pasta, rice, legumes, vegetables and fruit).
- Be moderate in protein intake (for example, lean meat, skinless chicken, fish and eggs).
- Select foods high in fibre (for example, wholegrain bread, fruit and vegetables).

Avoid:

- Fats (for example, margarine, butter, cream, cheese, peanut butter, oils, processed snacks and take-away foods).
- Foods high in sugar (for example, desserts, sweets and some processed breakfast cereals).

Carbohydrates provide energy

Think carbohydrate, think starch and sugar. Carbohydrates supply the body with energy. When starch and sugar are digested they are converted to glucose, which then enters the blood stream.

Make foods such as breads, cereals, pasta, rice, fruit and vegetables the major source of carbohydrates in your meals. The amount of sugar contained in *small* servings of foods such as ice-cream, many breakfast cereals, dried fruit and fruit loaves is generally acceptable.

Sugars

Sugars occur in different forms such as fructose in fruit and lactose in milk. The form sugar takes in our blood is called glucose. Glucose is also added to some lollies and medicines.

Sucrose is cane sugar – the sugar we usually eat. Honey is also a natural form of sugar.

Starch

Starch is stored by plants, especially grains, cereals, legumes and vegetables.

Chemically, starch is actually composed of clumps of glucose. Through cooking and digestion, these clumps (starch molecules) are broken down to a simpler form – glucose.

Carbohydrate management

When you eat carbohydrates such as starch and sugar your digestive juices break them down to become glucose, which is absorbed into the bloodstream. Because the glucose goes directly into your system to create energy, it is important to regulate carbohydrate intake (amount and timing) so you can manage your blood glucose levels.

The effect of carbohydrate on your blood glucose level depends largely on:

- the amount eaten
- the type of carbohydrate eaten
- your level of physical activity
- and your level of control over your diabetes.

Blood glucose response (Glycaemic index)

Some carbohydrate foods cause a large increase in blood glucose levels while others barely affect them.

Foods which have only a minor effect include legumes such as lentils and baked beans; pasta, stone fruits, wholegrain bread, yoghurt, custard and porridge.

Carbohydrate foods which cause a large increase in blood glucose include some rice, potatoes, biscuits, Rice Bubbles™ and Corn Flakes™.

However, be aware that over-consumption of any

carbohydrates may adversely affect your blood glucose level.

The good-better-best system

This is a system to discuss with your dietitian. It will show you the importance of selecting foods with a low glycaemic index (GI). Low GI foods are your *best* choices. By selecting a low GI food at each meal, you'll lower your daily blood glucose levels, increase the effectiveness of your insulin, lower your cholesterol and triglyceride levels, plus reduce hunger.

Ask your dietitian to review with you the importance of small serves of low GI foods, plus how you can reduce fatty foods and select low-fat protein foods.

Factors which influence the effect of carbohydrates on blood glucose:

1. *The degree of processing.* Highly processed foods usually increase your blood glucose levels, while less processed foods generally have less effect.
2. *The amount and type of cooking.* Raw foods tend to have less effect on blood glucose levels.
3. *Particle size.* Finely ground or milled grains have a greater effect; whole grains have less effect on blood glucose levels.
4. *Type of starch.* Different forms have different effects on blood glucose levels.
5. *Fat content.* In the short term, fat in food slows down the rate of digestion, but long term it actually increases blood glucose levels.

Carbohydrate spacing

By spreading your carbohydrate intake evenly over the day you'll achieve better blood glucose control. Include at least two or three carbohydrate foods in each meal. Snacks also should contain carbohydrate. Eat more carbohydrate if you are physically active.

Fat

Reducing fat intake is the most significant achievement of your eating plan. Over-eating fat and fatty foods can disrupt your diabetes control and produce health complications.

Saturated fat is the most damaging type of fat because it interferes with the action of insulin. Saturated fat is found mainly in animal foods, plus some oils. Examples include pork products and lard; cream and high-fat dairy products; sausages, processed meats and meat fat; chicken skin; take-away foods; coconut oil; palm oil and cottonseed oil.

Polyunsaturated fat aids circulation and reduces the risk of heart disease. It is found in seafood, nuts, seeds, lean meat, sunflower oil and safflower oil.

Monounsaturated fat is also beneficial to the blood circulation and helps reduce the risk of heart disease. It is found in olive oil, canola oil and avocado.

However, all fats will increase your weight if eaten in excess. For example, even if your margarine is made from canola oil, it is still a tub of fat!

How much fat should I eat to lose weight?

If you're female, no more than about 35 g daily (about nine teaspoons). If you're male, about 40 g daily.

This isn't just what you spread on bread, but includes all the fats and oils used in cooking. If you are attempting to lose weight, it is imperative you reduce your intake of fats and oils.

Even if you do not have a weight problem, it is still worth changing the type of fat you eat. For example, use canola or olive oil in cooking instead of lard or butter.

Health pyramid

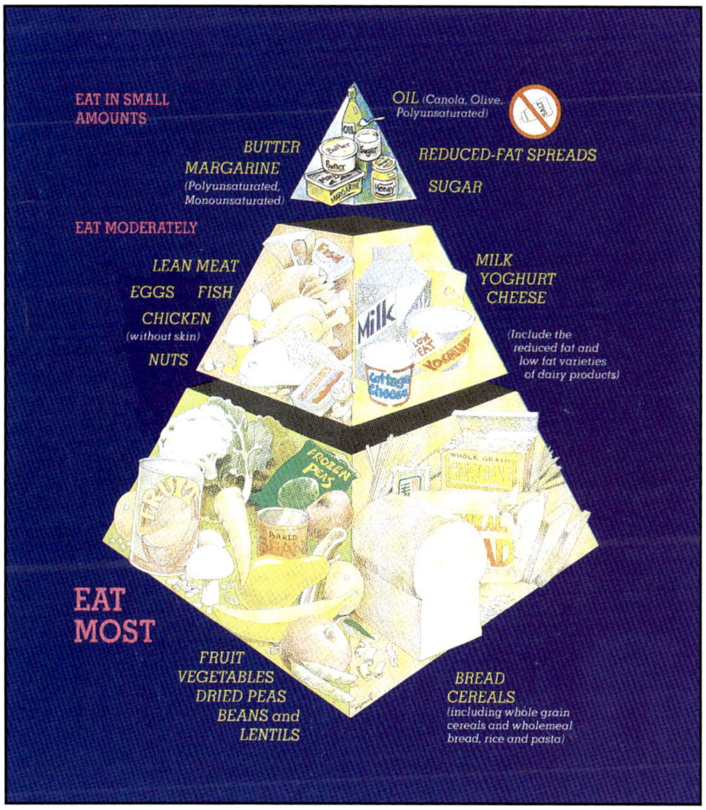
EAT IN SMALL AMOUNTS
OIL (Canola, Olive, Polyunsaturated)
BUTTER
MARGARINE (Polyunsaturated, Monounsaturated)
REDUCED-FAT SPREADS
SUGAR
EAT MODERATELY
LEAN MEAT
EGGS FISH
CHICKEN (without skin)
NUTS
MILK
YOGHURT
CHEESE
(Include the reduced fat and low fat varieties of dairy products)
EAT MOST
FRUIT
VEGETABLES
DRIED PEAS
BEANS and
LENTILS
BREAD
CEREALS
(including whole grain cereals and wholemeal bread, rice and pasta)

COURTESY AUSTRALIAN NUTRITION FOUNDATION

Healthy eating is the same for everyone, whether they have diabetes or not.

Protein

You need to include protein foods in your daily meal plan. Children and teenagers require more protein than adults. In Australia most adults eat much more protein than their bodies require. Too much protein can lead to weight gain, especially since protein foods (for example, meat) often contain large amounts of hidden fat. Eating too much protein may also contribute to kidney disease.

Choose small to moderate serves of low-fat protein foods such as lean meats, skinless poultry, fish, legumes, lentils, seeds and low-fat dairy products.

Surviving in the supermarket

It's easy to become confused when trying to choose the healthiest processed foods. Often the wording on food labels is open to misinterpretation.
For example:

- *light* may not mean low-fat
- *cholesterol-free* may not mean fat-free or even low-fat
- *no added sugar* does not mean sugar-free
- *natural* has no relevance to amount of fat or sugar
- *oven-baked* does not always mean low-fat.

To be sure of the ingredients you're buying, check the information on labels' nutrition panels. The example below is a typical breakdown of a product's nutrition content.

CANNED FRUIT – NUTRITION INFORMATION

Servings per can: 6		
Serving size: 125 g	Per Serving 125 g	Per 100 g
Energy	276 kj	221 kj
Protein	0.5 g	0.4 g
Fat	0.1 g	0.1 g
Carbohydrate		
- Total	15.6 g	12.5 g
- Sugars	11.3 g	9 g
Sodium	5 mg	4 mg
Potassium	238 mg	190 mg

Product labelling guidelines

- Compare similar products by checking the fat in the per 100 g column, and choose the product lower in fat. Generally products containing less than 10 g of fat per 100 g are good choices.
- Check the list of ingredients for the type of fat. Ingredients are listed in order of size.
- Small amounts of sugar in a product are acceptable. Sugar is included in the figure for total carbohydrate. Sugar is also shown as a separate figure underneath the total.

To develop or improve your ability in the interpretation of food labels, contact your health professionals.

Hints for reducing fat in your diet

There are two types of fat – invisible and visible.

Invisible fats – Some foods contain fats you can't see, so in many foods you may be unaware that there is fat present.

Watch out for:

- meats, especially processed and luncheon meats and sausages
- cheeses and even some light cheese, whole milk, yoghurt and dairy desserts
- nuts and seeds
- cakes, pastries and biscuits, ice-cream, chocolate (including 'lite' chocolate)
- many snack foods – potato crisps, Twisties™, corn chips, Cheezels™, muesli bars
- many take-away foods
- many gravies and sauces.

Visible fats – In some foods you can see the fat, so you can either avoid it or remove it. Visible fats include butter, margarine, oils, lard, dripping, cream, peanut butter, fats on meat (including bacon), skin on poultry, salad dressings and mayonnaise.

How to reduce your fat intake

- Grill, dry roast or steam meats.
- Use lean meats such as veal or skinless breast of chicken.
- Eat fish more often.
- Steam, boil or stir-fry vegetables (use a minimum of fat).
- Select low-fat biscuits.
- Use 'low-oil' salad dressings.
- Use skim milk and fat-reduced dairy products including cheeses such as 90 per cent fat-free slices and cottage cheese.
- Top vegetables and meat with low-fat cheeses or vegetable sauces.
- Prepare meat sauces, casseroles and soups ahead of time; refrigerate and remove fat before adding vegetables or thickening.
- Use fresh herbs rather than fats and oils on vegetables and meats for flavouring.

Alcohol and diabetes

Alcohol may interfere with your diabetes control so avoid it when your diabetes is not well controlled. Alcohol may cause hypoglycaemia if taken without food. Alcohol is also fattening as it contains 29 kilojoules (7 calories) per gram. It is recommend that overweight people and those who want to lose weight abstain from drinking alcohol. What's more, excessive alcohol intake causes liver, pancreas, brain and heart damage.

Guidelines for drinkers

- Have two or three alcohol-free days each week.
- Two average-sized drinks daily is acceptable.
- Select only dry wines, spirits or beer. Avoid sweet wines (dessert wines, and moselle), fortified wines (muscat and port) and liqueurs.
- For mixers use low-joule cordials or carbonated beverages, soda water and unsweetened mineral waters.
- Eat some carbohydrate foods while drinking to avoid hypoglycaemia (one exchange per two to three drinks is sufficient).

Hints for dining out

- Select restaurants with menus offering a variety of low-fat foods.
- Select restaurants renowned for speedy and efficient service.
- The action of each type of insulin varies greatly. By understanding how *your* insulin works, you can best decide how soon before a meal you need to take it.
- If you are unsure about ingredients or cooking methods, ask. Many establishments will prepare low-fat meals or modify menu items so they are lower in fat.

- Foods with descriptions such as sauteed, fried, crispy, butter sauce, pan-fried, creamed, escalloped, au lait and basted are likely to be high in fat.

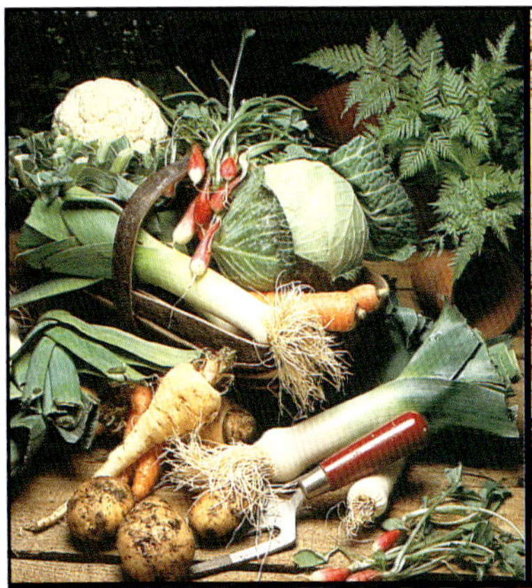

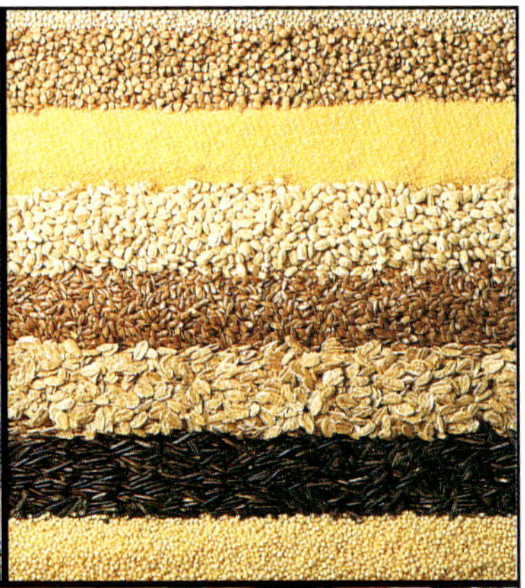

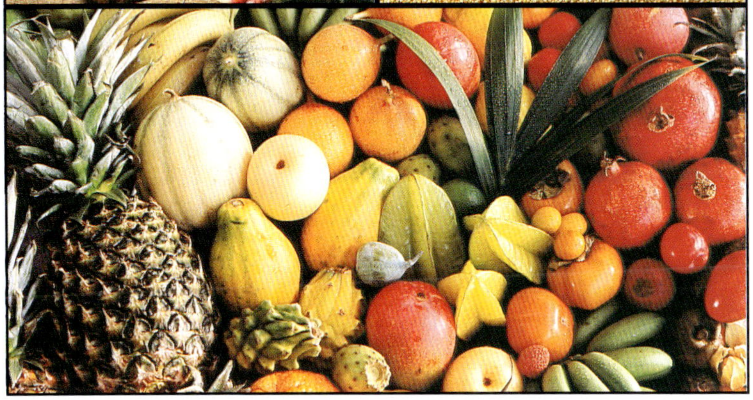

Menu suggestions

Entrée selections – consommé soups; seafood cocktails with the sauce on the side so you can choose how much to use; smoked salmon; oysters natural; salad (not Caesar); cooked vegetables or fresh fruit.

Main course selections – grilled fish; lean grilled meats; baked meats; roast chicken (remove the skin); Chinese dishes without a high fat content such as braised chicken and Chinese vegetables. When selecting pasta dishes, the entrée size may be more in keeping within your meal plan than the main course serving. Select tomato and fresh vegetable-based sauces rather than the cream or cheese sauces. There are many different ethnic foods on the market – why not try a few new ones?

Vegetable and salad selections – sauces, dressings, bacon and cheeses may add extra fat to vegetables and salads. Steamed, boiled or raw will have the lowest energy value. Lemon juice and vinegar are low-energy options to add flavour.

Dessert selections – many desserts have a very high saturated fat and energy content. Fresh fruit, ice- creams and sorbets are an excellent choice. Familiarise yourself with the nutrient content of desserts found in the frozen food section of the grocery store so that if you choose the dessert you'll have an idea of how to adjust your insulin.

Suitable selections can be made at some fast food family restaurants and take-away bars. For guidelines on what to select at these places, ask your dietitian.

Nutrition education

The more you know about food and its relationships to diabetes the easier it will be for you to choose appropriate meals.

Sample meal plan

Breakfast

breakfast cereal – porridge, oat or bran flakes with low-fat milk
bread or toast – wholegrain or fruit loaf – with a thin spread of polyunsaturated or mono-unsaturated margarine; fresh fruit; water, tea or coffee

Light meal

soup – lentils, beans, vegetables, pasta
bread roll (wholegrain) – spread thinly with margarine
salad or cooked vegetables; small serve of lean meat, skinless chicken or turkey, fish, eggs or low-fat cheese; fresh fruit; water, tea or coffee

Main meal

soup – as above if desired
starchy vegetables (corn, sweet potatoes, pasta)
other vegetables
small serve of lean meat, skinless chicken or turkey, fish, eggs or low-fat cheese
fresh fruit
water, tea or coffee

Between meal snacks

fresh fruit
low fat milk desserts (yoghurt, light ice-cream)
bread, fruit loaf, scone, roll – wholegrain thinly spread with margarine
muffins, cakes, biscuits (select low-fat recipes)

Carbohydrate exchange system

You may already be familiar with this system. If not, ask your dietitian about carbohydrate exchange and the relationship between a carbohydrate exchange and your blood glucose levels.

With guidance from your dietitian you can design an eating plan which defines the number of carbohydrate exchanges desirable to include at each meal/snack. If you are on insulin, your dietitian will explain the relationship between insulin action and carbohydrate spacing so that you can manage meal planning to give you a flexible lifestyle.

You'll learn about low-fat options and how to choose and prepare meals low in saturated fats.

For more information about food and nutritional needs, ask the dietitian at your diabetes education centre, local hospital, community centre or State or Territory diabetes association.

The Use of Tablets

◆ By the late Dr Pincus Taft ◆
Revised by Dr Pat Phillips

TABLETS have been available for the treatment of diabetes for more than 30 years.

During the 1970s there was a drop in popularity due to concerns about their safety but these days, with better understanding of their actions, potential dangers and side effects, tablets – or *oral hypoglycaemic agents* – now have a recognised place in diabetes treatment.

Because one of the major effects of tablets is to stimulate insulin production, they can be used only by people whose pancreas still produces some insulin.

For this reason they cannot be used in the treatment of type 1 (insulin-dependent) diabetes and are confined to people with type 2 diabetes, usually to those aged over 50 or who were overweight at diagnosis.

Tablets no substitute for diet

It is very important to note that use of tablets is restricted to situations where diet alone is unable to restore blood and urine glucose to normal levels or where the diet required to lower blood glucose causes weight to fall below the normal range for the person's age, sex and height.

Tablets cannot be used as a substitute for any eating plan.

Effectiveness of tablets

Because tablets promote natural insulin production and because insulin action in type 2 diabetes usually declines over time, it is often necessary to increase the tablet dosage to maintain ideal diabetes control.

In fact, after a long period, tablets may become ineffective in regulating blood sugar, but maintaining a sensible eating plan plays a major role in prolonging the effectiveness of tablets – often for many years.

The effectiveness of tablets is assessed in the same way as all diabetes treatments – by regular monitoring.

The aim of treatments is to relieve the person with diabetes of all symptoms while restoring blood glucose levels to normal, or as close to normal as possible.

Determining whether this effect is achieved will be confirmed by blood or urine glucose tests or a combination of both.

It is the responsibility of the person with diabetes to do these tests. (Details are explained in chapter 10, Self-monitoring of Blood Glucose, and chapter 11, Testing Urine).

The doctor will also carry out similar or additional tests from time to time.

Weight will also be carefully monitored because being underweight or overweight may call for a modification of meals or tablet treatment.

Should control be unsatisfactory or fail to improve in spite of attention to eating plan and adjustments to tablets or dosage, it may be necessary to transfer to insulin.

Choice of tablet and side-effects

Tablets belong to three chemical families – the more widely used *sulphonylureas*, and the less common *metformin* and *acarbose*.

There are several tablets to choose from the sulphonylurea family. They vary in dosage, potency and frequency of use. Side-effects can occur occasionally and include skin rashes, gastric and bowel upsets and, on rare occasions, jaundice.

Sulphonylureas can cause hypoglycaemia, as does insulin, where doses larger than necessary are prescribed or where food is omitted.

The second family group contains only one medication, metformin, which is thought to act differently. Metformin can be used alone or with a sulphonylurea.

The only significant side-effects are nausea and diarrhoea (especially if the dosage is increased quickly), and these occur more commonly than with the other drugs. However, metformin does not cause hypoglycaemia and some authorities suggest it may assist diet-induced weight loss.

The third group also contains one medication, acarbose, and has only one preparation.

Acarbose works differently from the sulphonylureas and metformin and can be used alone or combined with either of these.

AT A GLANCE

- **Tablets are inappropriate for people with type 1 diabetes.**
- **Tablets are not a substitute for a meal plan.**
- **Over time, tablets may cease to be an effective treatment.**
- **Sensible eating may prolong the effectiveness of tablets for years.**
- **Regular glucose testing monitors the effectiveness of tablets.**
- **Any of the three families of tablets may cause side-effects.**
- **Illnesses can effect the effectiveness of tablets.**

ORAL HYPOGLYCAEMIC AGENTS AVAILABLE

Chemical Name	Brand Name	Tablet Size	Daily Dose Range	Approximate Duration	Frequency (Times/day)	Administration (Times/day)	Potency	Side-Effects
Acarbose	Glucobay	50 mg 100 mg	150–600 mg	3 hours	3	With meals	Weak	Flatulence Abnormal LFT Skin rashes
Chlorpropamide (a)	Diabinese	250 mg	125–500 mg	36 hours	Once	With Meals	Strong	Weight gain Hypoglycaemia Jaundice Alcohol Flushing Hyponatraemia Skin rashes Blood dyscrasias
Gliclazide (a)	Diamicron	80 mg	40–320 mg	18–24 hours	1–2	With Meals	Strong	Weight gain Hypoglycaemia Skin rashes Blood dyscrasias
Glibenclamide (a)	Daonil Euglucon Glimel	5/2.5 mg 5 mg 5 mg	2.5–20 mg	18–24 hours	1–2	With Meals	Strong	Weight gain Hypoglycaemia Skin rashes Blood dyscrasias
Glipizide (a)	Minidiab Melizide	5 mg	2.5–40 mg	6–12 hours	1–2	With Meals	Strong	Weight gain Hypoglycaemia Skin rashes Blood dyscrasias
Metformin (b) (c)	Diabex Diaformin Glucophage	0.5/0.85 g 0.5 g 0.5 g	0.5–30 g	12 hours	2–3	With/After Meals	Weak	Hypoglycaemia is rare Anorexia Vomiting Diarrhoea Lactic Acidosis
Tolbutamide (a) (d)	Rastinon	0.5 & 1.0 g	0.5–3.0 g	8–12 hours	2–3	With Meals	Weak	Weight gain Hypoglycaemia Skin rashes Blood dyscrasias

Note: Oral agents should be used with special care in the elderly.
(a) Sulphonylurea (b) Biguanide (c) Care renal, liver and cardiovascular disease (d) Choice in renal disease

Acarbose slows the digestion of carbohydrates. This decreases the rate of glucose absorption from the gut and limits the rise in blood glucose before meals.

Acarbose should be started at a low dose and increased gradually to avoid uncomfortable flatulence or diarrhoea.

If acarbose is used with a sulphonylurea or insulin and hypoglycaemia occurs, glucose preparations are required to increase the blood glucose. This is because ordinary sugar or carbohydrate will not be digested and absorbed quickly because of arcabose's intended effect.

With each tablet option, the doctor will carefully assess the user's health to ensure safety. Pre-existing heart, liver and kidney disease may make them unsuitable. If they do not work satisfactorily, they will be stopped and insulin substituted.

Don't forget, other medications may affect diabetes medication and control (see chapter 13, Diabetes and Other Medications).

Using tablets during illness

Even in people who maintain successful control by balancing food intake and insulin, illness such as flu or gastroenteritis may upset the effectiveness of tablets.

These occasional illnesses can increase blood and urine glucose levels, causing a recurrence of diabetes symptoms – thirst, urinary frequency and vomiting.

Whether people with diabetes use tablets or insulin, they should see their doctor if illness or any other issue affects their control. In these cases additional treatment with insulin may be needed.

During pregnancy treatment with insulin may be required if an eating plan alone does not achieve control. (See chapter 20, Diabetes and Women's Health.)

Chapter 7

Diabetes and Exercise

◆ By Professor Don Chisholm ◆

AN understanding of the relationship between diabetes and exercise is of great importance in the proper management of diabetes for two main reasons.

First, it is important for people with diabetes who wish to play sport or engage in vigorous physical activity to be able to do so without running into serious problems. Second, there is evidence to suggest that regular physical activity may have important benefits for people with diabetes.

One of the major underlying problems associated with diabetes is the body's inadequate response to insulin. This is called insulin resistance.

We know that regular physical activity can improve insulin sensitivity and, to some extent, reverse insulin resistance.

Studies suggest that people with a relatively active lifestyle have only about half the chance of developing type 2 diabetes as those who are physically inactive. What's more, regular physical activity assists in weight reduction, a factor which is very important in the management of type 2 diabetes.

It is therefore appropriate to regard exercise as a vital part of the treatment of type 2 diabetes.

Insulin resistance is not a major feature of type 1 diabetes so, generally, regular exercise will not improve its inherent metabolic abnormality. However, regular physical activity may lead to a reduced insulin dosage and provide cardiovascular benefits.

In both types of diabetes there is a substantially increased risk of coronary artery disease and disease of other blood vessels in the body.

Regular physical activity has a number of effects that may reduce the risk of cardiovascular disease. These include a reduction in the bad type of cholesterol (LDL cholesterol) or an increase in the good type of cholesterol (HDL cholesterol), reduced blood pressure and a reduction in the clotting elements of the blood.

Although there is no absolute proof that years of regular physical activity reduce cardiovascular risk in people with diabetes, there is significant evidence to suggest that this is the case. Therefore most diabetes physicians believe that regular exercise is a desirable objective in the management of most people with diabetes.

AT A GLANCE

- **By taking appropriate precautions, most people with diabetes can exercise and play sport.**
- **Monitor yourself so you know what to do to avoid hypoglycaemia or hyperglycaemia.**
- **Blood glucose monitoring is vital to help you make appropriate adjustments to meal plans and medications, plus maintain blood glucose control during and after exercise.**
- **If you are middle-aged or older, have a thorough physical check-up, especially your feet, heart and eyes, before starting any exercise program.**
- **By taking a gradual and sensible approach, you can safely enjoy the benefits of regular physical activity even if you have some diabetes complications.**

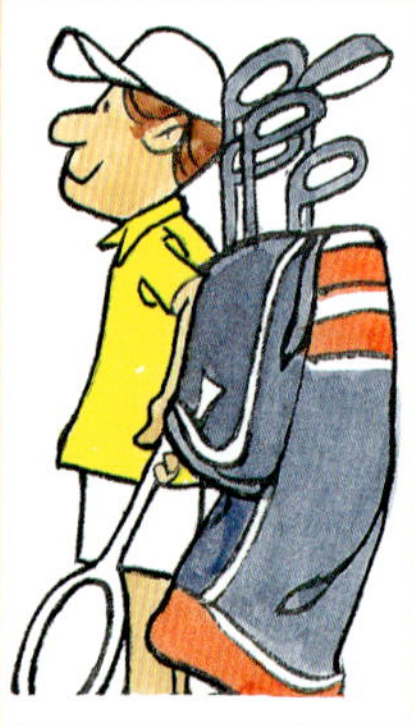

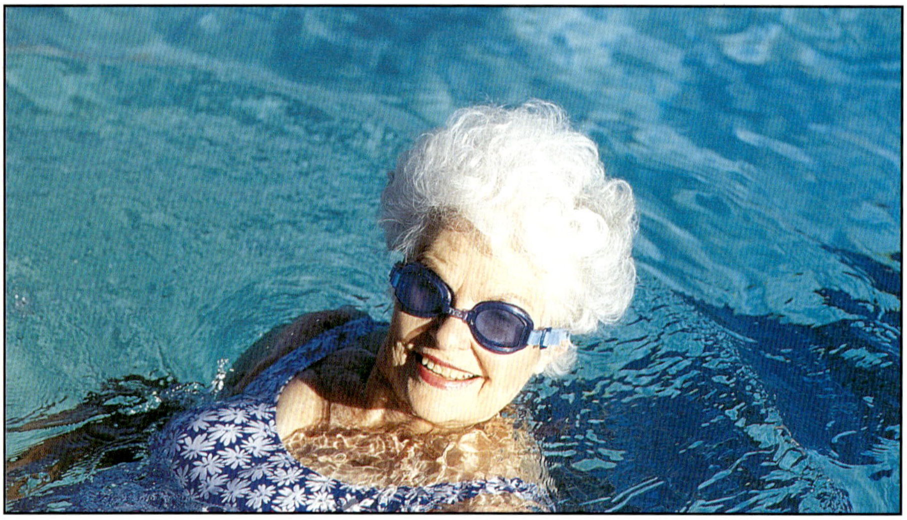

What happens during exercise in people without diabetes?

Exercise stimulates the body to use glucose. During moderate exercise, the amount of glucose used by the body increases by 200–300 per cent. In response to messages transmitted by hormones and from the nervous system, the liver increases its production of glucose to correspond exactly to the amount of glucose being used.

It means that people without diabetes can exercise for up to about two hours without taking any glucose or carbohydrate and without any significant fall in their blood glucose level.

The other important fact about exercise is that it greatly increases the body's response to insulin. In other words, it increases the body's insulin sensitivity. This effect is produced for about 12 hours by a single bout of exercise and even longer with regular exercise training.

The effect of exercise on blood glucose and the body's response to insulin are beneficial in the prevention and treatment of type 2 diabetes.

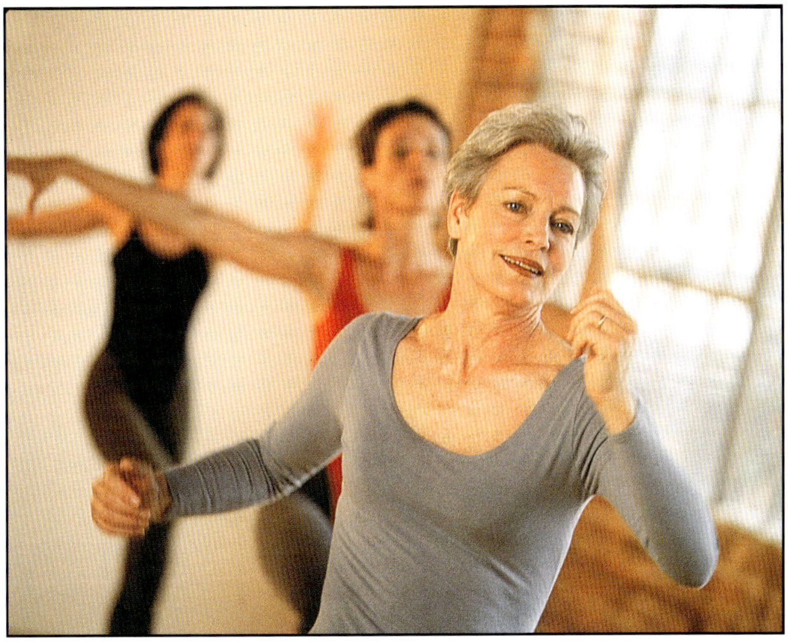

EXERCISE TIPS

- Take extra carbohydrate before and during exercise.
- Adjust insulin and medication.
- Take care of feet.
- Increase fluid intake to avoid dehydration.
- Wear sun block when exercising outdoors.

What happens in people with diabetes?

Exercise has the same effect on muscle in people with diabetes as in people without diabetes – the muscles use more glucose.

In people with diabetes, the liver's response is much more unpredictable. Generally, the liver produces less glucose than the muscles use, so the blood glucose level falls.

However, this is not always the case and the liver may put out the same amount of glucose or more than the muscles use. If the liver puts out more than muscles use, the blood glucose level will rise – as sometimes happens during exercise in people with diabetes, especially with short bursts of very intense exercise.

How to manage diabetes during exercise

The response of blood glucose levels to exercise in diabetes varies greatly from one individual to another.

The following advice is appropriate when initiating an exercise program, but it is important for everyone with diabetes to determine their own response to exercise and modify their intake of carbohydrates, insulin or tablets accordingly.

Some common management principles are:

Intake of extra carbohydrates before and during exercise

For those on insulin injections or sulphonylurea tablets, it is likely that there will be a substantial fall in blood glucose during exercise. It is advisable to take extra complex carbohydrates 30–60 minutes before exercise or extra simple sugars immediately before or during exercise.

In general, take about 15 g of carbohydrate (equivalent to one slice of bread or one-third of a can of ordinary lemonade) for each 20 minutes of exercise of moderate severity, such as brisk walking.

For exercise lasting more than an hour, it is unwise to try and take all the carbohydrate beforehand. Have some ordinary lemonade or take some other form of simple sugar at regular intervals during the exercise.

Although the blood glucose response to exercise varies greatly from one individual to another, it tends to follow the same pattern for a person doing the same exercise at the same time of day.

To determine your response so that you work out a management plan, check the blood glucose level immediately after, and six to eight hours after exercise. If the level has risen substantially by the end of the exercise, take a little less carbohydrate next time. If the blood glucose is unduly low at the end of exercise, take a little more carbohydrate on the next occasion.

In people who are not on insulin but are taking sulphonylurea tablets, there is also a risk that exercise will cause a reduction of blood glucose, with the possibility of a hypoglycaemic reaction. However, the fall in blood glucose is likely to be substantially less than in people taking insulin. This fall does not occur in people who are taking metformin tablets alone, or who are being treated with a modified meal plan (without tablets).

People with type 2 diabetes who are on tablets are often also trying to lose weight. They can take half the amount of extra carbohydrate suggested earlier during exercise and monitor the blood glucose response. If there is a substantial fall in blood glucose, reduce the sulphonylurea tablet dosage when exercising instead of increasing carbohydrate intake.

Adjustment of insulin dosage

If exercise is only brief, it may be preferable to adjust food intake rather than your insulin dose. For more prolonged exercise, reduce the dose of insulin operating at the time of exercise and take extra food.

However, keep in mind that response to exercise varies significantly between individuals. Determine your particular blood glucose response and modify your insulin dose accordingly, having discussed the adjustments with your diabetes health care team.

Adjustment of tablet therapy

People taking only metformin or acarbose tablets have virtually no risk of a hypoglycaemic or low blood glucose reaction. Generally they can continue the same tablet dosage.

People taking sulphonylurea tablets have a potential risk of a substantial fall in blood glucose during exercise. This may be prevented by taking extra carbohydrate during exercise, as indicated earlier. However, if the person is trying to lose weight and wants to avoid extra food intake, they can reduce the morning dose of sulphonylurea tablets on the day of exercise.

It is important you check the blood glucose response and modify what you eat or the number of tablets you take until you achieve a satisfactory blood glucose response.

Late hypoglycaemia occurring after exercise

As mentioned previously, a single bout of exercise may improve the body's insulin sensitivity for about 12 hours afterwards.

This means that there is a real risk of hypoglycaemia occurring in the 12 hours after exercise in people taking insulin treatment. This risk is substantial in people with type 1 diabetes, but is not so pronounced in people who have type 2 diabetes who are on insulin treatment or sulphonylurea tablets.

For example, it is common for someone with type 1 diabetes who plays a long game of afternoon tennis to have a hypoglycaemic reaction around midnight to 2am. Therefore it is usually wise to make a small reduction in the dosage of insulin operating during the 12 hours after vigorous exercise.

In other words, the person playing a long game of afternoon tennis would probably be wise to make a 10–20 per cent reduction in the evening doses of quick and intermediate acting insulin to avoid night-time hypoglycaemia.

Because there is so much variation between individuals, on the first couple of exercise sessions determine your blood glucose response before modifying your insulin dose.

Additional advice regarding insulin or suphonylurea tablets

If an insulin injection is given into a limb to be vigorously exercised, the insulin will be absorbed into the bloodstream more rapidly during the exercise, which increases the risk of hypoglycaemia. It is wise not to inject insulin into an arm or leg involved in exercise. Ideally, inject into the abdomen before exercise.

Be careful about exercise when the blood glucose level is already high. If the insulin dosage before exercise is reduced too much, or if some other problem has caused a rise in blood glucose so that the blood glucose level is already substantially elevated, exercise may produce a strongly adverse response.

If you start exercise when your type 1 diabetes is inadequately controlled, there may be a greater rise in the blood glucose level and a substantial increase in ketones.

If you plan prolonged and vigorous exercise such as marathon running or triathlons, you may need to substantially reduce your morning dose of insulin. Sometimes it is necessary to reduce the insulin dose to less than half the usual amount. People who undertake this sort of activity usually do a lot of training for the event – so the degree of insulin reduction and their response to exercise can be worked out over time.

Other important considerations

Recognition of hypoglycaemia

During exercise it may be more difficult to recognise the warning symptoms of hypoglycaemia.

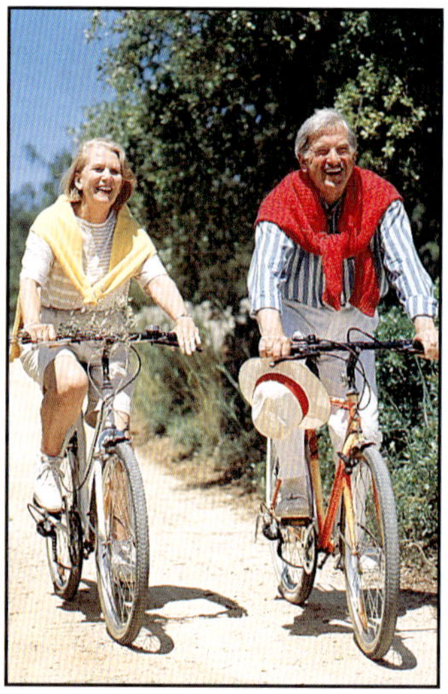

Warning symptoms like sweating, palpitations and tremulousness may be confused with normal responses to exercise.

Because of this, it is important that people with diabetes who exercise (especially those with type 1 diabetes) are careful to take the necessary steps to avoid hypoglycaemia – and that they immediately take some sugar if they notice any of the warning symptoms of a hypoglycaemic reaction.

Don't forget: always carry sugar in your pocket.

Need to reduce dosage of insulin or sulphonylurea tablets

With increased regular physical activity, people's response to insulin or sulphonylurea tablets also tends to increase. This means it may be necessary to reduce the dose of medication or the amount of exercise to avoid hypoglycaemia.

Risk of coronary artery disease

People with diabetes have an increased risk of coronary artery disease. Therefore, if you are aged 35 or more, have a thorough medical check-up before commencing any exercise program.

Depending on the individual's circumstances, this assessment may be a simple clinical examination, or may include an electrocardiograph or cardiac stress test.

Foot problems

Ulcers or other lesions on the feet are a serious potential danger for people with diabetes. It is imperative that people with diabetes who plan to increase their regular physical activity do so in a way that avoids foot damage. This is particularly true for middle-aged and elderly people. Often it is wise for them to avoid exercise, such as running, which causes stress to the feet.

Exercise which poses minimal weight or stress on the feet, such as riding an exercise bike, is ideal, although brisk walking in good footwear is also an excellent alternative.

It is wise for those in the middle to more mature age group to have a podiatrist's assessment to determine the state of their feet and the most appropriate type of footwear before starting an exercise program

Exercise in people with retinopathy

In any person with diabetes who has actively progressing retinopathy, exercise may present some danger as it may cause bleeding from blood vessels in the back of the eye. Sudden stress through anaerobic exercises like weight lifting are more dangerous than aerobic exercises like jogging. Avoid any vigorous exercise until your eye specialist reports if laser therapy or other treatment has stabilised or arrested progression of the retinopathy.

What type of exercise?

Aerobic versus anaerobic physical activity

Aerobic activity relates to exercises such as jogging or swimming which are associated with movement over a reasonably long period and during which the body uses a substantial amount of oxygen.

Aerobic activity is generally beneficial to the body and causes improvements in insulin sensitivity, blood glucose, blood pressure and lipids.

Anaerobic physical activity is usually a sudden, rapid stressful exercise such as weight lifting or 100-metre sprints. This type of activity produces fewer benefits and may be associated with a sharp rise in blood pressure. Anaerobic exercise is not generally recommended for people with diabetes.

Activities which may present special dangers

Because of the risk of a hypoglycaemic reaction causing mental confusion or coma, there are certain activities which may constitute significant danger to people with diabetes. These include motor racing, high standard mountain climbing, hang gliding, solo yachting and scuba diving. These activities should generally be avoided or approached with extreme caution.

Other potentially dangerous activities may be undertaken as long as the person recognises and accepts the risks. These activities include surfboard riding, long distance running, triathlons and cross-country skiing. It is strongly recommended that the person with diabetes is with a friend who understands the person's diabetes and knows how to deal with a hypoglycaemic reaction.

How much exercise is desirable?

So far there is no precise answer as there has not been enough study of the long-term effects of exercise in people with diabetes. However, 20 to 40 minutes of moderate exercise, three or four times a week, is very useful in exerting favourable effects on blood fats, blood pressure and heart function. About 40 minutes exercise four times a week is suggested as ideal, although recent studies suggest that even less physical activity still reduces the risk of cardiovascular disease.

Moderate physical activity means exercise that is strenuous enough to make you puff a bit but you would be able to carry on a conversation during exercise, taking a few puffs between sentences. This is about 50 per cent of maximum aerobic capacity.

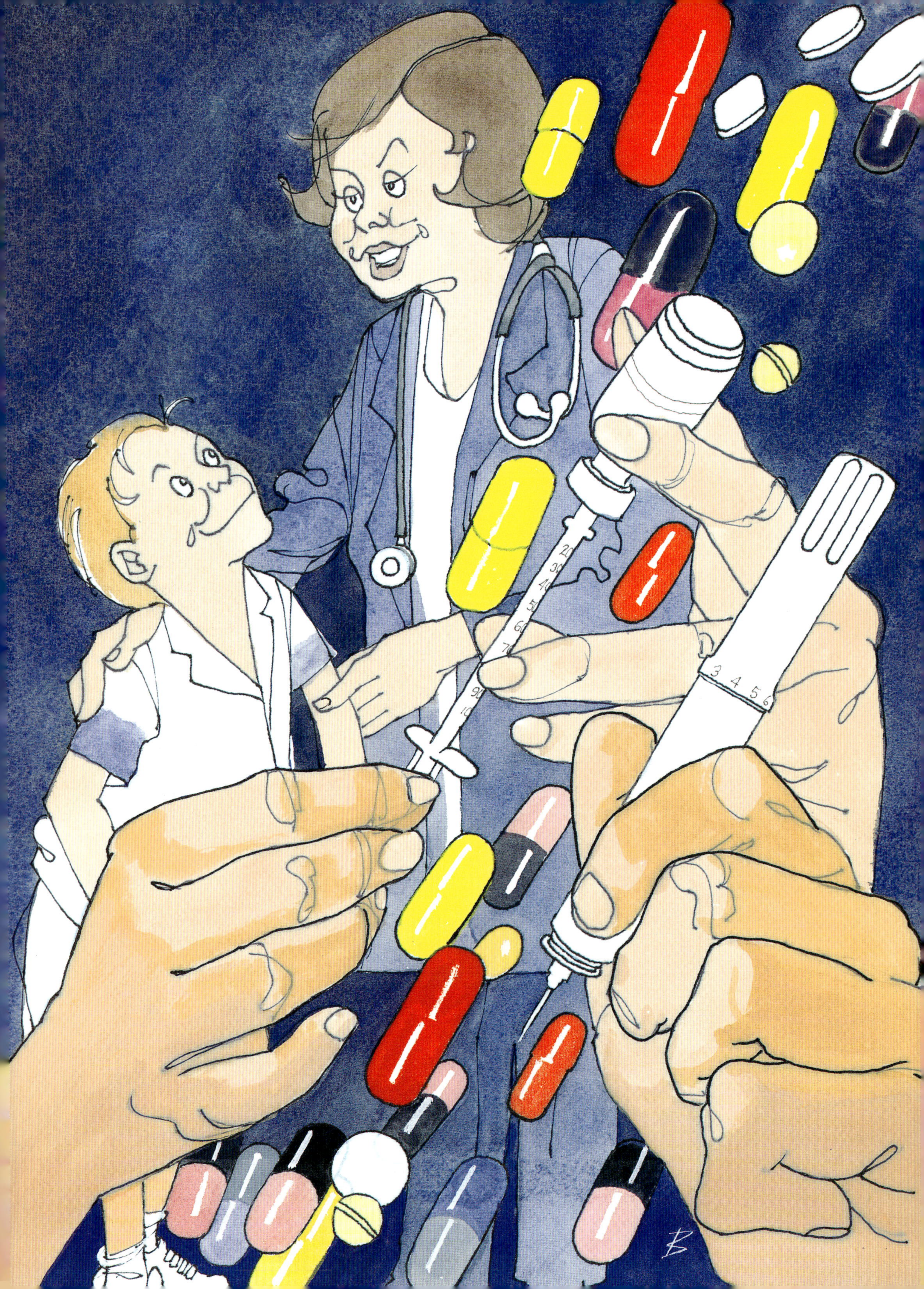
3 4 5 6

Chapter 8

Insulin and its Role

◆ By Dr Frank Alford ◆
Revised by Dr David O'Neal and Trisha Dunning

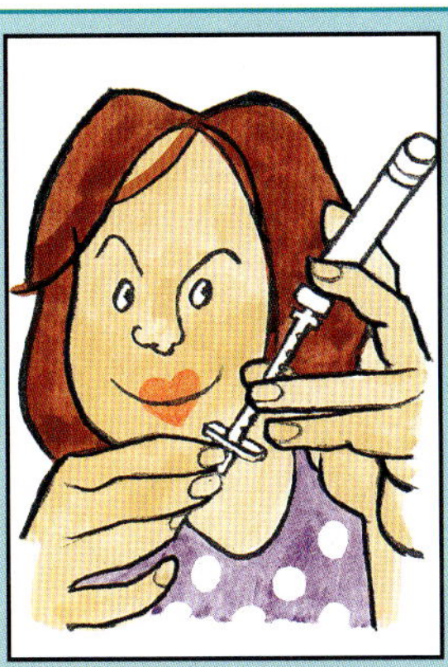

AT A GLANCE

- **Five types of insulin are available and you and your doctor will discuss which is right for you.**
- **Know your condition – have a good working knowledge of your diabetes.**
- **Know your insulin – remember its time of peak action and total duration.**
- **Test regularly – and monitor results.**
- **Record test results – and use your records to make informed decisions.**
- **Consider your diet – often a change of diet can be as useful as a change in insulin dosage.**
- **If in doubt, ask your doctor or diabetes nurse educator.**

INSULIN is a hormone produced by a gland called the pancreas. Insulin enables glucose in the blood to enter body cells such as muscles where it can be used for energy.

In people without diabetes, a perfect balance exists between glucose entering and leaving the blood, and blood glucose levels are maintained within a fairly narrow range.

In the case of diabetes, the pancreas does not make enough insulin and normal levels of blood glucose cannot be maintained. The body needs help and this may require the administration of insulin.

Because insulin cannot be given as a tablet, insulin injections are required.

All insulin preparations basically do the same job. They all lower blood glucose levels.

One unit of short-acting insulin will have the same capacity to lower blood glucose as one unit of long-acting insulin. The difference is in the amount of time it takes to do this.

The choice of which type of insulin is best suited to a person's particular needs and lifestyle will be made by the doctor and patient together.

The choice, and the education process that goes with it, are most important. The person with diabetes must know which insulin they use and what its properties are.

It is not advisable to switch randomly from one insulin to another, regardless of how similar their names or qualities may seem.

Getting the dose of insulin correct is vital. Too much insulin produces too great a fall in blood glucose. This leads to hypoglycaemia. Not enough insulin won't lower blood glucose levels sufficiently, resulting in poorly controlled diabetes.

Key points to remember are:

- *Type of insulin preparation used and daily dosage.*
- *The time your insulin has its maximum effect and how long it lasts for.* This is important because the time when the insulin preparation is having its greatest effect is also the time when the person with diabetes is most likely to have hypoglycaemia.
- *Regular timing of injections and meals.* It is important to appropriately match the timing of the insulin injections and the time of meals. Regular meals at regular times are important. It may also be

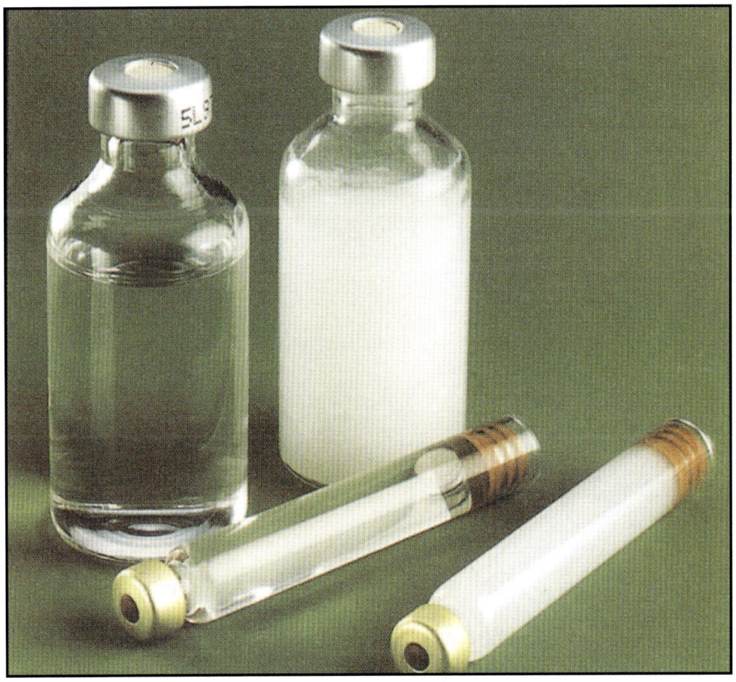

COURTESY BECTON DICKINSON

necessary to take snacks between meals on the advice of your doctor, diabetes nurse educator or dietitian.

- *Report to your health care professional any change in lifestyle, working hours, physical activity or meal times.* Each of these factors – plus stress and illness – can affect the control of diabetes or blood glucose levels.

The most important thing is to ask questions. It is vital that you have access to all information on diabetes and its treatment. If there is anything you are not sure about, ask your doctor or diabetes nurse educator and insist on answers you can understand.

Types of insulin preparations

The treatment of diabetes is based on learning about the condition and the ways to control it. Your initial discussion with your doctor or nurse educator about diabetes and the various types of insulin will probably seem confusing. Don't panic. No one can be expected to grasp all the information at one sitting.

Once you begin to become more familiar with insulin, you will be able to discuss it further. Once you feel more confident and in control, you will be able to determine the best ways to make your treatment fit in with your lifestyle.

The table gives examples of widely used types of insulin and how they work in relation to your day. You will see that they all have different brand names, but don't let this worry you. The actual type of insulin (generic name) always appears on the label, so as long as you know the type of insulin you need, the brand name should not confuse you.

There are different brands of insulin preparations made by various manufacturers. Almost all insulin used in Australia today is made in the laboratory and is exactly the same as human insulin. It is available in either short-acting insulin, with effects which last six to eight hours; medium, up to 24 hours; and long- acting, which can last up to 36 hours.

In addition, more recently a modified form of human insulin with a rapid onset and duration of about five hours has become available.

There are five types of insulin preparations currently available:

- rapid onset – short-acting
- short-acting
- intermediate-acting
- mixed (short and intermediate)
- long-acting.

Currently there is only one rapid onset – short-acting insulin available in Australia. It is specially modified human insulin known as lispro insulin (HUMALOG®). It is clear in appearance and its precise role is yet to be determined. Because of its rapid onset of action, it can be administered immediately before a meal. It has not been tested in pregnant women, but there does not appear to be any reason why it should not be used in pregnancy.

Short-acting insulin preparations – also known as soluble or neutral insulin – have their maximum effect from about three to six hours after injection, with the effects wearing off rapidly after about eight hours. They are clear in appearance.

Intermediate-acting insulins are cloudy and look like very delicate milk and have their maximum effect between 8 and 15 hours after injection. This means they work hardest in the mid-afternoon or early evening after a morning injection. A mid-afternoon snack to balance the insulin action may be needed.

Mixed short and intermediate-acting insulins contain a mixture of two insulins in various proportions. These are known as premixed insulins. For instance, mixtures of three parts short-acting to seven parts intermediate-acting insulins known as Humulin 30/70 or Mixtard 30/70 are available, as are other combinations.

Long-acting insulins have a gradual onset and last up to 36 hours. They are cloudy in appearance.

When are different insulin preparations used?

Short-acting insulins are used in standard day-to-day treatment, either several times a day on their own (usually with a pen device rather than a syringe), or fewer times a day, in combination with intermediate or long acting insulins. They are also used when control is needed quickly or when some complicated situation has arisen, such as acute infection or surgery.

Intermediate-acting insulins are usually used in standard day-to-day control, either once or twice daily.

Long-acting insulins are used with short acting insulins and given by pen devices.

However, their use may be associated with hypoglycaemia which may cause problems.

Strength of insulins

All insulin preparations carry a label to indicate their strength, on the basis of how many units of insulin there are in one millilitre (ml) of the solution. In Australia, this is 100 units per ml, signified on the label as U100.

U100 insulin has taken over in Australia from U40 and U80, but in some countries these strengths may still be available. This means you must take extra care to check the strength of the insulin when travelling overseas. U40 or U80 insulin should not be used with the standard Australian U100 syringe as the dose will be incorrect.

To be sure, no matter where you are, always check that the chemist and the doctor have given you the correct type of insulin. And always check the expiry date on the label.

Storage of insulin

The insulin (vial or cartridge) not in use should be stored in a refrigerator, but not in a freezer. Check expiry date and appearance before using.

Insulin is destroyed by heat, so must not be left in the car glove box or elsewhere where temperatures may exceed 30°C.

TYPES OF INSULIN COMMONLY USED
TIMES OF ACTION IN HOURS AFTER INJECTIONS

TYPES OF INSULIN		OVERALL EFFECT Hours	START OF EFFECT Hours	MAXIMUM EFFECT (Greatest Chance of Hypoglycaemia Hours	END OF EFFECT	APPEARANCE	SPECIES OF INSULIN
GENERIC NAME	TRADE NAME APRIL 1999						
Insulin Lispro	Humalog	Rapid onset/ short-acting	¼–½	1–2	4	Clear	Modified Human
Neutral (Soluble)	Actrapid Humulin R Hypurin	Short-acting	½–1	2–4	6–8	Clear	Human Human Beef
Isophane (NPH)	Humulin NPH Protaphane Hypurin	Intermediate	2	4–10	16–18	Cloudy	Human Human Beef
Insulin Zinc Suspension	Humulin L Monotard	Intermediate	2	6–12	16–24	Cloudy	Human Human
Isophane plus Neutral Mixed insulin	Humulin* Mixtard*	Mixed Short & Intermediate-acting	1-2	2–12 (Biphasic)	16–18	Cloudy	Human Human
Insulin Zinc Suspension (crystalline)	Humulin UL Ultratard	Long-acting Pens/Syringes	2–6	6–20	24–36	Cloudy	Human Human

**Available in various mixtures of neutral and Isophane 20:80, 30:70, 50:50.*

Finding the right dose

Treatment with insulin usually begins in a diabetes centre or hospital.

There you will be taught a number of things such as injection techniques, storage of syringes and needles, interpretation of blood and urine tests, and how to recognise and treat hypoglycaemia.

At this time you will work closely with your doctor and diabetes nurse educator. They will suggest an insulin dose for you to start on. This is fine in principle, but usually needs to be adjusted and fine-tuned when you are at home in your normal environment. Then your doctor can recommend the most appropriate dose for you.

Adjusting the dose

Some people are reluctant to change their daily dose of insulin without consulting a doctor or nurse, but there are situations in which it may be necessary to do so.

For instance, there could be a change of diet or increase in activity at work. You may have a minor infection or be under stress. All these things mean that your usual insulin dose will not provide the level of control it should. In such cases you will need to adjust the dose to keep your blood glucose at a satisfactory level. However, it is important not to change the dosage too much and risk hypoglycaemia.

You will need confidence and experience to do this, which will come in time. A general rule is that it is quite safe to vary your insulin by up to one-tenth of your regular dose. That is, two units if you are taking up to 20 units per dose; four units if you are taking 20–40 units per dose; six to eight units for a dose between 40–80 units.

Through your own experience and by keeping a careful blood glucose record, you will know whether larger variations can be made safely. Generally speaking, an increase in insulin will be necessary to counter illness such as infection, inactivity, an increase in food and, in some instances, extreme stress.

A decrease in insulin will be necessary after recovering from infection, with increased activity or when food intake is likely to be less than normal. Dosage should also be decreased if you've had hypoglycaemia for no apparent reason.

The menstrual cycle may also affect diabetes control and it is not unusual for women to need different doses of insulin before, during and after their periods.

Ideally, the insulin dose should be tailored to match regular blood glucose test results. Measurement of blood glucose levels is the best guide to glucose control. This is why it is so important to record the results of your regular blood glucose tests. If you have this information, you can use it to make the right decision at the right time.

A guide to interpreting blood glucose levels is in chapter 10, Self-monitoring of Blood Glucose.

Charts for varying insulin dosage are available. Ask your doctor or diabetes nurse educator to explain how to use them. However, there are some basic rules that you should follow:

- *Know your condition* – have a good working knowledge of your diabetes.
- *Know your insulin* – remember its time of peak action and total duration.
- *Test regularly* – and monitor results.
- *Record test results* – and use your records to make informed decisions.
- *Consider your diet* – often a change of diet can be as useful as a change in insulin dosage.
- *If in doubt, ask your doctor or diabetes nurse educator.*

Problems you may encounter

There are some problems associated with injecting insulin, but most are rarely encountered and, if so, are usually temporary.

One that can be avoided through knowledge and practice is incorrect injection technique. If insulin is injected into the skin instead of under it, it may cause a painful local reaction with redness around the injection site.

The correct technique is explained in chapter 9, Injections and Injectors.

Reactions brought on by incorrect technique occur immediately after injection. This is different from another rare problem, local allergy, which occurs in the first couple of months of using insulin, and goes away after one or two months.

The problems of loss of fatty tissue or hollows (fat atrophy) and the formation of fatty tissue or lumps (fat hypertrophy) are both rare today because of the use of purified insulins. These problems are usually avoided by changing the site of injection each day.

There are also two types of systemic, or generalised, immune reactions, both of which are very rare. They come either in the form of a skin rash with or without swelling, or as insulin resistance that is generally taken to mean a daily requirement of more than 200 units of insulin.

Insulin delivery systems

A number of devices are available to help you with the regular injection of insulin. These include disposable syringes and insulin pens. These devices are described in chapter 9, Injections and Injectors but, simple and convenient as they are, they neither lessen the need for a full understanding of insulin and how it works, nor the need for diligent blood glucose monitoring.

Some people use a mechanical infusion pump which uses short acting insulin, delivered at a low rate at night and between meals, and at a high rate at meal times. However, they are expensive to buy and maintain.

In a hospital setting insulin is sometimes delivered directly into the vein. This is known as insulin infusion. This usually involves a mechanical infusion device and requires careful monitoring by medical and nursing staff.

Chapter 9

Injections and Injectors

◆ By Dr Alan Stocks AM ◆

PEOPLE with type 1 or type 2 diabetes may need insulin treatment. Those with type 1 usually start insulin within the first year of diagnosis. Those with type 2 diabetes who need insulin usually start several years after diagnosis and may also be treated with oral medication and by modifying their lifestyle.

When people start using insulin they need to learn the correct injection and dosage techniques from the doctor or diabetes nurse educator. The learning process takes place in hospital or a diabetes clinic. When the person with diabetes goes home to get on with day-to-day life, daily injections will become routine.

The doctor or diabetes nurse educator is always available to give advice, but the daily management of your diabetes ultimately rests with you. Therefore it is vital to inject correctly and measure insulin accurately.

Insulin cannot be taken as tablets because it is broken down by digestion in the stomach. Experiments are under way with insulin that is inhaled into the lungs, similar to an asthma spray – and this may be available in the near future. At present, there is no alternative but to inject insulin and this can be done with syringes, pen injectors or a special infusion system.

Obviously no one enjoys having injections, but it can be made a lot less uncomfortable by using the right equipment and the correct technique.

Most people with diabetes prefer to use a pen injector rather than a syringe. However, some insulins are not marketed in penfill cartridges and can only be given with syringes.

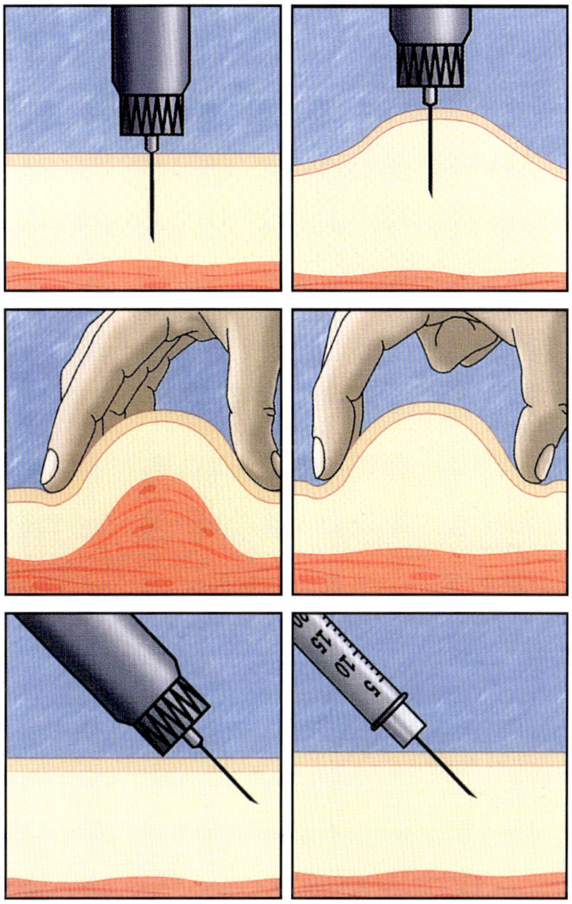

COURTESY BECTON DICKINSON

AT A GLANCE

- **The daily injection process will become routine.**
- **Your doctor or diabetes nurse educator will teach you the correct injection and dose measurement techniques, while answering any of your treatment queries.**
- **A wide variety of injectors and injections are available, each designed for a particular purpose and individual's needs.**
- **Bruising, lumps and other responses to injections can be avoided if you have the know-how.**

Types of syringe

Insulin syringes are all marked with a scale and there is only one strength of insulin available in Australia (U100). Insulin syringes are obtainable from state branches of Diabetes Australia on the National Diabetic Services Scheme (NDSS), or from chemists and some hospital diabetes clinics.

The most commonly used syringe has a total capacity of 1 ml, marked with 50 lines along its side – one line equals two units. The major divisions, 10, 20, 30 and so on are marked with a number and a longer line. Smaller syringes are also available with a total capacity of 30 units or 50 units. In both of these, the lines are at one-unit intervals. Major divisions for every five units are marked with a number and a longer line. All insulin syringes are disposable plastic items with fixed needles of 8 mm or 13 mm length. Most syringes now have a 30-gauge needle, but 28 and 29-gauge needles are still available. (The higher the gauge the finer the needle.) The needles also come in different lengths for people with different skin thickness. For example, 8 mm for those with thin skin; 13 mm for those with thicker skin.

Withdrawing insulin from the bottle

The recognised routine for withdrawing insulin from a bottle is as follows:

1. Wash and dry hands.
2. Gently swirl the bottle or turn it upside down to mix

and suspend the insulin (but do not shake the bottle). This is especially important with cloudy insulins, which should become an even suspension. If there are obvious particles that stick to the inside of the bottle, the insulin may have deteriorated and should be thrown out. Clear insulin should be exactly that – clear – and bottles with sediment floating in them should also be thrown out.

3. Remove the needle guard but don't touch the needle tip. Pump the syringe with air to be sure that the needle is clear and the plunger moves easily.
4. Withdraw the plunger to measure the same amount of air as the required dose of insulin.
5. Invert the insulin bottle. Holding it firmly, pierce the centre of the cap with the needle and inject air into the bottle. Draw the plunger down again and insulin will then flow easily into the syringe to replace the amount of air injected. It is not necessary to swab the top of the insulin bottle before use.
6. Tap the syringe barrel gently with one finger to send any air bubbles up into the bottle. This is sometimes difficult with plastic syringes but if only a few tiny bubbles remain this will not matter.
7. When the bubbles are expelled, adjust the plunger to measure the exact dose of insulin.
8. Withdraw the needle from the bottle. The syringe now contains the correct dose.
9. Inject the insulin.

Withdrawing a mixed dose

If you need to withdraw insulin from two bottles for a mixed dose:

Follow steps 1, 2 and 3 above, then:

4. Withdraw the plunger on the syringe to measure the same amount of air as the required dose of cloudy insulin. Inject this air into the cloudy insulin bottle but do not withdraw the insulin. Instead, with the plunger fully pressed down, remove the needle from the bottle. This leaves the positive air pressure inside the bottle.
5. Measure air in the syringe to equal the required dose of clear insulin.
6. Inject this air into the clear insulin bottle.
7. Withdraw the required amount of clear insulin and expel the bubbles.
8. Re-insert the needle into the cloudy insulin bottle and carefully pull down the plunger to withdraw the required cloudy insulin. If you accidentally withdraw too much cloudy insulin, do not press the plunger to return it to the bottle, as this will put clear insulin into the cloudy bottle. Simply remove the bottle, expel all insulin from the syringe, and start again from step 4.
9. Inject the mixture.

When drawing up mixed doses always draw up the two insulins in the correct order – if cloudy insulin is accidentally put into the clear insulin, the cloudy addition will affect the clear insulin.

Types of pen injector

Pen injectors have many advantages over syringes, mainly the speed and convenience of having the insulin in a disposable cartridge inside the pen. Cartridges of quick-acting and intermediate insulins plus mixtures with varying proportions of the two are available containing 1.5 ml and 3 ml of insulin.

Insulin zinc suspensions such as Humulin® L, Humulin® UL, Monotard™ and Ultratard™ are not marketed in cartridges. Details of insulins used in pens appear in Table 1 (page 28).

The Novopen I™ looks like a metal fountain pen but when the cap is unscrewed and fitted on to the other end of the pen, a small plunger appears and it becomes a syringe. It uses disposable cartridges containing 1.5 ml or 150 units of insulin.

Pressing the plunger down completely delivers two units of insulin and a double click is easily heard. Pushing the plunger down halfway causes a single click and delivers one unit of insulin.

As the cartridge empties, a red rubber bung can be seen moving up through a window on the side of the pen. When the leading edge of the bung reaches the coloured line on the side of the cartridge, there are 10 units remaining. When replacing the cartridge, it is important to hold the Novopen vertically, with the needle downwards so the ratchet device inside the lid falls into the new cartridge and comes to lie hard against the rubber bung. If it doesn't, depressing the plunger may not deliver insulin. Before using the pen, it is essential to check that it is delivering insulin by pressing the plunger until a tiny jet of insulin is expelled.

The Novopen II™ is no longer available and has been replaced by the Novopen 3™. This is larger and fatter than the Novopen I™ and uses a cartridge containing 3 ml or 300 units of insulin. The insulin dose, from 1–70 units, is set by twisting the end section of the pen anti-clockwise and a click is heard after each unit. The dose can be checked on a visual scale and the insulin can be injected by twisting the end clockwise back to zero or by pressing the plunger at the end of the pen, whichever you prefer.

When the leading edge of the bung is seen to reach the coloured line on the side of the cartridge, there are 50 units remaining.

If too large a dose has been dialled in error, pull the main body of the pen and the section which holds the insulin apart, and the silver part will show. While holding the two sections apart, push down on the plunger and the dial will return to zero. Release your hold and then redial your new dose. It is important to perform this manoeuvre before inserting the needle into the injection site, otherwise an accidental overdose may be given if your hand slips.

When replacing the cartridge, the piston must be wound back completely before inserting the new cartridge. It is then essential to dial and expel insulin until a jet of fluid appears from the needle.

The B-D pen is a plastic device, similar in size to the Novopen 3™ but uses a 1.5 ml cartridge. Twisting the end section of the pen clockwise sets the dose from 1–30 units, and a click is heard after each unit. As with the

Novopen 3™, the dose can be checked on a visual scale and the insulin can be injected either by twisting the end of the pen anti-clockwise back to zero, or pressing the plunger at the end of the pen.

If too large a dose has been dialled in error, continue dialling past 30 units and the plunger will return to zero without wasting the insulin; then you can start again.

As with the Novopen 3™, when replacing the cartridge the piston is wound back completely before inserting the new cartridge. It is essential then to dial and expel insulin until a jet of fluid appears from the needle.

A version of the B-D pen is available which uses a 3 ml cartridge but each click on the scale measures two units. It is useful for people needing large doses of insulin, and can deliver 2–60 units per dose. *An earlier 3 ml pen known as the B-D Plus™ was found to be dangerous when not used according to the manufacturer's instructions and has been withdrawn from the market.*

A new injector pen produced by Eli Lilly and called Humapen™ is now available. It accommodates a 3 ml cartridge and can deliver one unit increments. The container into which the cartridge fits is marked to indicate the number of units remaining, and this clicks into place when a new cartridge is loaded into it. The plunger can easily be pushed down.

The required dose of insulin can be dialled up, as with other pens to a maximum of 60 units. If too much insulin has been dialled, the dial can be wound down without wasting insulin. The insulin is injected by pressing down on the end of the plunger, and a moulded hand grip makes the injection process easier.

Questions about injector pens

Many people who have used syringes for years have doubts about pens and commonly ask the following questions:

1. *Are injector pens accurate?* Yes. Many trials of all the above pens show them to be highly accurate, even with small doses.
2. *Can you check the accuracy?* Yes. The conical cover of Novopen needles has flanges extending halfway down the tube. If you expel 20 units of insulin into the tube, the fluid level should reach the end of the flanges. If it does not, the pen is faulty.
3. *How do you know the pen is delivering insulin?* Before making an injection, dial up two units of insulin and expel it. The jet of fluid should be obvious and a tiny drop of insulin on the end of the needle indicates that it is full.
4. *What happens when the cartridge is empty?* When the cartridge is empty, the plunger cannot be depressed and the dose remaining to be given is indicated on the dial. A new cartridge should be inserted and the remainder of the scheduled dose given.
5. *With syringes, some people can draw back the plunger to be sure the end of the needle is not in a vein. How can they check this with a pen?* Unfortunately, this is not possible but, in practice, an accidental injection into a vein is rare. In fact, most people don't draw back the plunger of the syringe and it is not necessary for a pen injector.
6. *What can you do if the pen jams or won't work?* Such faults are uncommon but, in an emergency, use a syringe to withdraw insulin from a cartridge. It is not necessary to inject air into the cartridge first because the bung will be sucked forward as the insulin is withdrawn. When travelling, carry a spare pen plus a few syringes, just in case.
7. *How should the insulin cartridges be stored?* Insulin is remarkably stable at room temperature and pens can safely be carried around in a coat pocket or handbag. They should not be left anywhere where the temperature is likely to exceed 30°C.
8. *Why does a drop of insulin appear at the end of the needle after the injection has been completed and the needle withdrawn?* This is because the 29 and 30-gauge needles are so narrow it takes a while for all the insulin to pass through them. It is wise to leave the needle in place for five seconds after completing the injection; even then, a tiny drop may still appear, but it is only a fraction of one unit and is not important.

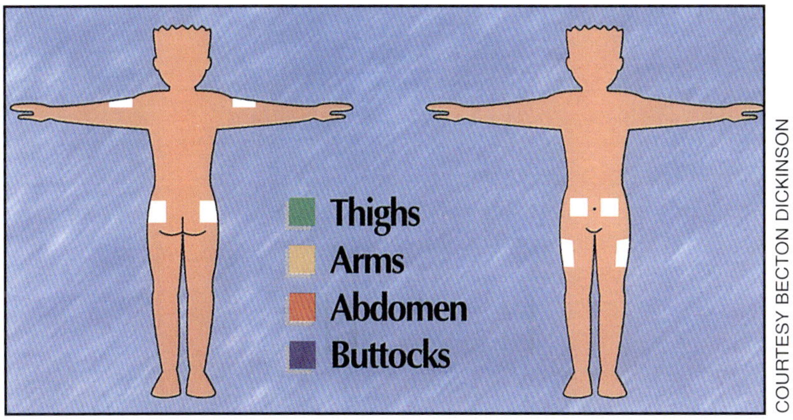

Key insulin injection sites

9. *How often should the needle be changed?* The manufacturers recommend single use only but, in practice, most people re-use needles until they become blunt (easy to tell, as they don't slide easily and painlessly through the skin). People who do re-use needles simply replace the cap. Multiple use for one person is safe but of course needle sharing is not!
10. *Why are some insulins like Monotard™ and Humulin-L™ not marketed in cartridges?* Longer acting (cloudy) insulins are a suspension of crystals and the longer the action the larger are the crystals. The insulin manufacturers believe that it is too difficult to keep the large crystals in suspension in a cartridge and dosage inaccuracies could occur due to incomplete mixing. All cloudy insulins should be

Table 1

Insulin Cartridges available in Australia

	Brand Name	Company	Cartridge Size		Colour of Cap (Novo) or Label (Lilly)
			1.5 ml	3 ml	
Quick-acting					
	Actrapid	Novo Nordisk	+	+	Yellow
	Humulin R	Eli Lilly/Aza	+	+	Yellow
	Humalog (LisPro)	Eli Lilly/Aza	+	+	Purple
Intermediate					
	Protaphane	Novo Nordisk	+	+	Green
	Humulin NPH	Eli Lilly/Aza	+	+	Green
Mixtures					
	Mixtard 50/50	Novo Nordisk	0	+	Grey
	Mixtard 30/70	Novo Nordisk	+	+	Brown
	Mixtard 20/80	Novo Nordisk	0	+	Pink
	Humulin 30/70	Eli Lilly/Aza	+	+	Brown
	Humulin 20/80	Eli Lilly/Aza	+	+	Orange

re-suspended before each injection by gently tipping the pen up and down a few times. Violent shaking is unwise, as the insulin crystals can be damaged.

Automatic injectors

Some people find automatic injectors of great benefit if they are not confident about giving themselves injections. These devices have a mechanically controlled spring which thrusts the needle through the skin quickly.

Some also depress the plunger automatically, but these are not recommended because there is a risk the insulin will be injected too closely under the skin.

Devices such as the Busher injector insert the needle mechanically but the plunger has to be pushed by hand to make the device less liable to error.

There are some claims that automatic injectors give painless injections but this may not be true. Some require special syringes and these may not conform to the Australian Standard for insulin syringes.

Jet injectors

Jet injectors have the supposed advantage that it is not necessary to insert a needle as the injection device fires a jet of insulin through the skin at high speed.

Such devices are extremely expensive, need frequent sterilisation by boiling in distilled water, are too bulky to be easily carried around, and drawing up the insulin is more complicated than with syringes. Injections are usually – but not always – painless and bruising at the injection site occurs just as often as with ordinary syringes and pen injectors.

Jet injectors may be useful for people with diabetes who cannot bring themselves to inject with a needle, but cannot be recommended for the majority of people with diabetes.

Devices for people with poor eyesight

For people using syringes there are several devices which enable safe and accurate measurement of doses for the partially sighted or blind. The B-D Magni-Guide™ clips on to an insulin bottle and ensures that the needle of a standard insulin syringe will puncture the rubber cap of the bottle in the centre. It also magnifies the markings on the syringe to three times normal size for easy reading of scale and improved dose accuracy.

Pen injectors are the safest device for people who are partially sighted or blind and who wish to continue giving their own injections, as the dose does not have to be measured from a bottle.

Choosing the site of injection

The best places for injections are those where a loose fold of skin can be pinched up. These are the abdomen, upper outer thighs and the buttocks.

It is difficult to give an insulin injection into the arms as insulin absorption may be variable and lumps and hollows may occur. It is best to use unexposed areas on the abdomen, buttocks and upper thighs.

The injection should not be given into the same area day after day as this can cause fatty lumps to develop. These are not only unsightly but the absorption of insulin is delayed, reduced and unpredictable, causing unstable blood glucose control.

Therefore, it is necessary to vary the site, but in a calculated and systematic way. If, for example, you use the abdomen, vary the site by about 2 cm each day, moving along an imaginary line running up and down. You can give the injections as far up as the rib margin; down to the top of the pelvic bone and round to the side as far as you can see. The only area on the abdomen which should not be used is 2.5 cm (1 inch) around the navel.

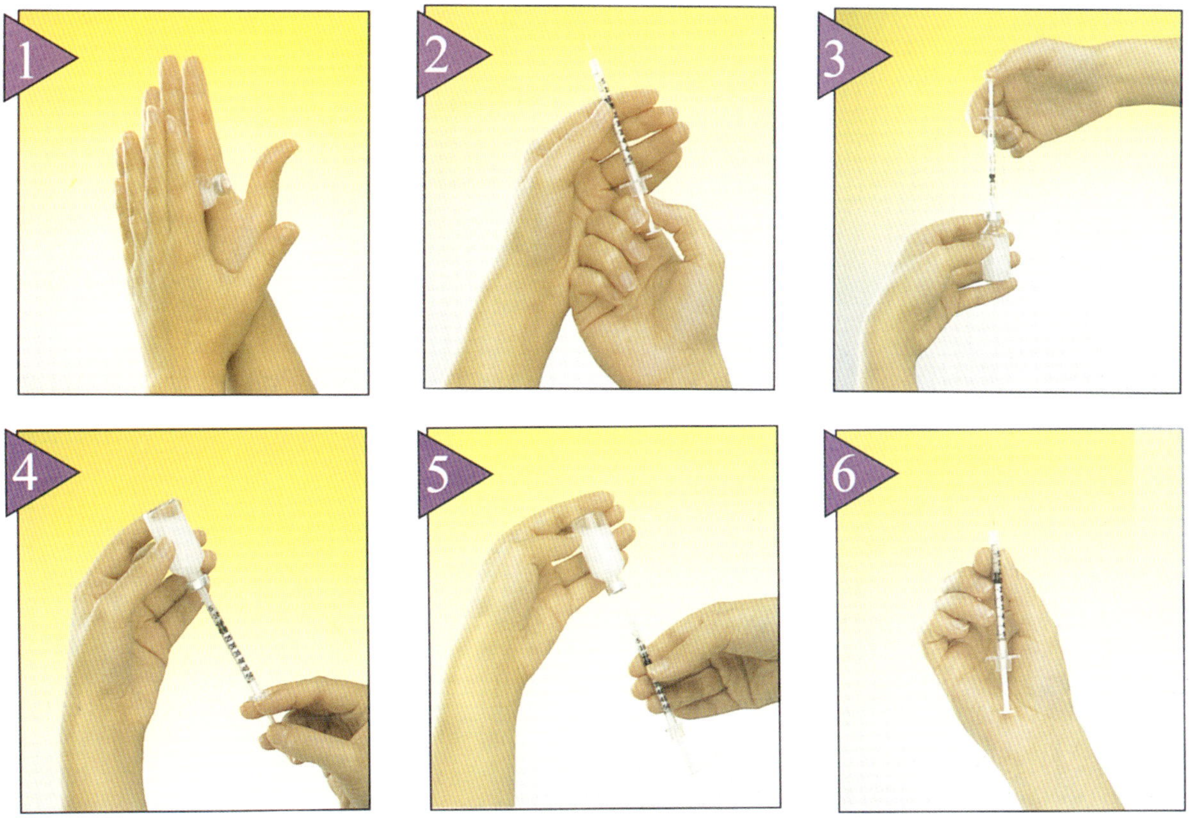

COURTESY BECTON DICKINSON

Figure 1: *If you are using a cloudy insulin gently rotate the bottle to make sure that the insulin is evenly mixed (never shake the bottle).*

Figure 2: *Remove the white cap covering the plunger, then carefully remove the orange needle cap by gently twisting and pulling.*
Pull back the plunger of the syringe to measure the amount of air equivalent to the amount of insulin you require.

Figure 3: *With the bottle standing upright, insert the needle straight through the centre of the rubber cap of the insulin bottle and push the plunger completely in. This pushes the air into the bottle, making it easier for you to draw up the insulin out of the bottle.*

Figure 4. *Turn the bottle upside down. Make certain that the point of the needle inside the bottle is well beneath the surface level of the insulin.*

Pull back the plunger until you have measured your correct dose of insulin.

Figure 5: *Remove the needle from the bottle and expel any air bubbles. Flick or tap the syringe at the bubble with your finger. When the air bubble goes to the top of the syringe, push the plunger up to expel the bubble.*

Figure 6: *Check you have your correct dose of insulin. You are now ready to give your insulin injection.*

It should be possible to place 8–10 injections on each line and to fit in at least 10 lines, 2 cms apart, across the abdomen. Imagining the abdomen squared off like a grid, it should be possible to fit in up to 100 injections before using the starting spot again. This will prevent fatty lumps developing. You can use a similar grid-like pattern on the thighs.

Where not to inject

Insulin should never be injected into the inner side of the arms, the inner side of the thighs or groin creases because in these locations large nerves and blood vessels are near the surface. To reduce the risk of bruising avoid areas that show networks of fine veins.

If fatty lumps have already developed, don't inject insulin into the lumps. Use other sites until the lumps go away.

Giving the injection

The technique of giving an injection will be discussed and demonstrated by your doctor or diabetes nurse educator. There are two standard routines:-

A. One method is to hold the syringe between the thumb and middle finger, leaving the index finger free to push the plunger. Pinch up an area of skin with your other hand.

   Insert the needle at a slight angle off the vertical. Slowly push in the plunger to inject the insulin dose. Withdraw the needle after five seconds, then release the pinched up area and press firmly.

B. 1. Alternatively, if the injection site is dirty, it should be cleaned with soap and water. It is not necessary to swab the area with spirit or alcohol as this increases the likelihood of a painful injection.
   2. Hold the syringe like a pencil between the fingers.
   3. With the other hand, pinch up a fold of skin, 2–3 cm across. Hold the syringe at an angle of about 90 degrees to the skin
   4. Insert the needle to the full length.
   5. Let go the fold of skin and grasp the bottom of the syringe. This releases the other hand to

operate the plunger. Thin people using a 13 mm needle should maintain the pinch of skin while injecting the insulin, to avoid injecting into muscle rather than the fat under the skin. This is not a problem when using 8 mm needles.

6. Gently raise the plunger to check that the needle is not lying in a blood vessel. If blood appears in the syringe when the plunger is raised, withdraw the needle and start all over again.

   NOTE: Only a very gentle upward pressure is needed. If the plunger does not withdraw easily, it is most unlikely that the needle tip lies in a blood vessel.

7. If no blood appears in the syringe, inject the insulin slowly.
8. Wait five seconds then withdraw the needle and press firmly over the injection site. Do not rub the site. If bleeding or bruising occurs, press firmly for two or three minutes.

If a disposable needle or syringe is used it should be disposed of safely. It should be placed in a metal or plastic sharps container, available from Diabetes Australia, some chemists and local councils.

Local skin reactions

These are rare when injections are given correctly but include:

- Stinging which may occur at the injection site when you first start treatment; when insulin is cold; when injecting through alcohol from a swab or when the insulin is injected into the skin (leaving a lump) rather than under the skin.
- Mild local allergy which may cause tender itchy red lumps at the injection site. This usually occurs during the first few weeks of treatment but these days is extremely rare as insulin is purer than years ago. This problem usually solves itself after a few weeks and it is not necessary to change the type of insulin being used. If it is distressing, apply an antihistamine cream before injecting.
- Hollows (fatty atrophy) – the wasting of fatty tissue under the skin is a problem rarely encountered since the introduction of highly purified insulins. It is more common among women than men; more common when long-acting insulins are used and much more common when insulin is injected cold. Insulin should always be injected at room temperature. Store the bottle of insulin being used at room temperature rather than returning it to the refrigerator after each injection.
- Lumps (fatty hypertrophy) – repeated injections of insulin into one area will produce a fatty lump at the injection site. Although they may be unsightly, of greater importance is that absorption of insulin from fatty lumps is inefficient and unpredictable so may cause unstable blood glucose control. If you change the injection site after a lump has formed, the resulting more rapid absorption of insulin from the new site may cause unexpected hypoglycaemia. Lumps usually disappear slowly over several months when you stop injecting at that site.
- Bruising sometimes occurs, no matter where the insulin is injected. It is sensible to avoid obvious networks of veins. If you experience a stinging sensation as the tip of the needle touches the skin, you are injecting through a pain receptor. These are more likely to occur over the top of surface veins and it is wise not to persist with this injection but to shift the needle tip by 1–2 mm and find a spot where no stinging occurs.

General reactions

- General allergy to insulin which affects the whole body is very rare but if it occurs it may produce a skin rash, fever, joint pains and difficulty breathing. Report any of these symptoms to your doctor immediately.
- Insulin resistance is very rare since the introduction of highly purified insulins.

Self-monitoring of Blood Glucose

◆ By Trisha Dunning ◆

IN order to go about their everyday lives, people with diabetes must know what their body is doing. Effective control of diabetes is about maintaining a satisfactory blood glucose balance in the bloodstream. You can achieve this balance by a combination of meal plan, exercise and, if needed, tablets or insulin.

Regular monitoring of your blood glucose levels enables you to determine the required dose of insulin or tablets and the amount of food and exercise needed to create that balance.

Monitoring blood glucose does not require complex equipment and is a relatively simple procedure easily fitted into your regular routine.

After your diagnosis, a member of your diabetes health care team will teach you how to monitor your blood glucose and explain why it is such a vital management tool. If you need follow up advice, simply ask your diabetes nurse educator, general practitioner or diabetes specialist.

AT A GLANCE

• Regular monitoring of blood glucose levels need not be a hassle and plays an active part in your ability to maintain a happy, enjoyable life. • Keep asking questions about blood glucose testing and keep practising blood testing until you feel confident and comfortable about your technique. • There are at least 10 good reasons why you should regularly monitor your blood glucose, including measuring the effectiveness of your treatment and preventing or delaying the onset of complications. • Several factors – including equipment faults and human error – may influence the reliability of your test results. • Record your results in a record book and take them to your diabetes advisers on each visit.

Reasons for blood glucose monitoring

The main reasons for testing blood glucose are to:

- monitor the effectiveness of your diabetes treatment to help you and your diabetes advisers adjust your medication and meal plans
- define unacceptable control as indicated by blood test results
- detect unstable or brittle diabetes
- show the relationship between blood glucose, food, exercise and medication
- diagnose hypoglycaemia, including nocturnal (night-time) hypoglycaemia
- help you manage illness or convalescence at home
- monitor your response to any new treatments, for example, if you start tablets or insulin injections
- provide continuity of care after you go home from hospital following an illness or operation
- establish your renal threshold – the reliability of urine testing for glucose
- help achieve ideal diabetic control during pregnancy
- assist people with nerve damage (neuropathy) to recognise hypoglycaemia
- help you achieve an acceptable blood glucose range, a factor which helps prevent or delay diabetes-related complications.

Frequency of testing

You will establish how many tests are needed and your target blood glucose range in consultation with your diabetes advisers. Each will depend on your personal treatment goals, state of health, age and type of treatment (meal plan, tablets or insulin).

If you have any problems which make testing difficult (such as arthritis in the fingers or problems with your eyesight), discuss them with your diabetes advisors. There are aids available, such as meters with enlarged numbers and talking meters, which help overcome these problems.

Some recommended testing schedules

Blood glucose is usually tested before meals and, in some cases, two hours after eating, to show how well your body utilised glucose in the food.

Some common schedules are:

- *three or four tests each day* – when diabetes is unstable or if treatment is being altered; and (usually) in young people with type 1 diabetes.
- *daily or twice-daily tests* – changing the time of day at which the test is done, when diabetes is stable.
- *one or two tests each week* – when diabetes is stable, especially for those not requiring medication.
- *every two hours* – during periods of illness. When you are ill it may be necessary to test this often.

Blood glucose range

In Australia, the units used to measure blood glucose are called millimoles (one teaspoon of sugar is the equivalent of 30 mmol of glucose). The following table is a guide to blood glucose levels (see page 32).

During pregnancy, levels of 3 to 7 mmol/L are required to ensure healthy outcomes for mother and baby.

Because hypoglycaemia is not tolerated well by elderly people, a higher blood glucose range between 8 and 15 mmol/L may be acceptable to reduce the risk.

However, if hyperglycaemic symptoms such as urinary frequency or tiredness occur, the blood glucose level may be too high.

What influences blood glucose levels and test results?

Several factors can affect blood glucose levels, causing them either to increase or decrease, depending on individual circumstances.

Factors which *increase* blood glucose levels:

- *Food* – time of last meal, quantity and type of carbohydrate and fibre eaten.
- *Illness* – such as flu or an operation (physical stress on the body).
- *Pregnancy* – in women with diabetes and gestational diabetes.

Factors which *decrease* blood glucose levels:

- *Exercise* – type (weight bearing or non-weight bearing) and its relationship to meal times, medication and insulin injection site. Weight bearing exercise such as walking can increase the uptake of insulin and increase the risk of hypoglycaemia. Exercise helps the body use glucose and fat and therefore assists in weight control.
- *Medications* used for diabetes control – tablets and insulin.
- *Alcohol* – depending on amount consumed and its relationship to food intake.
- *Emotional stress* – medications used to treat stress may mask perception, especially of hypoglycaemia, but they usually cause high blood glucose levels.

Factors which may *increase* or *decrease* blood glucose:

- *Pregnancy* – in women with diabetes and gestational diabetes.
- *Childhood* – erratic swings in blood glucose are usual.
- *Adolescence* – hormonal factors during adolescence can affect results.
- *Disease* – such as kidney, liver and pancreatic disease and other endocrine disorders such as thyroid disease.
- *Testing technique results* – the accuracy of the monitoring technique, including not washing hands before testing if sweet substances such as jam have been handled.

Testing Techniques

There are two types of blood glucose testing.

- **Testing using Visual Comparison Method**

The technique for testing blood glucose levels involves pricking your finger and placing a drop of blood on a strip impregnated with enzymes which react with the glucose in the blood. After a specified time, you read the strip and compare its colour to colour blocks on the strip container. However, blurred vision and disturbances of colour vision may interfere with one's interpretation of the colour changes. Discuss any of these difficulties with your doctor or diabetes nurse educator.

Risk of hypoglycaemia	less than 3 mmol/L – if insulin or diabetes tablets are used, but does not apply to people controlled by meal plans alone
Normal	3–8 mmol/L
Ideal control	3–6 mmol/L before meals up to 8 mmol/L 2 hours after meals
Satisfactory control	6–7 mmol/L before meals 11mmol/L after meals
Unacceptable control	7 mmol/L or more before meals 11 mmol/L or more after meals

Table 1 (page 34) shows the four main types of blood glucose test strips which can be used without a blood glucose meter. Because it is sometimes difficult to match the colour on the strip with the colour block on the container, ask your diabetes advisers to indicate on the strip container the colour range you aim to achieve. Colours outside that range are either too low or too high. In time you will become more accurate at matching the strip colours with the colour blocks. Alternatively, use a blood glucose meter.

Record your results in a record book and take it to your diabetes advisers on each visit. Remember, if your testing technique is not accurate – or your tests not precisely timed – the results will be incorrect.

The key points to remember about testing are:

- get a good drop of blood
- time accurately
- remove blood correctly
- if using a meter clean, calibrate and check it regularly.

Care of strips – Strips can be damaged if exposed to heat, light or moisture. Keep the container tightly capped, with the packet of chemicals (the desiccant) inside. Store at room temperature. Check the expiry date stamped on each container before use. These strips have acceptable accuracy over a wide range of blood glucose values provided the timing is accurate and they are used in accordance with manufacturers' directions.

- **Testing using a blood glucose meter**

Before you buy a meter, examine the range available to determine which one best suits your needs. Always make sure you fully understand how to use and maintain the meter.

If you use a meter, it is vital to use the correct strips for that meter and to ensure it is correctly calibrated and regularly checked with glucose control solutions.

Factors to consider when choosing a blood glucose meter

1. Costs:
   - consider the initial outlay for the meter and other necessary equipment such as a fingerprick device – most meters come in kit form with strips and fingerprick devices included
   - ongoing costs for meter maintenance, such as batteries, control test solutions and the cost of the strips.
2. Ease of operation:
   - suitability for your lifestyle
   - size and portability
   - ease of handling
   - time required to complete each test.
4. The availability of back-up service should repairs or servicing be necessary.
5. Availability of a health fund rebate on the purchase cost of meters. Check with your fund before you buy. A doctor's letter could be required to confirm you need a meter to monitor your diabetes.
6. Special offers. Occasionally pharmaceutical companies offer special prices and trade-in discounts. Check with your Diabetes Australia office and check issues of *Conquest* magazine.
7. Before buying a meter overseas, check the cost and availability of strips and back-up service in Australia. Also be aware the display values may not be in mmol/L.

Types of blood glucose meters available

The two types of meter available are light reflectance meters and electronic devices.

Light reflectance meters

Strips for this type of meter usually need to be wiped or blotted before insertion into the meter and can also be read by comparing the colour change on the strip with colours on the side of the strip container. Examples include the Reflolux S™, Glucometer™ and Meridian™ meters.

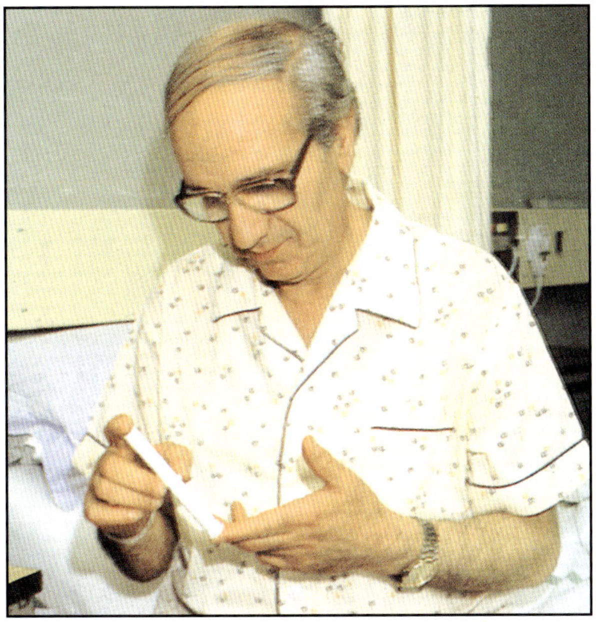

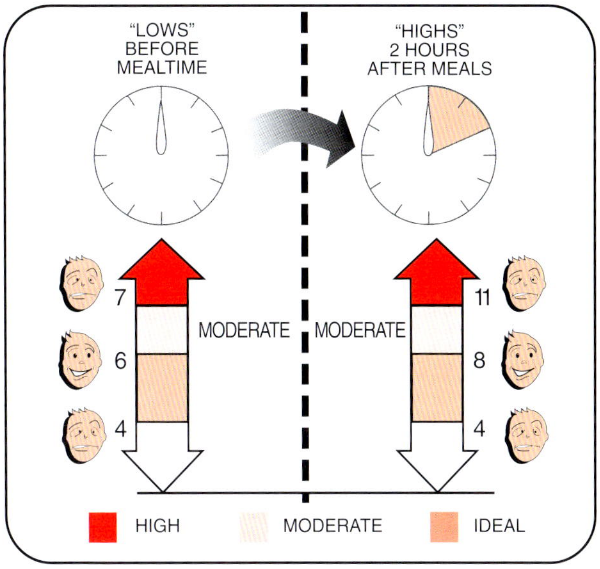

Target values are lower before meals than afterwards.

Electronic devices

Electronic devices are gradually replacing light reflectance meters. With most electronic devices, the strip is inserted into the meter before the drop of blood is applied. The timing for the reaction to occur is automatic and a reading is given without the need to blot or wipe the strips. Examples include MediSense Precision™ and the BM Advantage™.

Quality control

Most meter manufacturers provide glucose fluids to check that the strip and meter are working correctly. The fluid checks, your technique, the meter and the strip act as a control of the quality of results. You should get values within a certain range, depending on the type of meter. If your values lie outside the required range, something is wrong with the strip, the meter or your technique. Conduct regular checks. You may choose to do this once a week, each time you use a new page in your record book, or each time you open a new bottle of strips. Always check if the quality control fluid has passed its expiry date.

Reasons for inaccurate results

Inaccurate blood glucose readings may occur in the following circumstances.

Meters

- using the wrong strip for the meter
- using an incorrect calibration or code
- using the meter incorrectly, for example, not being exact with the recommended testing times, or placing the strip in the meter facing the wrong way
- insufficient blood on the strip will give a falsely low reading with some meters
- using an unclean meter with a spot of blood or lint from cotton wool on the window (more likely with light reflectance meters)
- if the battery is old, the meter may not display a result.

TABLE 1

Types and characteristics of blood glucose test strips currently available in Australia (April 1999) which can be used without a blood glucose meter to estimate the blood glucose levels

STRIP NAME	COLOUR BLOCK RANGE	COLOURS	TIMING	COMMENTS
Boehringer Mannheim 20-800	10 colour blocks:	Beige and blue green	Blood is wiped from the strip after one minute and colour compared at two minutes	Two colours can cause confusion
Hypoguard Supreme	10 colour blocks:	Blue	No wiping. Colour compared after 30 seconds on reverse side of strip.	One colour decreases confusion Values also given in mg/dl which can cause confusion
Ames Glucostix	9 colour blocks:	Green, apricot and pink.	Blood is blotted after 3 seconds and the strip read at 120 seconds	Values given in mmols/L and mg/dl which can cause confusion
Betacheck	14 colour blocks:	Blue, pink, mauve	Blood is wiped at 30 seconds and read at 90 seconds	

Light reflectance meters and visual testing

- blood wiped from the strip too soon can give low readings
- blood left on the strip too long can give high readings
- too forceful wiping of the blood off the strip gives low readings
- incomplete removal of blood from the strip makes interpretation difficult
- touching the pad of the finger on the test strip leads to patchy colour development and difficulty in reading
- strips used after the expiry date may not be accurate
- failure to wash hands before testing, especially if sweet substances have been handled, can cause high readings.

If in doubt, repeat the test. If still in doubt, perform a control test or have your meter tested or serviced. It is not useful to compare meters because, in most cases, results obtained will be different. This can lead to confusion about which meter to believe.

How to obtain a drop of blood for glucose testing

Your diabetes advisor will explain the correct technique for carrying out an accurate blood glucose test. If in doubt, keep asking questions and practising the technique until you feel comfortable with the procedure.

It is important to assemble all the equipment needed before you commence the test, that is:

- blood test strip and meter, if used
- fingerprick devices: lancet
- cotton wool or tissues (depending on the test method)
- wrist watch with a second hand or display (depending on the test method)
- record book
- sharps disposal container.

- Wash and dry hands thoroughly.
- Squeeze blood towards the tip of the finger.
- Prick with the fingerprick device on the side of the last segment. (An automatic fingerpricking device is recommended.)
- Squeeze towards the end of the finger until a large drop of blood forms. Hang the hand downwards if you experience difficulty and warm the hands before testing.

Complete the test according to the system chosen. Do not use the same finger for every test and do not prick the pads of the fingers. The ear lobes may be used, although it is difficult to apply the blood to the strip without assistance.

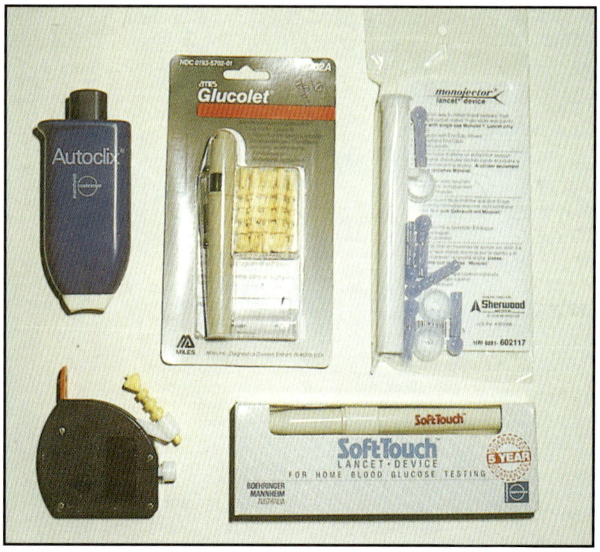

The latest devices make finger pricking easier and cause less discomfort.

The feet should never be used except in the case of infants, where blood can be obtained from the heel.

Equipment should be cleaned, disposed of and stored correctly after use.

Automatic fingerpricking devices available

Fingerpricks cause minimal discomfort if you use an automatic device. The most commonly used devices in Australia are:

- Ames Glucolet™
- Autolet II – Austral Scientific™
- BD Autolance™
- BM Soft Touch™
- Comfort Touch™
- Mini Autolet™
- Unistick™.

They are all simple to operate. Some are spring-loaded and durable, given reasonable care. All have clear operating instructions and allow you to obtain an adequate drop of blood.

The Glucolet™ and Soft Touch™ have two different sized caps; one allows deeper penetration of the lancet and is used if the fingers have very tough skin.

Most people prefer to use a device rather than the lancet alone. Manufacturers recommend lancets are used only once then discarded into an appropriate sharps disposal container.

Safe disposal of used lancets

Fingerprick lancets are manufactured for one use only (like syringes and pen injector needles). We recommend you use an Australian Safety Standards-approved sharps container to store used lancets before disposal. Sharps should be kept out of children's reach. Some local councils supply inexpensive sharps containers and will collect full containers for disposal.

Ask your Diabetes Australia office or your diabetes advisers if there are local arrangements for disposal.

Testing Urine

◆ By Trisha Dunning ◆

AT A GLANCE

- **Urine testing can help your control over your diabetes management.**
- **Establish whether the urine threshold is normal before considering urine testing.**
- **Finding out your renal threshold lets you understand what the results mean.**
- **If you use insulin, measure your blood glucose as urine testing won't provide enough information to determine any required changes in medication dosage.**
- **Urine tests – and other tests used in diabetes management – are not only your early warning system but a valuable management tool in diabetes control.**

ALTHOUGH blood glucose testing is more accurate than urine testing and generally is preferred, urine testing can be a useful additional tool in diabetes management.

The amount of glucose in the urine reflects the amount of glucose in the blood. The kidneys form urine by filtering water and waste substances out of the blood. The urine and waste products pass out through the bladder.

The kidney constantly monitors the concentrations of substances in the blood and when excessive amounts are present, they pass into the urine. For example, if the blood is deficient in salt, the kidney will retain as much as possible in the blood. If there is too much salt, the kidney will allow as much as possible to escape into the urine.

There are three substances which should not appear in the urine under normal circumstances – glucose, ketones and protein. All three can be detected by testing the urine with special testing sticks.

The kidneys usually will not permit glucose to pass into the urine until the level in the blood rises above 10 mmol/L, as in Figure 1. This is known as the renal threshold for glucose. (Renal means to do with the kidneys.)

The threshold is a spill-over point. In other words, the kidney – like a dam – holds back normal amounts of glucose in the blood but, when the renal threshold is reached, glucose spills over into the urine.

A person with a normal renal threshold who has glucose in the urine will usually have recently had a blood glucose level over 10 mmol/L (Figure 2), but the renal threshold can vary from person to person.

The renal threshold can be higher in some people than in others and also can increase with age. Some older people with diabetes therefore have high levels of glucose in their blood, even though their urine is completely free of glucose (Figure 3).

Some people may be born with – or develop – a low renal threshold, meaning their kidneys allow glucose to escape from the blood into the urine when the blood glucose is normal (Figure 4). Pregnant women sometimes develop a low renal threshold at around six or seven months gestation and show glucose in the urine even though blood glucose levels are normal. The threshold returns to normal after the birth.

Establishing the renal threshold is important for all people who test their urine so that they can understand what the results mean.

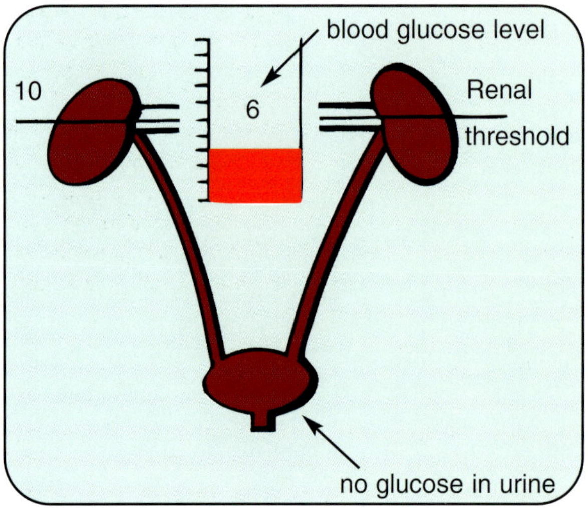

Figure 1: Usually the renal threshold is around 10 mmol/L. No glucose overflows into the urine.

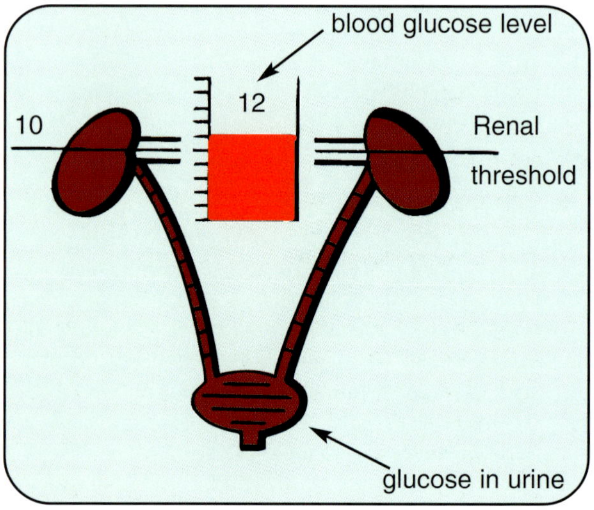

Figure 2: In diabetes the blood glucose may rise above the threshold. Glucose overflows into the urine.

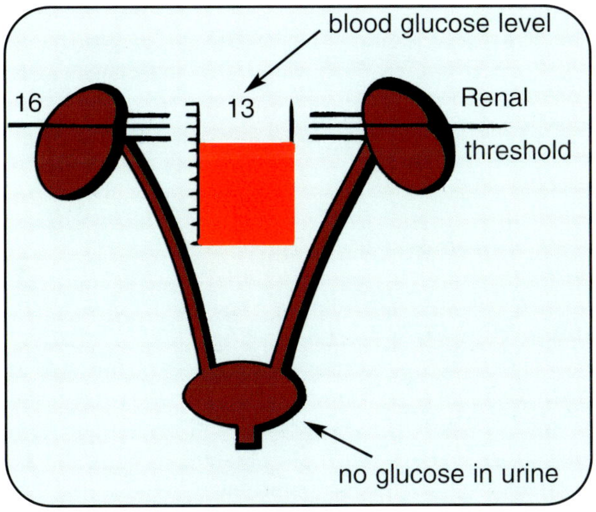

Figure 3: ***High renal threshold*** *– With a high renal threshold blood glucose levels can be higher than normal but no glucose overflows into the urine.*

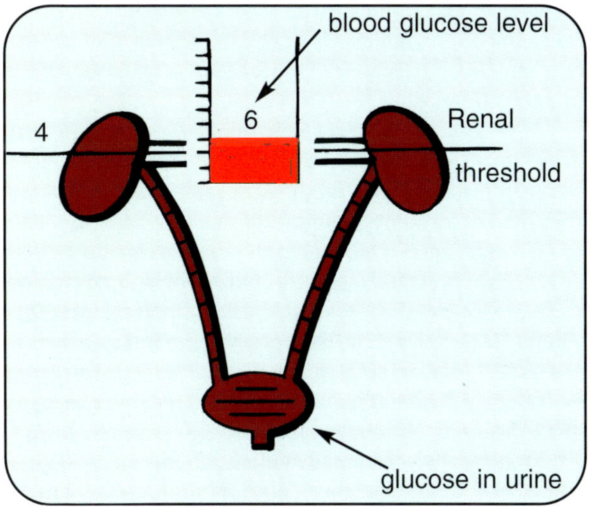

Figure 4: ***Low renal threshold*** *– With a low renal threshold blood glucose levels can be normal but glucose overflows into the urine.*

A low or high renal threshold will render urine testing useless as a means of assessing the level of glucose in a person's blood (Figure 3 and 4).

People with a low renal threshold may believe they have high levels of glucose in the blood when the urine shows glucose, while people with a high renal threshold may be deluded into believing everything is all right because there is no glucose in the urine.

Taking this into account, it is important that the person with diabetes and the diabetes advisor know whether the renal threshold is normal before considering urine testing.

All methods of testing urine for glucose are based on a scale of glucose concentration. The scale is different from the scale used to measure blood glucose and cannot be used to determine the blood glucose level. For instance, the presence of 2 per cent glucose in the urine usually does mean a high blood glucose level; the presence of only 0.5 per cent glucose in the urine does not necessarily mean a moderate level of glucose in the blood. It could, in fact, be quite high. Many factors can affect the glucose concentration in both the urine and blood.

Testing for glucose

The most common methods of testing for urine glucose are:

- Diastix™ and Clinistix™ strips. Accurate timing with a watch is essential to get a proper reading and care must be taken not to use the strips after the expiry date has passed.
- Ketodiastix™ is a combined strip and allows the person to test for ketones (keto) and glucose.
- Testape™ and Clinitest™ tablets have largely been replaced by Diastix™ but a few people still use these methods to test for urine glucose.

Urine test strips must be stored correctly and the container should be dated once opened as the strips usually only last four to six months after opening.

Testing for ketones

The presence of ketones in the urine, known as ketonuria, indicates that the body has switched from glucose to fat as a source of energy for the body cells. Ketones are more likely to develop in people with type 1 diabetes.

The presence of moderate or heavy ketones in the urine, plus large concentrations of glucose, is a serious sign and you should contact a doctor immediately because you may be developing keto-acidosis (see chapter 14, Sick Days – Feeling Unwell?).

When a healthy person with diabetes gets out of bed in the morning and has a trace of ketones in the urine, there are two possible explanations.

If the urine contains only ketones and no glucose, it suggests you had low blood glucose levels during the night because of too much insulin, too much exercise or not enough food the previous evening. If the trace of ketones is accompanied by a large amount of glucose in the urine, the most likely explanation is you had a deficiency of insulin during sleep.

Medical opinion differs on how often a person with diabetes should test their urine for ketones. It is essential for people with type 1 diabetes to test for ketones during any acute illness such as flu or other infection.

The doctor or diabetes nurse educator will explain the various urine testing systems and different characteristics of each product and help you decide which one is best for you if you monitor your urine. (For example, when using Ketodiastix™, the presence of moderate to large amounts of ketones will give falsely low readings for glucose.)

Testing for protein

People with diabetes rarely test their urine for protein. The doctor usually does this for them. The presence of more than a trace of protein may suggest kidney damage, possibly due to years of high blood glucose levels. Testing the urine for protein is particularly important during pregnancy as the presence of protein may indicate the very serious condition of toxaemia of pregnancy. However, the presence of protein does not always mean kidney damage. It may indicate a urinary infection.

It is possible to detect very small amounts of protein in the urine – referred to as *microalbuminuria*.

Until the recent introduction of speed dipsticks which test for microalbuminuria, laboratory tests of 12 or 24-hour urine specimens were necessary. The continued presence of microalbuminuria indicates damage to the kidneys. Tests for microalbuminuria should be performed at least every 12 months.

Both high blood pressure and poor control of diabetes produce microalbuminuria. Effective treatment of high blood pressure and improved diabetes control will reduce the amount of microalbuminuria. People who are found to have microalbuminuria should, therefore, try to achieve the best possible diabetes control and normal blood pressure.

When to test

It is important to realise that the bladder is merely a storage place for urine and urine present could be a mixture of water and waste products stored there recently or for two or more hours. In this case, the old urine could have glucose in it, the newer urine no glucose. However, the test would show glucose even though the blood glucose level may have dropped back to normal. Some doctors recommend that the bladder be emptied one and a half to two hours after a meal and the urine tested 15 to 30 minutes later. Others recommend testing just before the next meal.

Glucose from food increases blood glucose to its highest level after about one hour. The blood glucose level then falls progressively until the next meal. In other words, the lowest blood glucose level occurs before meals and the highest level one to two hours after meals. Frequency of testing will vary from once daily to five or six times daily, depending on the circumstances.

For example, a person whose type 2 diabetes is controlled by food or by a meal plan alone or with tablets may need to test only once daily. In this case, test about two hours after a meal and choose a different meal each day – after breakfast on the first day, after lunch on the second, and so on.

These tests should prove negative for glucose but, if not, test your urine more frequently and consult your doctor or diabetes nurse educator.

In the presence of some illnesses such as flu or bronchitis, people with type 2 diabetes will need to test urine as often as five or six times a day (see chapter 14, Sick Days – Feeling Unwell?). However, blood glucose testing is preferable during illness.

Interpreting the tests

The test before breakfast shows the effectiveness of the previous day's insulin or tablet in controlling your blood glucose. The test before the evening meal measures the effect of that morning's medication and the other tests help fill in the picture throughout the previous 24 hours.

Recording results

Charts for recording results of urine tests are available in book form. Accurate records are needed to enable your doctor to make decisions about your treatment. Your diabetes adviser will tell you the preferred method of recording the chart, either in colours, percentages or negative trace, +, ++, +++, ++++ according to the scale on the strip container.

Urine tests may sound complicated if you have just been diagnosed, or are the parent of a child recently diagnosed with diabetes, but this is not the case. In time, testing becomes routine.

Remember, these tests are your early warning system. Take notice of the signals they send.

The preferable option for people with type 1 diabetes and people with type 2 diabetes treated with insulin, is to measure blood glucose. The information provided by urine testing is not adequate when working out changes in the doses of insulin or diabetes tablets.

Chapter 12

Hypoglycaemia and Hyperglycaemia

◆ By Dr Tim Welborn ◆

HYPOGLYCAEMIA means a low blood glucose level ('hypo' rhymes with low).

People with type 1 diabetes need to be watchful not only of avoiding low glucose levels but of dealing with them if they occur.

Some people with type 2 diabetes who are on tablets or insulin can also experience hypoglycaemia.

Most people with diabetes know the symptoms of high blood glucose levels because usually they were present at the time of diagnosis.

AT A GLANCE

- **This chapter describes the symptoms of low blood glucose and the symptoms of high blood glucose and explains how to treat each separate problem.**
- **Learn to recognise the symptoms of hypoglycaemia plus the simple treatment of eating sugar and teach those around you to do the same.**
- **Repeated prolonged attacks of severe hypoglycaemia may cause nervous system injury and brain damage and should be avoided at all costs.**

Hypoglycaemia (low blood glucose)

The symptoms of a low blood glucose level usually appear quickly, say, over about 10 to 15 minutes.

It is important to recognise them because the remedy is simple – just eat sugar or carbohydrate.

When the blood glucose level falls to less than 3.0 mmol/L, usually there are early warning symptoms. The brain sends messages to the adrenal glands which pour out adrenaline, causing:

- a feeling of anxiety and unease
- palpitations or rapid heart beat
- sweating
- shakiness
- hunger
- a pins and needles feeling around the mouth or in the hands.

These symptoms, which are adrenaline-related, can also occur with anxiety or apprehension, for example, when going into a big examination or heading to face an important football match.

People can usually banish the early warning symptoms by eating sugar or some other form of carbohydrate.

If they ignore or misinterpret the symptoms, or fail to notice them, the condition can progress to involve brain and nerve function.

This is a more serious stage of hypoglycaemia which causes clumsiness and disturbed moods such as irritability, or aggressive behaviour and inappropriate responses.

It is important to have someone around, such as a relative, spouse or workmate, who can identify this stage and treat it to prevent progression to coma or even fits (convulsions).

The symptoms of hypoglycaemia in children are often overlooked or misinterpreted because it is normal for children to occasionally be irritable, aggressive, poor performers at school, excessively hungry or oddly behaved.

People taking diabetes tablets (oral hypoglycaemic agents) may not show the classic symptoms of hypoglycaemia. Instead, their symptoms may be tiredness, headaches or dizziness – symptoms which may be mistaken for having another cause.

If hypoglycaemia symptoms are difficult to recognise, check the blood glucose more often and discuss the problem with your doctor.

The most common causes of low blood glucose in a person with diabetes are:

- lack of sufficient carbohydrate intake
- too much insulin given
- excessive activity
- aiming at perfect diabetic control
- excessive alcohol.

Insufficient food intake can be due to eating less or missing a meal, even to poor digestion (as can occur with the anxiety of a big examination).

Sometimes excessive alcohol blunts awareness of the body's warning systems, such as the symptoms of low blood glucose. Some people with diabetes are particularly susceptible to alcohol-induced hypoglycaemia because alcohol stops their liver from releasing glucose.

Excessive insulin can occur through mistaken over-dosage. Some people have been known to give themselves a double dose without realising it.

Older people on tablets may also experience hypoglycaemia through missed meals or inadvertent over-dosing on their medication.

Increased physical activity burns up blood glucose during the activity, but there is also increased insulin sensitivity for 6–12 hours after vigorous physical exertion.

Some people who seek improved control, for example, women wishing to become pregnant, are more prone to hypoglycaemia because their blood glucose levels are much lower so less warning occurs when blood glucose levels fall, say, from 5 mmol/L to 3 mmol/L.

Because treatment of low blood glucose levels is so

	Hypoglycaemia (low blood glucose)	Hyperglycaemia (high blood glucose)
Cause	Too much insulin Too little food Food not digested (anxiety, nausea) Excessive exercise Alcohol	Not enough or omission of insulin dose or tablets. Too much food Failure to test urine or ignoring positive tests Infections and illnesses Injury and stress
Onset	Good health immediately before Rapid onset	Ill health for hours or days Gradual onset
Symptoms and signs	Hunger, sweating, pallor, nervousness, headache, dizziness, palpitations Tingling sensation in tongue and lips Weakness Progressing to: • Confusion, mood change, belligerence • Clumsiness, slurred speech • Drowsiness • Unconsciousness or coma • Convulsions and fitting	Excessive thirst, excessive passage of large volumes of urine, dramatic weight loss, weakness, lack of energy over a period of days. Progressing to: • Nausea and vomiting, abdominal pains, increased breathing • Smell of ketones (acetone) on breath • Drowsiness and dehydration • Unconsciousness or coma
Urine	Negative for glucose, providing the bladder has been recently emptied	Glucose ++++ Large ketones
Blood	Low blood glucose, usually less than 3 mmol/L	High blood glucose usually higher than 15 mmol/L
Treatment	• Immediate glucose, sweets or sweet drinks by mouth • Alternatively carbohydrate food of any sort, biscuits, bananas etc. • If uncooperative, try honey or syrup placed inside the cheek • Do not attempt to give solid foods by mouth • If unconscious, Glucagon injection either subcutaneously or into muscle will generally improve symptoms of hypoglycaemia in 10–15 min. • If unconscious, lie on one side and ensure a good airway and lift the chin to enable more easy breathing • If fitting or convulsing, lie on one side, restrain excessive movements, prevent falls (from bed) until the fit subsides	• Test blood glucose levels every two to four hrs and record the results. Test the urine for glucose and ketones • More than the normal dose of insulin is usually required • Seek advice concerning small doses of short-acting insulin, eg, Soluble/Actrapid™/ Humulin R™/Humolog™ insulin four units every hour for adults subcutaneously • If vomiting occurs contact the doctor concerning treatment • Maintain at least the normal dose of insulin • If symptoms do not respond, hospitalisation is necessary as an emergency
Glucagon is the first line of defence for a child		

important, everyone with diabetes plus those who live or work with them should study the procedure.

Above all, prevention is better than cure. All people on insulin should carry a supply of quick-acting carbohydrate or glucose, whether it is in glucose tablets, sugar lumps, jelly beans or barley sugar.

Prevention tips

Keep quick-acting carbohydrate or glucose in the car if you drive, in your drawer at work or in your pocket when on the move.

Be alert to the symptoms so you can spot hypoglycaemia early and prevent progression to more severe stages.

Monitor blood glucose levels regularly

If you drive, be especially careful about identifying symptoms and, if in any doubt, check your blood glucose level.

If you recognise or even suspect hypoglycaemic symptoms, take action!

How to treat a hypo ...

Treat early symptoms by eating one or two dessertspoonfuls of glucose or table sugar; a can of ordinary (not diet) lemonade or other sweet drink; a biscuit; slice of bread, banana or honey.

Within 10 minutes the symptoms should improve, but it is important to take some long-acting carbohydrate such as bread or a biscuit to ensure the improvement continues.

If the symptoms progress to irritability or confusion it is vital someone around you gets you to eat or drink sugar.

It can take up to an hour to fully recover, even if the blood glucose levels have returned to normal, so avoid driving or working near machinery.

How to treat severe hypoglycaemia

If the person with hypoglycaemia is drowsy, goes into coma or has convulsions, this is a medical emergency.

The first step is to restrain the person from self-injury by lying them on one side. If a relative or associate is trained in the technique, this is the time to administer an intramuscular injection of glucagon (1 International Unit) to the outer thigh. (It works almost as quickly given subcutaneously, like insulin).

Otherwise call an ambulance or get the person to a casualty unit or hospital emergency centre. In hospital, staff will give an emergency intravenous glucose injection.

Repeated prolonged attacks of severe hypoglycaemia may cause nervous system injury and brain damage and should be avoided at all costs.

People on insulin – and some on tablets – will experience mild hypoglycaemia occasionally.

Since the introduction of human insulin, some people report the absence of adequate early warning signals and say they go straight into confusion, slurred speech or other symptoms of disturbed brain function.

It is all the more important for these people to regularly monitor their blood glucose levels, being particularly attentive to meal and snack times.

Glucagon

Glucagon is a hormone made by the pancreas.

Release of glucagon by the pancreas causes the liver to release glucose from stored starch (also known as glycogen). Glucagon release is part of a healthy person's response to low blood glucose levels.

This response can be blunted in those who have had diabetes for many years.

An injection of glucagon is useful in treating severe hypoglycaemia when the patient cannot – or will not – take oral glucose or other carbohydrates.

An injection of glucagon should cause sufficient glucose release from the liver to bring a person out of hypoglycaemic coma within 10 minutes. The person will regain consciousness, become cooperative and should eat something.

Glucagon is available as a dry powder in a sealed bottle with a partner solution that is injected into the bottle to dissolve the powder.

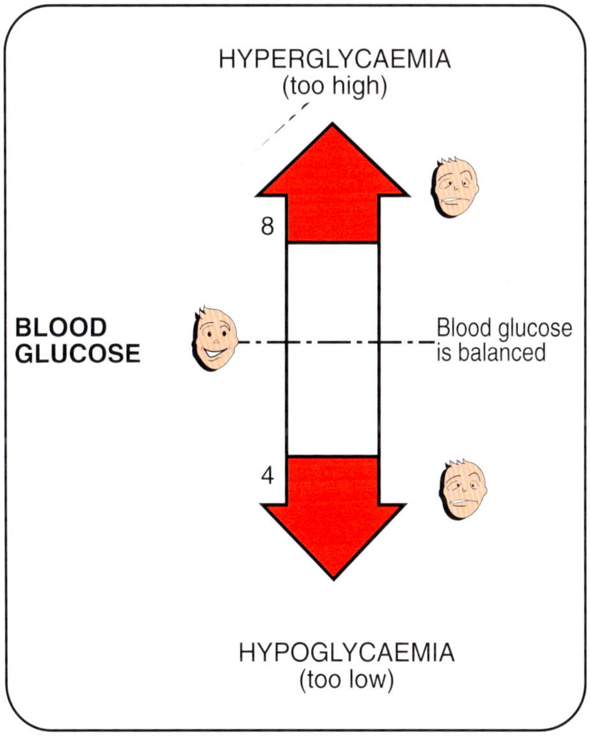

Mix the fluid with the powder by swirling, draw up the entire amount of dissolved glucagon and inject the glucagon intramuscularly or subcutaneously.

After a hypoglycaemic attack always ask why the episode happened and take necessary precautions to prevent it happening again.

Once you have used your glucagon, obtain new stocks by prescription from your doctor.

Hyperglycaemia

This means an excessively high blood glucose level. The onset of hyperglycaemia is gradual and can take hours or days.

The symptoms of very high blood glucose level are:

- extreme thirst
- passing large volumes of urine, frequently
- weight loss
- weakness
- blurred vision.

If you have type 1 diabetes, which means you have no natural insulin secretion, severe hyperglycaemia can become even more serious with the following manifestations:

- ketones on the breath
- deep breathing
- abdominal pain
- drowsiness
- coma.

On the other hand, many people with diabetes can have mild hyperglycaemia, recognisable by some dryness of the mouth, passing urine once or twice overnight, indolent skin infections or genital irritation, and unusual tiredness.

Causes of hyperglycaemia are insufficient insulin, either a mistaken dosage or not giving the injection, or that the insulin has deteriorated for some reason or other and forgetting to take the usual tablets (if medication is used). Dietary indiscretions are a common cause. Infection or other intercurrent illness can precipitate hyperglycaemia. Mental stress can trigger the sympathetic nervous system and, as a result of this, the liver manufactures excessive glucose that enters the bloodstream. Stress hormones can also cause resistance to insulin action. Finally, some people have true insulin resistance for a number of reasons, often requiring exhaustive testing in the hospital situation.

Severe hyperglycaemia in people with type 1 diabetes must be recognised and the insulin dosage increased. If necessary, ring your doctor or nurse about this. It is usually quite safe to give frequent small doses of short-acting insulin, 3–6 units every hour as required, by subcutaneous injection. If you know how to give intramuscular injections, small doses of short-acting insulin every hour are very effective (see chapter 14, Sick Days – Feeling Unwell?). Contact your doctor or diabetes nurse educator if blood glucose levels don't respond within four hours. Hyperglycaemia in someone with type 2 diabetes on tablets is often temporary and, although the dose of tablets is sometimes increased, this is not always effective. Medical advice should be sought if symptoms persist.

Intake of fluids is very important where there are symptoms of high blood glucose. Drink as much water or low-calorie fluids as possible to keep up with the fluid that is lost by passing urine. Don't take fluids that contain sugar because this will make the symptoms and the hyperglycaemia much worse.

If vomiting prevents fluid intake and makes eating difficult, this is a real emergency, and a doctor should be notified. An injection can be given to stop the vomiting.

Summary

This chapter has dealt mainly with the emergency treatment of hypoglycaemia and hyperglycaemia. Lesser degrees of low and high blood glucose levels can exist in people with diabetes and cause unrecognised problems. It is important, therefore, to check blood glucose profiles at regular intervals and to have these on record when you visit your doctor or diabetes nurse educator. This gives the best chance of being able to discuss management and obtaining useful advice. Low blood glucose levels can give 'early warning' that the insulin dosage should be adjusted. Similarly, many people run rather high blood glucose levels, putting them at risk of complications (see chapter 15 – The Long Term Complications of Diabetes). In such people, adjustment of insulin and fine tuning ('the right insulin at the right time') should help them get back on the tramlines.

Chapter 13

Diabetes and Other Medications

◆ By Clinical Professor Gillian Shenfield ◆

DIABETES can occur at any age and is a life-long condition. It is therefore only to be expected that people with diabetes will, at various times, have other medical disorders.

Everyone in the community gets coughs, colds and chest infections. Kidney and bladder infections are extremely common and, as we get older, many of us get arthritis, high blood pressure and heart circulation problems.

The combination of diabetes and high blood pressure is dangerous, so many people with diabetes take medicines to lower their blood pressure.

Medications may affect diabetes in different ways. Space prevents us addressing every possible interaction so we will only consider the most common ones. It is important to realise that these interactions will not necessarily occur with everyone with diabetes who takes the medication described.

To avoid problems, your doctor or pharmacist must know you have diabetes. They can then assess the suitability of medications you may need for other conditions. If you have doubts about medication interactions, ask for advice from an expert such as a member of your health care team.

In the tables in this chapter we call medications by their proper or generic names. In the case of an individual drug, we also include its most common trade name. For example, oats, a generic food, are also known under trade names such as Uncle Toby's Oats™ .

Generally, the potential for highest risk occurs when a medication is stopped or started or the dose is changed. For example, you might be prescribed a new tablet for blood pressure or a different dose of arthritis tablet; or stop taking a sulphonamide antibiotic.

Watch for changes and take extra care with your blood tests when starting, stopping or modifying the dose of any medication.

However, long-term treatment with other medications and diabetes tablets is unlikely to cause trouble.

New medications can interact with diabetes in all sorts of ways so it is impossible to generalise, but the following explanations will alert you to some of the most common potential problems.

TABLE 1: Common medications that may increase blood glucose

Medication	Mechanism	Likely to have effect with: Insulin	Tablets	Meal Plan
Antibiotic syrups for children	Contain sugar	++	N/A	N/A
Antihistamine syrups for children*	Contain sugar	++	N/A	N/A
Corticosteroids	Oppose insulin action	++	++	++
Cough mixtures in syrup*	Contain sugar	++	++	++
Diuretics	Block insulin secretion	+	++	++
Nifedipine (Adalat™)	Delays insulin action	+	++	++
Oral contraceptives	Oppose insulin action	++	++	++
Phenytoin (Dilantin™)	Blocks insulin secretion	+	++	++
Phenothiazine tranquilisers	Not known	++	++	++

* Over the counter medications
++ = greater effect
\+ = some effect
N/A = not applicable since usually children require insulin

AT A GLANCE

- **Make sure each doctor or pharmacist you consult knows you have diabetes and is aware of all the medications you use.**
- **Never take a new medication without determining if it may affect your diabetes and, if so, what precautions you should take.**
- **Be aware that problems are most likely to occur at times of dose change or when you stop and start medications. At these times, take extra care.**

TABLE 2: Common medications that may lower blood glucose

Medication	Mechanism	Insulin	Tablets	Meal Plan
		Likely to have effect with:		
Alcohol	Stops liver producing glucose	+++	+++	++
Allopurinol (Zyloprim, Allorin/Progout)	Increases amount of sulphonylurea in blood	N/A	+	N/A
Angiotensin converting enzyme inhibitors	Increases insulin action	++	++	N/A
Antacids	Increases absorption of sulphonylureas	N/A	+++	N/A
Antifungal drugs	Increases amount of sulphonylurea in blood	N/A	+++	N/A
Aspirin™	Increases amount of sulphonylurea in blood	N/A	+++	N/A
Beta-blocking medications	Oppose action of adrenaline	+++	++	N/A
Clofibrate (Atromid-S™)	Not known	+	+++	N/A
Monoamine oxidase antidepressants	Interfere with adrenaline action	+++	+++	N/A
Non-steroidal anti-inflammatory medications*	Increase amount of sulphonylurea in blood	N/A	+++	N/A
Oxytetracycline	Slows insulin removal	+++	++	N/A
Quinine	Increases insulin secretion	+	++	++
Sulphonamide	Increases amount of sulphonylurea in blood	N/A	+++	N/A
Warfarin	Increases amount of sulphonylurea in blood	N/A	+++	N/A

* Over the counter medications
+++ = greatest effect
++ = greater effect
+ = some effect
N/A = not applicable

Medications that may raise blood glucose

Table 1 lists some commonly used medications that may cause blood glucose to increase. It indicates the likely effect (where known) and also shows the likelihood of it happening to people with diabetes, whether they are on insulin, on tablets or on a meal plan alone.

These three groups can have different reactions because the medication may directly affect the diabetes or interact with the treatment for diabetes. The column for tablets refers to the sulphonylureas. No significant interactions with other drugs are recorded for metformin.

Various medications for children are made up as sweet syrups, and large volumes may cause blood glucose to rise.

For different reasons, diuretics – used to treat blood pressure or ankle swelling – may have a similar effect.

In some people with type 2 diabetes, simply stopping a diuretic allows them to manage on a meal plan alone, with no need of tablets for blood glucose control.

Phenytoin (Dilantin™), used to treat epilepsy, is an example of a medication taken over a prolonged period. Problems are only likely to arise if phenytoin is stopped, started or the dose is changed.

Women with diabetes can take oral contraceptive pills. Oral contraceptives may slightly increase blood glucose, requiring an increased dose of diabetes tablets or insulin. However, many women find that contraceptive pills taken during a menstrual cycle actually stabilise their blood glucose control.

Medications that may lower blood glucose

Table 2, in the same format as table 1, shows medications most likely to lower blood glucose. Where interaction problems occur, they are mostly in people taking tablets (usually sulphonylureas) to treat their diabetes. This is because many medications raise the amount of sulphonylurea in the blood, increasing their effect – which is to lower blood glucose.

This occurs either by reducing the rate at which sulphonylureas are removed from the body or by displacing them from the carrier proteins to which they are usually attached in the blood. This type of interaction obviously won't occur in people treated by insulin or meal plans alone.

Medication is unlikely to decrease blood glucose in anyone treated solely by a meal plan.

Alcohol, although not strictly a medication, is included. Not only does alcohol directly affect blood glucose, it affects people's ability to detect hypoglycaemia and their judgment about appropriate action. In moderation, alcohol is unlikely to cause hypoglycaemia. However, if taken without food or in large quantities, it can lower blood glucose in anyone with diabetes, irrespective of treatment.

Alcohol interacts with some of the sulphonylurea tablets (especially chlorpropamide and tolbutamide) and may cause flushing, an unpleasant effect causing your face to become hot and red. You may also feel sick.

If you only drink alcohol occasionally, these issues are of little significance and cause no permanent harm. If you drink regularly and have flushes, ask your doctor to change you to another tablet.

Beta-blocking drugs are used to treat high blood pressure or heart disease. Their actions vary but they can all decrease blood glucose, meaning that you'll need to decrease your dose of insulin or tablets.

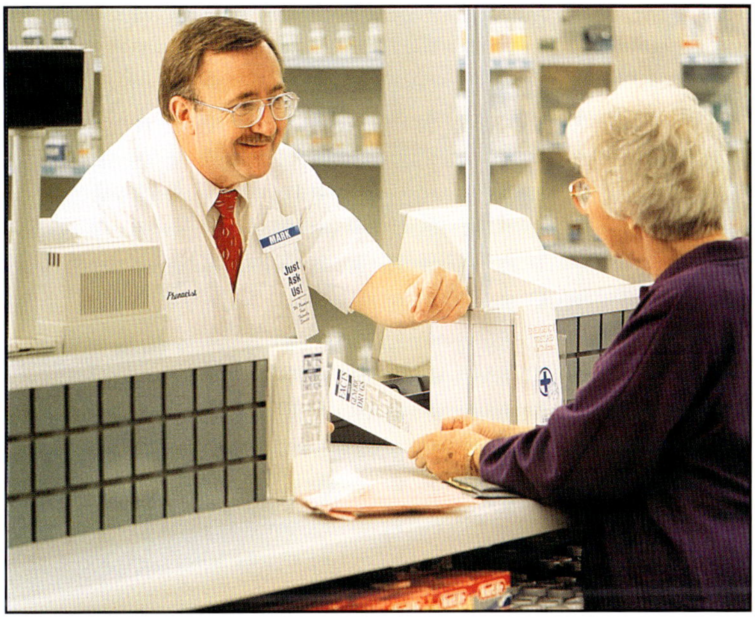

Antacids are used to treat indigestion and have recently been shown to increase the rate at which sulphonylureas are absorbed in the body. Therefore, they may rapidly reduce blood glucose. This will be a problem only if you delay eating. Avoid it by allowing two hours between taking antacids and sulphonylurea tablets.

In some people with diabetes, taking medication for other health problems will have no effect on blood glucose. Others will be particularly susceptible to interactions and may need a changed dose of insulin or diabetes tablets.

Quinine is often prescribed for night cramps in the legs and feet and in normal doses has little effect on blood glucose. However, it is also an ingredient in tonic water and the combined effects of that, plus gin and the tablets for cramps, might lower blood glucose, especially if you have not eaten much food.

Common examples of antibiotics which contain sulphonamide, and can therefore decrease blood glucose, are Septrin™ and Bactrim™. These may cause problems for people taking sulphonylurea tablets. Sudden decreases in blood glucose may occur one or two days after starting the antibiotics.

Other antibiotics (except for oxytetracycline) don't have this effect. However, blood glucose may decrease as the infection comes under control.

Medications that alter response to glucose or insulin

The beta-blocking medications block some of the actions of the naturally occurring hormones, adrenaline and noradrenaline. These hormones act in the body to oppose insulin effects so, if their potency is reduced, insulin will have a greater than normal effect.

Not only do beta-blockers reduce blood glucose, they interfere with the body's normal responses to hypoglycaemia.

Many of the warning signs of hypoglycaemia – sweating, fast pulse and anxiety – are due to the actions of adrenaline. But if you take beta-blockers, these signs and symptoms are absent. Your blood glucose can drop considerably without the usual warning that gives you time to take some form of sugar.

Adrenaline is also one of the substances that helps blood glucose recover after hypoglycaemia. If the action of adrenaline is blocked, you will take much longer to recover. People with diabetes, especially those on insulin, should therefore use beta-blockers with caution.

Some of the newer beta-blocking agents eg. atenolol (Noten™, Tenormin™) and metoprolol (Betaloc™, Lopressor™) have a so-called *selective* action and only oppose some of the effects of adrenaline. They are less likely to cause problems.

Smoking

Cigarettes are usually not considered medications but they are certainly drugs because they contain highly active foreign substances that enter the body and affect its functions. Smoking is not recommended for anyone, particularly people with diabetes, since it increases the risk of damage to the heart and circulation.

People with type 1 diabetes absorb insulin at a reduced rate for 30 minutes after smoking. Smokers with diabetes need an average 15–20 per cent more insulin than non-smokers, while heavy smokers may need 30 per cent more. Any change in smoking habits can produce alterations in the amount of insulin getting into the bloodstream.

If you are a heavy smoker and suddenly give up the habit, your body could suddenly absorb up to 30 per cent more insulin, causing a decrease in blood glucose. This is not a reason to keep smoking, but does indicate need for care when changing long-entrenched habits.

Interactions with complications of diabetes

The complications of diabetes are described elsewhere in this book. Some of them, such as heart disease, may need treatment with special medications. In some cases you may need to avoid substances that aggravate a problem or confuse the process of diagnosis.

For example, before a diagnosis of impotence can be attributed to diabetes, the doctor first eliminates blood pressure tablets as the cause because this medication, including methyldopa (Aldomet™) and various beta-blockers, may also cause impotence.

Autonomic neuropathy can cause low blood pressure. If you have this condition, avoid medications that lower blood pressure, including angina treatments such as isosorbide (Isordil™, Isotrate™), nifedipine (Adalat™) and felodipine (Agon™, Plendil™).

If you have low blood pressure, do not use nitrate patches and ointments (Nitro-bid™, Nitrodise™, Transiderm Nitro™) until you have discussed the matter fully with your doctor.

If you do use nitrates (usually for angina and heart disease) do not use Viagra to help with erectile problems (see chapter 19, Sexual Problems in Men) since Viagra can interact with nitrates and cause very low blood pressure. Discuss this with your doctor.

Sometimes diabetes impairs circulation to the hands and feet, making them cold and numb. If you have these symptoms, do not take medications that may reduce the circulation such as beta-blockers or migraine tablets containing ergot.

Over the counter medicines

It is important to realise that medicines bought without prescription (called over the counter medications) in pharmacies or at supermarkets can interact with your diabetes just as much as medications obtained by prescription.

An increasing number of medicines are being made available for direct purchase and those currently available in this way are marked with an asterisk in tables 1 and 2. Some antihistamine syrups and some cough mixtures which contain syrup can be bought, as can antacids and, of course, aspirin and some of the non-steroidal anti-inflammatory drugs used for arthritis. Tables 1 and 2 indicate how these medicines might have potential for interfering with your diabetes control.

Remember also that the many herbal and 'natural' medicines that are freely available in supermarkets and pharmacies may also contain sugar or have potential to interact with diabetes. It is not possible to list them here but it is important to be aware that even the most harmless seeming substance can sometimes have an effect on blood glucose.

Ask your pharmacist about any purchase you make and whether it contains sugar or might in some other way interact with your diabetes. Read the information on the labels and inside the packets of anything you purchase and, if there is only limited information or you are not sure if there might be a problem, do not take it until you have obtained further advice.

Conclusion

This is not a complete list but is intended to give you some indication of the difficulties that may occur with medications and diabetes.

Diabetes involves the whole body so it is necessary to think about the whole system when using medications for other conditions.

Sick Days – Feeling Unwell?

◆ By Dr Kerry Bowen and Melba Mensch ◆

BEFORE you developed diabetes your body's insulin production was sufficient to prevent the blood glucose from rising above normal levels.

Back then, putting your body under stress through illness or injury prompted your pancreas to produce extra insulin to match and counteract the increased production of stress hormones such as adrenaline and cortisol.

When you are unwell through illness or injury, it is likely your body's increased production of stress hormones will cause blood and urine glucose to rise to higher levels than you would normally experience. Be prepared to remedy this undesirable situation because the high test results are a warning that your regular medication for controlling blood glucose is not doing its job.

Type 1 diabetes and sick days

With type 1 diabetes you are at significant risk of developing a condition called keto-acidosis when you are ill. Because your pancreas makes minimal insulin, your body must rely on injected insulin to keep the blood glucose level within reasonable limits.

Insulin acts to stop blood glucose from rising to an excessive level (see chapter 8 – Insulin and its Role). Insulin also stops your body from releasing too much fat from storage at any one time and then turning the fat into substances called ketones. Large quantities of ketones in the blood increase blood acidity and, if this is not corrected, keto-acidosis (acid blood full of ketones) can occur. This can be life-threatening if left untreated.

To prevent keto-acidosis during illness, you may need to increase your insulin dosage in response to a sustained rise in your blood glucose level. People with type 1 diabetes are likely to show ketones on urine testing when they are ill, even though they may be receiving their normal dose of insulin.

If you have type 1 diabetes and are ill, it is important to test your urine for ketones every two to four hours. If you show moderate to large ketones on the test, it is important to inform a doctor and drink plenty of fluids.

If you have a very high blood glucose level during illness, you are likely to pass much more urine than usual. If you don't replace the fluid you will become dehydrated. Diarrhoea or vomiting can also cause dehydration, as can a high fever which causes excessive sweating. Be sure to drink enough to replace fluids you are losing.

Type 2 diabetes and sick days

Even if you have long-established type 2 diabetes requiring insulin injections – as opposed to tablets and diet alone – it is likely your pancreas still produces some insulin. Because your body needs so little insulin to prevent it breaking down excessive fat to convert into ketones, it is unlikely you will show more than a trace of ketones in the urine, even if when you are ill. Nevertheless, if you use insulin injections and are unwell, it is still important to test for ketones regularly throughout the day.

AT A GLANCE

- **Keep blood glucose test strips at home (and urine test strips for ketones if you are using insulin); check regularly that they have not passed the expiry date and that you know how to use them. If you are not sure how to use your blood and/or urine test strips correctly, ask a diabetes nurse educator, your doctor or a pharmacist.**
- **When you're ill, test your blood and urine more frequently than usual. Tests may have to be performed as often as every two hours if you are not improving quickly. Remember, you are looking for raised glucose levels in the blood and ketones in the urine. Ring your doctor if these remain high or increase over the course of several hours.**

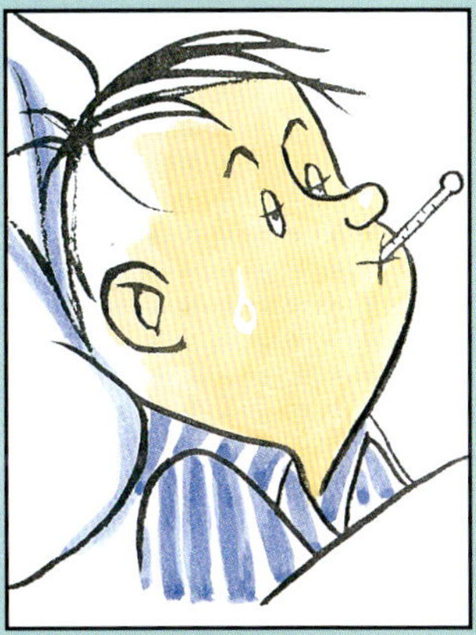

- **Have a supply of quick-acting insulin available.**
- **Always continue injecting your insulin when you are ill, but seek advice from your doctor or diabetes nurse educator about dosage changes.**
- **Have an adequate supply of suitable foods and fluids available and follow the general recommendations given in this chapter.**
- **Drink plenty of fluids; if you can't keep these down or have persistent vomiting or diarrhoea, seek immediate medical advice.**
- **Keep by the phone a list of contact numbers for your doctor, hospital and ambulance.**
- **Seek medical advice if you are ill and not getting better.**
- **If possible, have a friend or relative come and keep an eye on you.**
- **Persisting high blood glucose levels and/or ketones mean you need to talk to a doctor immediately.**

Since there is a risk of developing very high blood glucose levels (greater than 20 mmol/L) during an illness – whether you use tablets or insulin – you cannot afford to ignore persistently high blood glucose levels as they can cause serious illness if not addressed properly.

When to call a doctor

Regardless of the type of diabetes, if you are unwell and your blood glucose levels are higher than usual, test your blood glucose level every two to four hours. Test your urine for ketones as well. If your blood glucose remains unusually high, it is a warning to take immediate action. A prompt phone call to your doctor or diabetes nurse educator may well mean the difference between having the problem sorted out over the phone or being admitted to hospital.

If you are nauseated or vomiting, you may be unable to keep down medicines, food or fluids.

If there is someone with you, ask them if your breath smells sweet (like apple cider). This is a sign you have large amounts of ketones in your blood.

If any of these things occur, it is important to notify your doctor immediately and ask for advice; you may need to be admitted to hospital.

If you can't contact your own doctor, try other family doctors, physicians or diabetes specialists in your area.

If there is no medical assistance close by, phone your nearest hospital emergency department or diabetes education centre. Ask for the doctor on duty.

If this approach is unsuccessful and you are calling during business hours, ring your city's major general hospital, and ask the switchboard operator to put you through to the diabetes unit doctor or medical registrar on call for diabetes and endocrinology.

If ringing after hours, ask to speak to the doctor in charge of the emergency department. If none of these doctors are contactable, go to the local hospital's emergency department or call the ambulance service for assistance.

Be aware of these options in case you need to seek urgent help.

Do I still need my insulin when I am sick?

YES. Your body still needs insulin because you are under stress. The blood glucose level can rise to higher than normal levels even if you eat nothing during the day. Therefore, it is important that you do not miss your usual daily insulin injections. Sometimes your doctor will advise you by telephone to give extra insulin in between your usual insulin dosages if your blood glucose levels or urine ketone levels are not decreasing.

If you normally only use the premixed or intermediate/long-acting (cloudy) insulin, make sure you have a small supply of a quick-acting (clear) insulin (Actrapid™, Humalog™, Humulin R™ or Insulin 2™) on hand because your doctor may advise you to take some quick-acting (clear) insulin.

When you are ill you will need to check your blood glucose levels every two hours to ensure any extra insulin administered is not reducing your blood glucose to such an extent that you run the risk of hypoglycaemia. Although unlikely, this is a possibility to guard against by having glucose-containing foods or fluids handy.

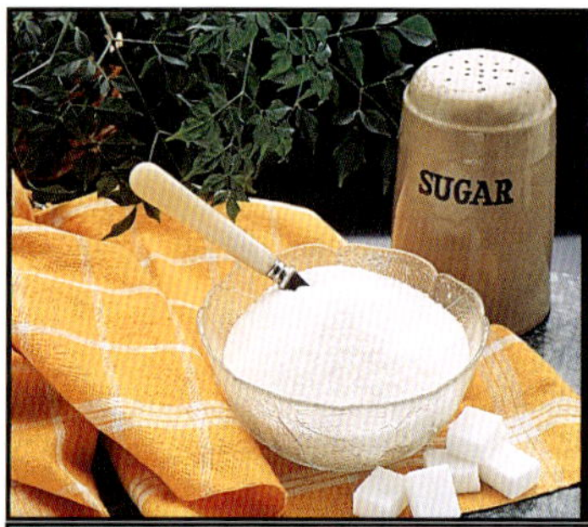

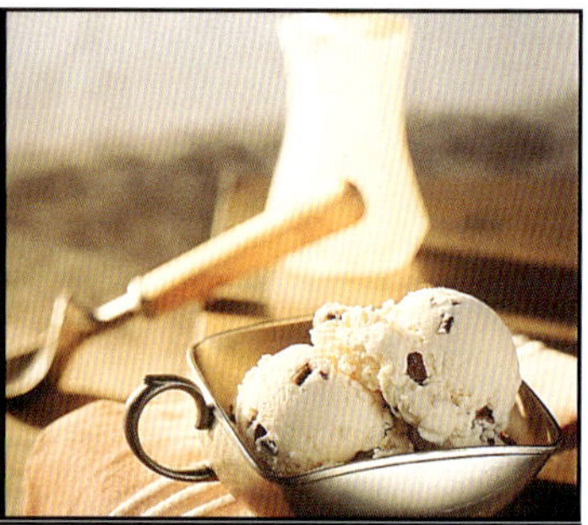

Light foods for when you are unwell	Amount to equal 1 carbohydrate exchange
Lucozade™	90 ml
sweet jelly	¼ cup
lemonade sweetened	⅓ can
other sweetened carbonated beverage	⅓ can
honey	1 tablespoon
sugar	1 tablespoon
custard with added sugar	⅓ cup
egg flip (sweetened)	1 cup
Lighter food options	
bread or toast	1 slice
crumpet	1
English muffin	½
plain biscuits	2
ice-cream	1½ scoops
soup	1 cup
fruit juice	½ cup
canned fruit	½ cup
grated apple	1
rice or bread pudding	⅓ cup
porridge	½ cup
fruit	1 piece
banana	½
diet yoghurt	1 carton
boiled rice	⅓ cup

What if I'm not hungry when I feel sick?

Sometimes you don't feel like eating food when you are ill. Nevertheless, when you feel sick it is important you continue to drink plenty of fluids and to eat carbohydrate if your blood glucose is falling.

Fluids

If you cannot eat or feel nauseated, take sweetened fluids to ensure adequate carbohydrate and fluid intake. Sip fluids slowly, taking small amounts frequently until you can tolerate light foods:

- lemonade or cola drinks (sweetened not diet)
  (1/3 can = 1 CHO exchange)
  (these may be better tolerated if flat)
- Lucozade™
  (90 ml = 1 CHO exchange)
- ginger ale (sweetened not diet)
  (1/3 can = 1 CHO exchange)
- lemon with honey
  (1 tblspn honey = 1 CHO exchange)
- black tea with sugar
  (1 tblspn sugar = 1 CHO exchange)
  To obtain extra fluids and make them easier to drink, the above may be diluted with extra water.
- Gastrolite™ or other re-hydration fluids (check food labels for carbohydrate content)
  Add water according to the instructions on the packet.

Drink extra fluids as well as the above. You may select diet drinks, broth, clear soups or Vegemite™ mixed with water. If your ketone levels are high, ensure you take extra fluids.

If you are vomiting or have diarrhoea, it is very important to include some salty fluids such as mineral water, broths or Bonox™ to replace any salt you may be losing. Be aware that some individuals find milk or milk products and fruit juice cause vomiting.

Dehydration is a life-threatening condition which can occur rapidly in any sick child or adult with diabetes. The dehydration occurs because the body loses water not only in urine, bowel actions and vomiting, but also through perspiration and breathing.

To help prevent or reduce dehydration, ensure sufficient fluids are taken to replace those being lost. About 150–200 ml of fluid for every waking hour should suffice, with proportionately less for children (see chart below). If ketones are present, extra fluid may be required. If you have any concerns, contact your doctor immediately.

Remember, dehydration can be life-threatening if not treated.

Fluid intake suggested for different age groups:

Age	ml/kg/day
3 months	140–160
6 months	135–155
9 months	125–140
1 year	125–135
2 years	115–125
Children above 2 years	1000–1500 ml/day
Adults	1500–2000 ml/day

Additional fluids will be needed to meet diarrhoea losses in gastroenteritis.
Source: Feeding Guide – Westmead Childrens' Hospital. 2nd edn, 1993.

Foods

When you are sick you can reduce or omit meats and fats from your meal plans. However, ensure that you include carbohydrate source foods – smaller snacks every two to three hours instead of three regular meals.

When you start to feel better you may like to return to normal meal plans by selecting from your list of favourite light foods.

SAMPLE MEAL PLAN
15 CARBOHYDRATE EXCHANGES

Breakfast (3 exchanges)
½ cup fruit juice (may dilute if better tolerated)
1 slice toast (lightly butter if desired)
2 teaspoons honey
2 teaspoons sugar in tea or coffee
If hungry, exchange an extra slice of toast for the honey and sugar

Morning tea (1 exchange)
½ cup fruit juice
or 2 plain biscuits
tea, coffee or low-joule drink for extra fluids

Lunch (3 exchanges)
1 cup soup
1 slice bread or toast (lightly spread if desired)
¼ cup sweetened jelly
tea, coffee or low-joule drink for extra fluids

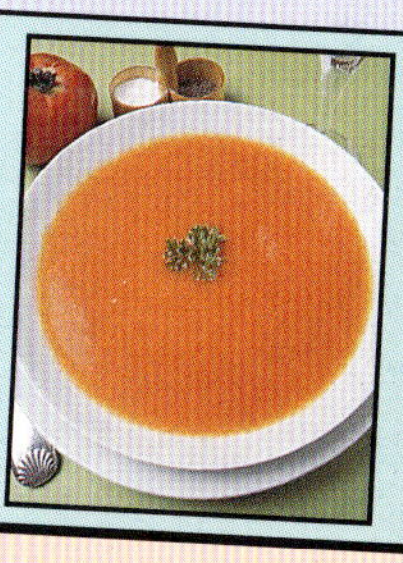

Afternoon tea (1 exchange)
⅓ cup sweetened yoghurt or custard
or 1 plain biscuit and ¼ cup fruit juice
tea, coffee or low-joule drink for extra fluids

Evening meal (3 exchanges)
1 cup soup
low-fat meat, chicken, fish if desired
⅓ – ½ cup boiled rice or potato or 1 slice bread
½ cup ice-cream or custard
tea, coffee or low-joule drink for extra fluids

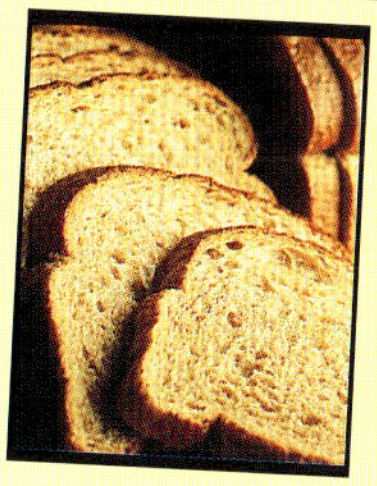

Supper (1 exchange)
1 slice bread or toast
or ⅓ can sweetened beverage

If your appetite is small, you might prefer foods from the above list. Because these foods contain sugar, the serving size to equal one carbohydrate exchange is smaller.

When vomiting, diarrhoea or fever occurs, it is necessary to replace salt and fluids. Therefore, try to have some extra Bonox™, Bovril™, clear broth, salty soup and other fluids.

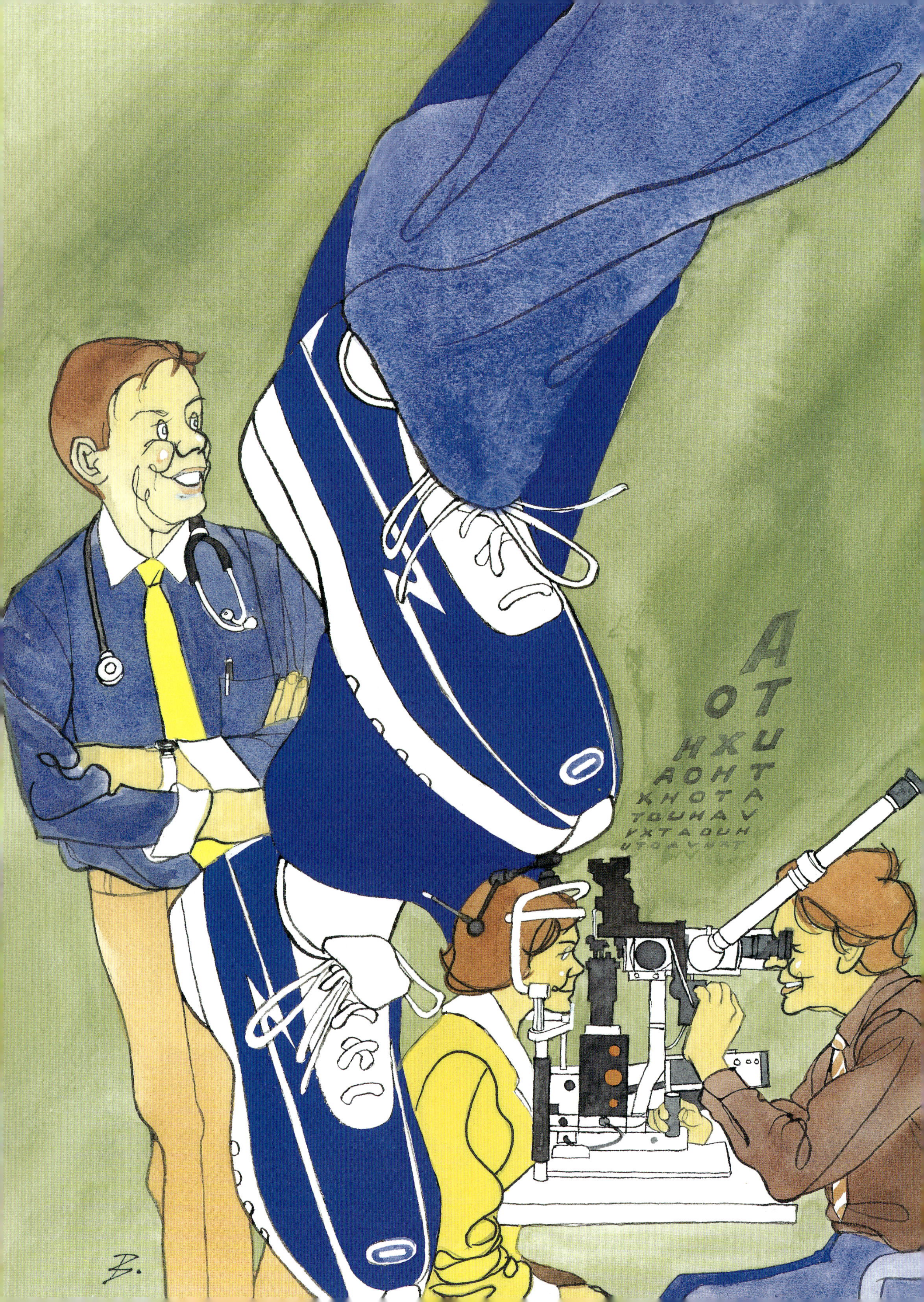
A
O T
H X U

Chapter 15

Long Term Complications of Diabetes

◆ By Dr Warren Kidson ◆

ALTHOUGH there are several long-term complications of diabetes, some complications can develop after only 6 or 12 months of high levels of glucose in the blood.

Important risk factors for complications are set out below and in Table 1 (page 54).

Family history

Some people inherit genetic protection from some of the complications of diabetes while others inherit increased susceptibility. However, an individual's susceptibility to complications cannot be determined.

High blood glucose levels

A high level of glucose in the blood is the most important factor causing long-term complications of diabetes.

When the levels of glucose in the blood are high, glucose can attach itself to different protein molecules throughout the body, damaging the proteins or changing their function. For example, glucose attached to the clotting factors of the blood increases the likelihood of the blood sticking to roughened areas of arteries, eventually blocking that artery.

When glucose attaches itself to the strengthening fibres in the blood vessels or joints throughout the body, these tissues become stiffer causing the arterial blood pressure to rise. Cholesterol enters the arterial wall more easily, accelerating the rate of artery blockage. Similarly, joints – particularly those in the hands and shoulders – can become stiff or painful.

The Diabetes Control and Complications Trial

The Diabetes Control and Complications Trial of improved blood glucose control in 1,441 people with type 1 diabetes in North America was published in 1996 and showed the benefits of tight blood glucose control with increased frequency of insulin injections (intensive insulin therapy). These factors can halve the development rate of eye, nerve and kidney damage and can even halve the deterioration rate of these complications compared with people treated with two insulin injections a day and higher blood glucose levels.

However the Diabetes Control and Complications Trial showed intensive insulin therapy led to some weight gain and more frequent hypoglycaemia.

The weight gain and increased hypoglycaemia may be less of a problem if you use the pattern recognition method of insulin dose adjustment, or if you adjust the dose of insulin responsible for the high or low blood glucose. This is better than using the top up or sliding scale method of insulin dose adjustment used in the Diabetes Control and Complications Trial, where a dose of quick-acting insulin is adjusted immediately after a high or low blood glucose reading.

Tobacco smoking

Tobacco smoking is the second single most important factor in the development of complications of the eyes, kidneys and blood vessels. It is extremely unusual for a person with diabetes to have a leg amputated due to blocked blood vessels unless they smoke.

AT A GLANCE

How to reduce your chances of complications:

- **Keep blood glucose levels between 4–8 mmol/L and lower than 11 mmol/L for most tests.**
- **Taking insulin injections more often may help control blood glucose – talk to your doctor.**
- **Do not smoke.**
- **Have regular physical exercise, keep your weight down to your healthy body weight, and keep your blood fats under control.**
- **If your blood pressure is high, have your doctor treat it.**
- **Have your blood pressure checked regularly plus occasional laboratory tests to check your blood fats, kidney function, and average blood glucose control.**
- **Have your eyes checked regularly by an eye specialist (ophthalmologist or optometrist) or by your diabetes specialist.**
- **Examine your feet regularly. From time to time have your doctor check them for blood vessel blockage, nerve damage, ulcers, ingrown toenails and tinea.**

High blood pressure

Untreated high blood pressure accelerates the blockage of arteries and increases the risk of heart attack, stroke, peripheral vascular disease and retinopathy.

Modern medications not only treat high blood pressure but, in many cases, give kidneys added protection from diabetic kidney damage.

Overweight and high blood fats

High blood fats and being overweight tend to accelerate the build up of fat in the lining of the blood vessels, accelerating the blockage of arteries.

Recent trials of cholesterol-lowering medication showed the medication can reduce the rate of heart attack by 50 per cent in people with diabetes.

Physical fitness

Regular physical exercise and physical fitness protect against many of the complications of diabetes and make weight reduction easier.

Alcohol

Excess alcohol consumption aggravates nerve damage and causes high blood pressure, high blood fats and excess weight gain.

SPECIFIC COMPLICATIONS

Eye damage (retinopathy and cataract)

These eye complications are described elsewhere in chapter 16, Diabetes and Eyes. It is important for people with diabetes to have regular eye checks by an eye specialist (ophthalmologist or optometrist) or a diabetes specialist.

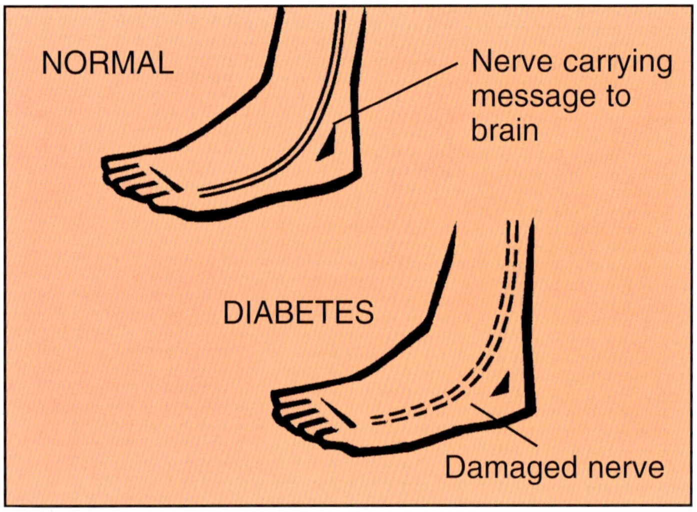

Diabetic nerve damage stops messages travelling from feet to the brain and warning of damage.

Blood vessel blockage (vascular disease)

Blood vessel blockage in the heart, brain or legs can occur in people without diabetes but, unfortunately, it occurs far more commonly in people with diabetes.

Blood vessel blockage in the heart (ischaemic heart disease)

This is caused by progressive narrowing of the coronary arteries which nourish the heart muscle. As the lining of the blood vessel thickens, the flow of blood is reduced and the heart muscle cannot function properly as it is deprived of oxygen and nourishment.

The symptoms are intermittent chest pain, generally brought on by exertion and relieved after a few minutes rest. This is due to a partial blockage of a heart or coronary artery and is called angina.

Unfortunately, people with diabetes are often unaware that they have narrowed blood vessels in the heart until they block completely, causing a heart attack (coronary occlusion or myocardial infarct).

The usual symptom of a heart attack is a heavy, pressing pain across the front of the chest, sometimes going into the neck or down the left arm. Unlike the intermittent pains of angina, the pain of a heart attack may last several hours and is not relieved by rest.

Summon medical help immediately if chest pain does not disappear completely within three to five minutes. This is a medical emergency.

Provided the amount of heart muscle affected is not large, healing usually takes place and the person can return to normal activity.

Blocked or diseased heart arteries are often surgically bypassed or sometimes opened up with a balloon and kept open by insertion of a round mesh of metal called a stent.

Blood vessel blockage to the brain (cerebrovascular disease)

A blockage of an artery in or leading to the brain can lead to a stroke or cerebrovascular accident. The symptoms are usually loss of speech, paralysis down one side of the body, loss of vision, coma or confusion.

Rehabilitation, including physiotherapy and speech therapy, often assists the person who has had a stroke to return to an active life.

A partial blockage of a blood vessel in or leading to the brain can cause symptoms such as temporary loss of speech, temporary paralysis, temporary impairment of vision, confusion or convulsions (transient ischaemic attack or TIA). This situation needs urgent medical attention because anti-clotting treatment or surgery to clean out the arteries in the neck can prevent a subsequent stroke.

Blood vessel blockage in the legs (peripheral vascular disease)

Symptoms are generally pain in one or both calf muscles during or after walking. Later, ulcers of the toes and feet may appear. In some cases, persistent pain occurs in the legs and feet.

Occasionally, blood vessels can be cleaned out, or bypassed, by surgery. Generally, however, in people with diabetes the blockage occurs in blood vessels that are so small, surgery is impossible.

If the blockage is severe, gangrene may develop in the toes and the feet, necessitating surgical treatment, usually amputation of the foot and leg below the knee.

Kidney damage (nephropathy)

Diabetic kidney damage is usually due to changes in small blood vessels leading to the filtering system of the kidney or to the smaller blood vessels within the filtering system itself. It is a completely painless process and cannot be detected, even by a physical examination by a doctor.

Detection of early kidney damage, however, is possible by testing the rate at which the kidneys are leaking a protein called albumin into the urine. The urine is tested with a special test strip in the laboratory.

If kidney damage is detected, high blood pressure medications called *ACE inhibitors* help protect the kidneys from further diabetic kidney damage.

Nerve damage (neuropathy)

Nerve damage is usually caused by high levels of glucose in the blood, but is occasionally caused by excessive alcohol consumption.

If the nerve damage extends to the nerves in the trunk of the body, the most common symptom in men is sexual impotence (see chapter 19, Sexual Problems in Men). Impotence can also be due to blockage of the blood vessels supplying the penis.

People with nerve damage can also lose the early warning symptoms of hypoglycaemia so that severe hypoglycaemia may occur without warning, causing episodes of confusion, convulsions or coma.

Nerve damage in the abdomen can also cause paralysis of the valve at the bottom of the stomach. This may lead to vomiting or to delay in the food passing out of the stomach into the intestine, leading to marked swings in blood glucose levels from low to high. This condition can be treated with medications such as metoclopramide, cisapride, or erythromycin.

Very rarely, nerve damage in the abdomen can lead to intermittent diarrhoea, particularly at night, and to faintness or dizziness on standing up out of bed or a chair. Nerve damage can also lead to incomplete bladder emptying, which can then lead to recurrent infections of the bladder and kidneys.

Nerve damage in the legs causes numbness, coldness of the legs, a tingling, pins and needles sensation in the feet and burning pains in the legs and feet, usually more noticeable in bed at night. Nerve damage in the legs and feet can lead to a loss of sensation in the feet, causing accidental damage because the person cannot feel any pain. This can develop into ulcers on the bottom of the feet that can penetrate to the bone, leading to osteomyelitis and chronic infection in bones and joints. This may necessitate amputation if not treated vigorously from the earliest time of infection, ulceration or the slightest discharge in the feet or toes. Always seek urgent medical advice for even the mildest looking foot infection.

Numbness or tingling plus a pins and needles sensation in the hand is more often due to compression of a nerve as it runs through a bony tunnel in the wrist, a condition relieved by a simple operation. This problem is relatively common in people with diabetes.

Nerve damage is detected by testing for different types of sensation in the feet and legs and by testing the knee and ankle reflexes.

It is very important for people with diabetes to examine their feet at least every second or third day.

If you have nerve damage in the feet, do not walk barefooted and do wear properly-fitted shoes that rub neither feet nor toes.

Foot damage

The combination of vascular disease and nerve damage makes the feet susceptible to damage. It is important to examine your feet every day to look for ulcers and infection if you have altered feeling in your feet due to nerve damage. Your doctor will test the pulses in your feet and legs occasionally.

Infections of the vagina, bladder and kidneys

People with diabetes have a higher chance of developing infections of the vagina, bladder and kidneys than people without diabetes. Bladder and kidney infections are more common in women because of the short length of the urethra, the tube taking urine from the bladder to the outside of the body. Germs can be massaged backwards up this tube in women during sexual intercourse and it is wise to empty the bladder after sexual intercourse to flush out any germs before they multiply.

The urine and vaginal secretions of people with diabetes often contain increased amounts of glucose, particularly if the level of the glucose in the blood has been high. This provides an excellent source of food on which germs (bacteria and fungi) can grow.

If the nerves to the bladder have been damaged by diabetes, the bladder may not empty completely when passing urine, leaving some urine inside the bladder where germs may multiply. Symptoms of bladder and kidney infections are:

- passing of small amounts of urine at more frequent intervals, day and night
- a burning discomfort or pain when passing urine
- backache is also an occasional symptom of kidney infection.

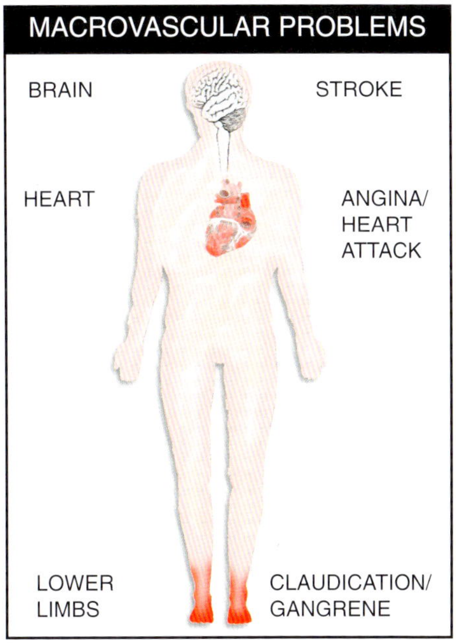

Macrovascular problems affecting the large blood vessels to the brain, heart and lower limbs.

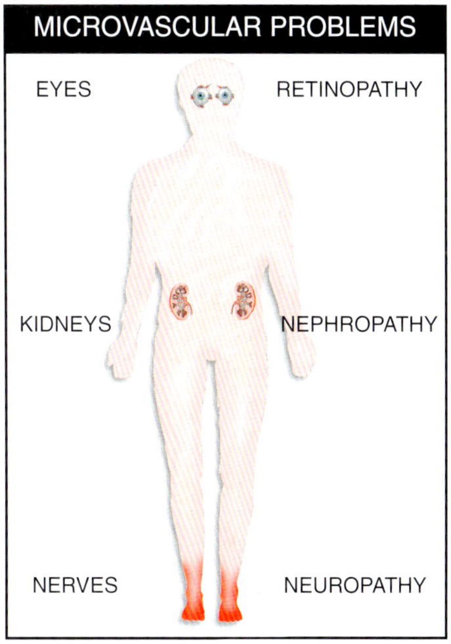

Microvascular problems affecting the small blood vessels in the eyes, kidneys and nerves.

TABLE 1: Danger factors for complications

Factors responsible for damage	Complications of diabetes				
	Blood vessel blockage in heart, brain and legs	**Eye damage**	**Kidney damage**	**Nerve damage**	**Infections of vagina, bladder and kidneys**
High blood glucose	+	+++	++	+++	+++
Tobacco smoking	+++	++	++	+	MN
High blood pressure	+++	++	+++	MN	MN
High blood fats and cholesterol	+++	MN	MN	MN	MN
Excess alcohol	MN	MN	MN	++	MN
Overweight	++	+	MN	MN	MN
Duration of diabetes	++	+	+	MN	MN

+++ = greatest effect
++ = greater effect
+ = some effect
MN = minimal or no effect

Infection of the bladder is called cystitis. Infection of the kidney is called pyelonephritis, but both infections usually occur together. These infections are diagnosed by a microscope examination of a specimen of urine and by a urine culture test. Infections are usually treated effectively by antibiotics taken by mouth.

Prompt treatment of bladder and kidney infections is important as these infections, if allowed to continue, may result in chronic kidney damage.

Symptoms of vaginal or penis infection are itching of the penis, vagina or vulva, often associated with discharge from the vagina on to the pants. This can be treated by pessaries and creams. Occasionally a course of oral tablets for the person with diabetes and their sexual partner is needed to clear the fungus from the bowel while it is also being cleared from the vagina or penis. Lowering high blood glucose levels to normal often helps the treatment.

Dental problems

If the blood glucose level is high, there may be a reduced flow of saliva, the infection-fighting white blood cells will be paralysed and the mouth will have a high glucose level. All these factors increase the risk of gum infections and dental caries (tooth decay).

Brush teeth once or twice daily after meals and have teeth and gums checked annually by a dental professional (see chapter 18 – Diabetes and Oral Health).

MINOR COMPLICATIONS OF DIABETES

Hollows in the fat tissue (fat atrophy)

Fat atrophy is the loss of fat between the skin and muscle at injection sites. It is probably due to an individual reaction by the fat tissue to certain types of insulin. This problem is now extremely rare since the introduction of highly purified insulins and human insulins.

Lumps of fatty tissue (fat hypertrophy)

Fat hypertrophy – the opposite of fat atrophy, also occurs at injection sites and is an increase or accumulation of fat between the skin and muscle. It is probably the result of injections being given too often in one spot. Insulin injected into these fatty lumps or bumps is erratically absorbed and blood glucose control becomes less predictable.

The cure is to avoid injecting into the fat bump and to rotate injection sites over a greater area than previously used (see chapter 9 – Injectors and Injections).

Insulin allergy

Insulin allergy causes redness, pain or itching, generally at the injection sites, although the itching may occur over the entire body. This complication usually develops in the first month or two on insulin and disappears within six to eight weeks. It is now extremely rare since the introduction of highly purified insulins and human insulins.

Skin redness or sores (necrobiosis lipoidica diabeticorum)

This is a rare condition on the fronts of the shins causing thinning of the skin and loss of underlying fat at the front or side part of the leg between knee and ankle. It does not appear to be related to blood glucose control and is very difficult to treat. It may appear after many years of diabetes but occasionally develops even before the diabetes. We believe it is caused by an immunological reaction.

Swelling of the ankles and face (insulin oedema)

Fluid retention causes swelling in the ankles and sometimes the face. Usually it only occurs when blood glucose levels are controlled after being very high for several months. We don't know the cause, but it usually gets better by itself after two to six weeks and does not usually respond to anti-fluid tablets (diuretics).

Xanthoma and xanthelasma

These are conditions due to an excess of cholesterol or fats accumulating in the skin. They usually consist of red or yellowish spots around the elbows and knees, occasionally in the palms of the hand, on the chest or above or below the eyelids. They usually indicate excessive fat in the blood but may indicate poor blood glucose control or excess alcohol consumption.

Diabetes and Eyes

◆ By Associate Professor Paul Mitchell ◆

EYE damage is a common complication of diabetes but, happily, through better prevention and treatment, it is less likely to cause blindness than in the past. The good news is that blindness caused by diabetes is decreasing.

Figures compiled in Newcastle show diabetic retinopathy was the cause of blindness in 7 per cent of people registered for the blind pension in the past decade, compared with almost 12 per cent for the previous 15-year period. UK figures from 1986 show that diabetic retinopathy, as a cause of blindness, was down to 3 per cent of the total.

While these figures are encouraging, Australian ophthalmologists (medically qualified eye specialists) still encounter many people with diabetes who lose their vision – in most cases unnecessarily.

There are several reasons for this. Many people with diabetes and their doctors may not strive to keep the blood glucose levels low enough and seem satisfied with what we now believe is less than adequate control.

This attitude is particularly common in people with older onset diabetes, that is, diagnosed after age 30. Too often people believe that type 2 diabetes is 'just a touch of sugar'. This is not the case and some people with type 2 diabetes actually achieve better control – and feel better – on insulin.

Another reason is that many people with diabetes do not visit their ophthalmologist for regular eye checks until their vision is impaired. Tragically, some older people do not visit an ophthalmologist until their second eye has become affected or vision has failed in both eyes.

While ophthalmologists and optometrists can help people affected by retinopathy, this is not the best time to start treatment. The ideal situation is to detect the earliest stages of retinopathy when vision is affected and to monitor its progress carefully. This enables the eye doctor to liaise closely with the person's diabetes doctor, especially if the early eye damage seems accelerated.

This is also a good time to look for other factors which could be important, such as high blood pressure.

The chance of retinopathy

Retinopathy is common in people with diabetes and is strongly related to the length of time they have had diabetes.

In all the Australian studies, about one in three people with known diabetes has some evidence of retinopathy and, of these, another one in three has retinopathy which has either damaged vision or threatens to do so. After five years, around 50 per cent, or one in two, has some retinopathy present, although this does not mean that all are at risk of losing their sight.

Retinopathy which damages or threatens to damage vision takes longer to develop but is seen in about 15 to 20 per cent of people after 10 years, and about a third of people after 20 years of diabetes. While the risk seems slightly higher for people on insulin, it is still substantial in people treated by food or tablets.

The development of some retinopathy may therefore seem almost inevitable after a long duration of diabetes, but the effect on vision is mostly preventable or can be decreased considerably with treatment.

AT A GLANCE

- **Educating people with diabetes, their doctors and the general public is important in the battle to prevent diabetic blindness – a battle we appear to be winning.**
- **Because diabetes can seriously and permanently affect vision, it is important to see your eye specialist regularly and well before you notice symptoms.**
- **Keep your diabetes well controlled.**

Effects of diabetes on vision

There are three ways diabetes can affect vision.

1. *Retinopathy* causes damage to the small blood vessels in the back of the eyes and may result in loss of vision due to obstruction, leak or haemorrhage.

   The most severe loss of vision comes from proliferative retinopathy in which abnormal blood vessels grow from the optic nerve or other vessels because large areas of the eye circulation have been blocked by the diabetic process.

   The 'new' vessels are not helpful and tend to bleed and scar. While occurring in all age groups, it is most common with type 1 diabetes that has been present for a long time, often more than 20 years.
2. The most frequent cause of loss of vision is *maculopathy,* a condition in which a leak occurs from blood vessels near the eye's centre of vision, leading to swelling and slow loss of reading vision. *Maculopathy* can occur in all age groups but is more common in people with type 2 diabetes.
3. *Cataract* is an opacity or opaqueness which forms in the lens of the eye and is a common cause of decreased vision. Cataracts tend to develop earlier in people with diabetes, but they can be removed surgically and a new lens implanted. This is done exactly the same way as for people without diabetes, usually with good results.

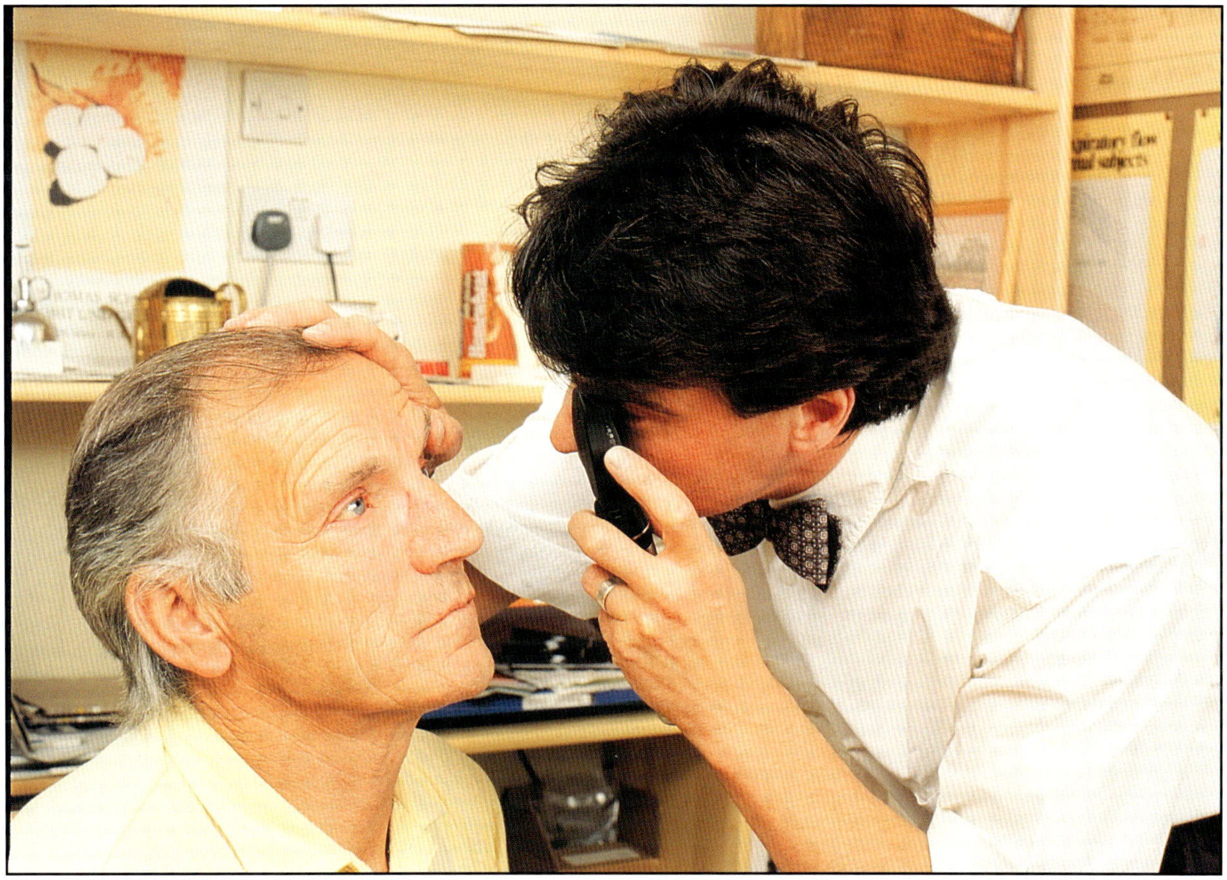

Who should examine?

The examination should be done by an ophthalmologist or optometrist who will check your vision and screen your retinas carefully after dilating your pupils with drops.

It is important the pupils are dilated with eye drops because it gives the examiner a good view of the retinas.

Some diabetes centres use a camera to photograph the back of the eye and an ophthalmologist checks the photos later.

When examinations should be done

Significant retinopathy threatening vision may be present in many people with diabetes before they notice any effect on vision. Because of this and the beneficial effect of early laser treatment for vision-threatening retinopathy, regular retinal screening of all people with diabetes is recommended.

- For people with diabetes diagnosed before age 30, retinal examinations should start no later than after five years of diabetes and generally from age 10 onwards.
- For diabetes diagnosed at or after age 30, the examination should be made at the time of diabetes diagnosis to detect any significant eye damage at that time.
- For both groups a subsequent examination is recommended every two years if no signs of retinopathy are found, and once any lesions are detected, a review is needed every 12 months or less.

There are some high-risk groups – people with high blood pressure, kidney damage or poor diabetic control – who may need closer follow up. Retinopathy can progress through a pregnancy, so it is recommended that women with diabetes are examined before they start a pregnancy and followed through it if there are any signs detected.

If retinopathy is found shortly after the diagnosis of diabetes – usually in type 2 diabetes – it can progress more rapidly, despite good control, and therefore close monitoring is needed.

If you notice any change in vision, see your eye specialist immediately.

Testing for retinopathy

Your eye specialist or his staff will test your distance vision carefully – with glasses if you wear them, and may either change the lens or use a pinhole to obtain the best vision. The specialist may also check your eye pressures as raised eye pressure or glaucoma is seen more commonly in people with diabetes. Your pupils will then be dilated with drops, a process which can take up to an hour.

Once your pupils are dilated, the doctor will use an ophthalmoscope or other instruments with fairly bright lights to screen your retina for any signs of diabetic retinopathy. While mildly unpleasant, this examination only lasts a few minutes.

If there is some evidence of eye damage, the doctor may recommend a test known as a fluorescein angiogram. In this test, dye is injected through a vein in the arm and a series of photographs taken as the dye passes through the blood vessels in the body and eyes.

Dye can be seen in the vessels of the retina and will show up the damaged areas in greater detail.

This test is usually only carried out when significant retinopathy is present. Nausea occurs in about one in four people. One interesting effect is that the skin remains yellow for a few hours – and urine for a day afterwards until the dye is passed out of the body.

Action if retinopathy threatens vision

If the eye doctor finds signs of proliferative retinopathy or maculopathy, or if these stages appear imminent, he will probably recommend laser treatment.

This treatment has been effective in many major trials and is now routine in all centres in Australia. The procedure is usually carried out in an outpatient department or doctor's rooms and usually takes about 15 to 30 minutes per session.

Laser treatment for maculopathy is usually not painful. But proliferative retinopathy affects large areas of the retina and treatment can be painful. A local anaesthetic through the lower eyelid – not into the eye – may be suggested to prevent the pain, although many people seem to cope well without it.

Some people find sunlight too bright for a week or so afterwards and wear dark glasses to reduce the glare.

A number of treatments may be required over a few weeks and vision may be blurred for a period.

The control of diabetes and retinopathy

There is increasing evidence that poor diabetic control increases the risk of retinopathy and its progression.

Further trials are under way to look at the relationship but, in the meantime, it is best for people with diabetes to strive for as tight control as possible.

Once severe retinopathy has occurred, good control may not influence its course significantly. This is presumably because the changes that have occurred in the retina are already too advanced and, to some extent, are independent of the diabetes. If improved control does have a beneficial effect, this will probably be a few years down the track.

The onset of the complications of diabetes emphasises the need to control diabetes as well as possible in the first few years, before any complications such as retinopathy have occurred. It also helps explain why retinopathy continues to progress despite insulin treatment in people found to have retinopathy at the time of diagnosis.

No medications have been found conclusively to be helpful in preventing or delaying retinopathy. Studies are being conducted to try and find a medication which may slow down the progression of retinopathy.

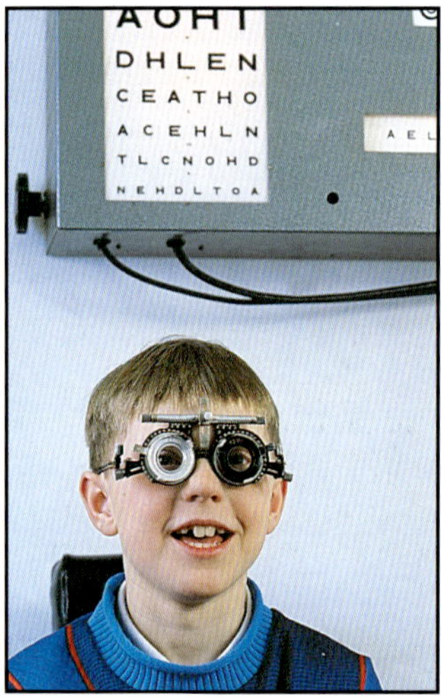

People with high blood pressure seem to have an increased risk of retinopathy so this must be treated as it could well delay or prevent retinopathy.

For further information on diabetic retinopathy contact Diabetes Australia on 1800 640 862 to obtain your copy of the NHMRC retinopathy guidelines.

Chapter 17

Foot Care and Foot Wear

◆ By Angela Evans ◆

WE tend not to think about our feet – other than as funny or smelly – until something goes wrong with them.

Then we appreciate how much we use and rely on our feet to carry us about, covering hundreds of thousands of kilometres in a lifetime.

Some complications of diabetes are due to a lack of knowledge, others to lack of adequate care. People with diabetes who develop foot problems are often unaware that the problems are linked to their condition or that there are simple procedures which can prevent the problems altogether.

Foot problems are associated with persistently high blood glucose levels. Therefore, it is important to keep blood glucose levels consistently within the normal range as this alone helps prevent many of the complications of diabetes, including foot problems.

Medical research shows that long-term control of diabetes – regular exercise, a low-fat diet, no smoking and moderate alcohol intake – greatly reduces the risk of all problems.

People with diabetes need to be aware of four considerations in foot maintenance which should be checked annually or more often as advised by their podiatrist, general practitioner or diabetes nurse educator. These are:

- nerve damage
- blood vessel damage
- foot shape
- self-care.

Nerve damage

Nerve damage (peripheral neuropathy) occurs after long-term poor diabetes control. It puts the feet at risk of serious damage because nerves serve as a warning signal to stop injury occurring.

Normal, healthy feet have nerves that give good sensation to every part of the feet and legs. It is because of these nerves that we are able to feel things such as sharp objects, ill-fitting shoes, a corn, in-grown nail or hot water bottle.

Pain or discomfort from such things is transmitted by the nerves to our brain, alerting us to immediate

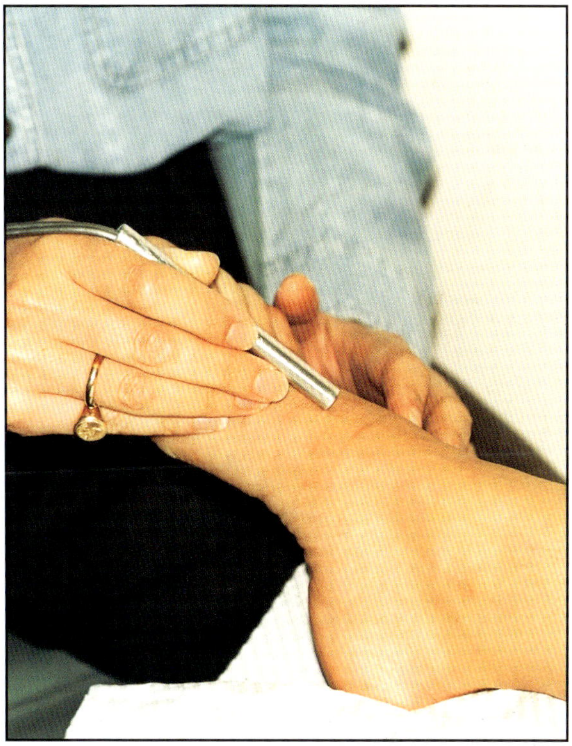

danger and protecting us from injury. If these nerves don't do their job, we are not alerted to potential danger and the feet may be damaged.

It is important to know how well your nerves are functioning so that you can take extra care to avoid injury. Your podiatrist, doctor or diabetes nurse educator will carry out tests to determine your level of sensitivity.

Some people with diabetes report uncomfortable feelings in their legs and feet. Called paraesthesiae, the feelings have been variously described as pins and needles, numbness or burning and are often worse at night.

If you have these uncomfortable feelings, contact your doctor because you may need a review of diabetic control or additional treatment.

Many people report such sensations before they know they have diabetes. Often the feelings disappear when the diabetes is brought under control.

AT A GLANCE

- **The needs of every person with diabetes are individual. It is essential to visit a podiatrist or doctor for complete foot assessment.**
- **You can then be advised specifically on the necessary foot care. This assessment should be performed at least annually.**
- **Foot problems can be a serious complication of diabetes but, with early assessment, regular check-ups and proper care there is no reason why they cannot be overcome.**
- **You can have healthy feet with diabetes – it is up to you. Remember the old adage about feet: One pair must last a lifetime.**

Apart from high blood glucose levels, heavy alcohol use and a diet lacking vitamin B may further damage the nerves and these, too, need to be addressed.

Blood vessel damage

Also known as clogging or narrowing of the arteries, this condition means that less blood is able to flow through the blood vessels. This is especially important for the feet where the arteries are small and the longer the clogging continues, the narrower the arteries become, meaning that the feet receive insufficient blood to keep them healthy.

Factors that are bad for your blood vessels include:

- smoking
- lack of regular exercise
- high blood pressure
- high blood fats
- high blood glucose levels.

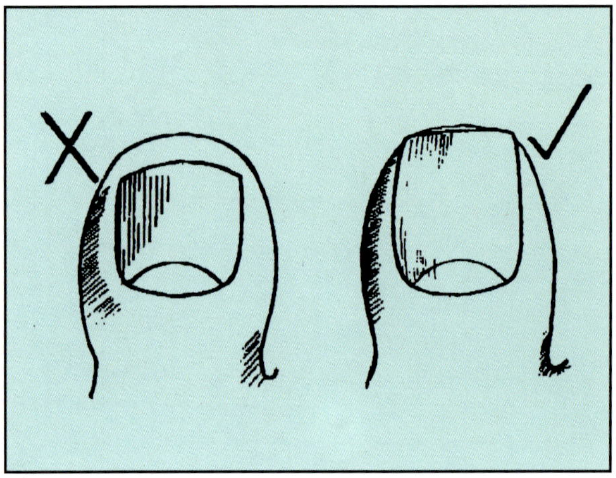

Nails should be cut straight across, not too short and never down the sides.

If the feet lack a healthy blood supply, they are more prone to infection following any injury that breaks the skin. People with a reduced blood supply to their feet must take great care of their skin, which is an important protective barrier against infections. Dry skin cracks easily providing an opening for infections, but you can avoid dryness with regular use of an effective moisturising cream.

In people with diabetes the effects of foot infections may go far beyond feet and cause high blood glucose levels. High blood glucose levels lower the body's resistance to infection. It is important to seek medical attention if blood glucose levels are high – especially if you have a foot injury and possible infection.

Foot infections can be difficult to detect because some of the signs are not obvious. So seek help early.

Signs of poor blood supply include:

- sharp leg cramps after walking short distances or up stairs
- pain in the feet, even at rest (often in the early hours of the morning)
- feet feeling cold
- feet looking a reddish-blue colour
- cuts which are slow to heal.

If you have any of these symptoms, see your podiatrist, doctor or diabetes nurse educator.

Most of the causes of blood vessel damage can be controlled by changes in your lifestyle and, in some cases, medication. Take action early to avoid serious blood vessel damage and prevent problems.

Foot shape

The feet are mechanical and consist of numerous bones, ligaments and muscles which perform simultaneously to carry and propel our bodies when we stand or walk.

Some people's feet do not work properly and become a funny shape; others may inherit an unusual foot shape. Whatever the reason, people with oddly shaped feet:

- have problems finding shoes which fit
- may find exercise difficult
- develop more corns and calluses.

People with diabetes with misshapen feet and nerve damage are the most likely to develop ulcers from too much pressure over some areas of the feet. Pressure can be due to difficulty in fitting a shoe on an irregularly shaped foot (with a bunion or a hammer toe). Or it may be due to the foot not working properly and overloading some weight bearing areas at the ball of the foot.

A callus or a corn is a symptom of too much pressure on one area and can be avoided with some changes. These include padded inner soles or orthotic supports to make the foot work more efficiently and reduce pressure areas.

Pressure areas on the feet are enemies of all people with diabetes, especially those with nerve and blood vessel damage. Seek your podiatrist's help to get rid of calluses or corns before they become ulcers as these can become infected, risking the leg. For feet belonging to people with diabetes, prevention is your best friend.

Self-care

Once you know the level of sensation and blood supply of your feet plus the importance of reducing pressure areas, issues of foot care and foot wear are a lot easier.

People with totally insensitive feet, poor blood supply and misshapen feet must be extremely careful if they are to avoid limb-threatening problems.

For these people, on a daily basis the feet need to be:

- well washed and gently dried
- moisturised with a suitable cream
- checked for trouble spots such as redness, swelling, cuts, pus discharge, splinters or blisters, being especially careful to look between toes, around heels and nail edges and at the soles of the feet – if you have difficulty with vision you will need someone else to check for you
- covered with a clean sock or stocking without rough seams
- protected in a shoe which fits well and has been checked for stones, pins, buttons or anything else which could cause damage.

If you have good sensation in your feet, adequate blood circulation and regular shape, good foot care is generally the same as that recommended for everyone.

Hygiene is always important. Make sure feet are dried well after a bath or shower, particularly between the toes, where moisture can encourage tinea infection.

If the skin is dry, use a good moisturiser.

Socks or stockings should be clean, with natural fibres such as wool or cotton providing better ventilation than synthetics.

Shoes are worn to protect the feet and must fit well and be appropriate for the activity you are undertaking. Your podiatrist can advise you on the best shoe for your requirements.

You may have read or heard that people with diabetes should never walk barefoot or cut their own nails. This is true for anyone who has lost sensation in their feet as they could step on something sharp, cut their foot and not be aware of it. If this person also has a reduced blood supply, this could lead to infection and even turn gangrenous. In such a case the wearing of well-fitting shoes could have prevented a disaster.

It is risky for anyone with poor blood circulation or limited sensation to cut their own nails. Thick or ingrown nails need special podiatry care. Cut your own nails only if you:

- can see clearly
- reach your feet easily
- have nails of normal thickness that are easily trimmed
- have good blood circulation.

Nails need to be cut straight across, not too short and never down the sides. Rough edges can be safely filed with an emery board.

Other mechanical foot and leg problems include sore leg muscles, recurrent ankle sprains, flattened or high arch and knee pain. These problems may need investigating by a podiatrist skilled at assessing the alignment of foot and leg. Although these difficulties are not directly related to diabetes, they can restrict exercising, which often affects blood glucose levels.

Things to avoid

Corn-cure chemicals are not only wrongly named, they are dangerous. Corns are due to excess pressure, so see a podiatrist to find out why this is happening and how it can be prevented.

Radiators and hot water bottles can cause burns, especially to someone without good sensation in their feet. Keep a safe distance from radiators and use a knee rug if still cold.

Hot sand, pavers or bitumen in summer can burn the feet if sensation is lost and shoes are not worn. Sunscreen creams (SPF 15+) need to be regularly applied to the skin of legs and feet when outside. Skin cancer is just as great a risk as sunburn.

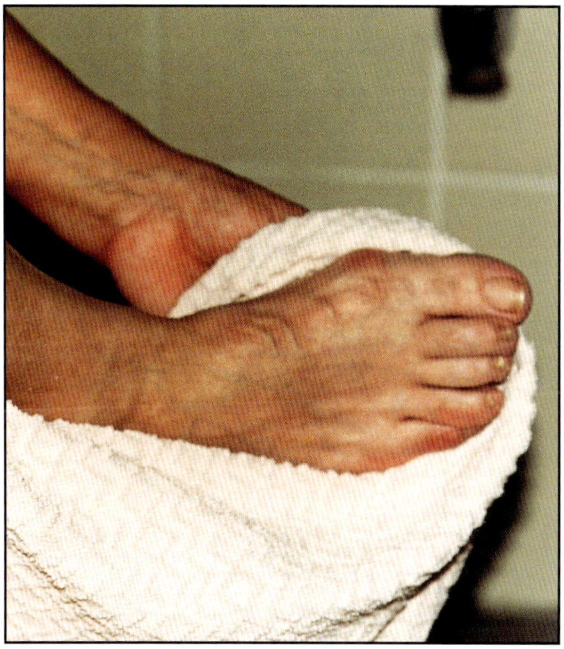

Foot first aid

If you have normal sensation in your feet you will feel injuries as they occur. If sensation is reduced you may only find injuries during your daily foot inspection.

If you find an injury:

- wash and dry the area
- apply good antiseptic
- cover with a sterile dressing.

It is important for you always to have dressings and antiseptic on hand. Your podiatrist, pharmacist, doctor or diabetes nurse educator will be able to advise you on the most suitable products.

If there is not improvement within 24 hours, seek professional help to avoid complications.

Diabetes and Oral Health

◆ The Diabetes Education Series ◆

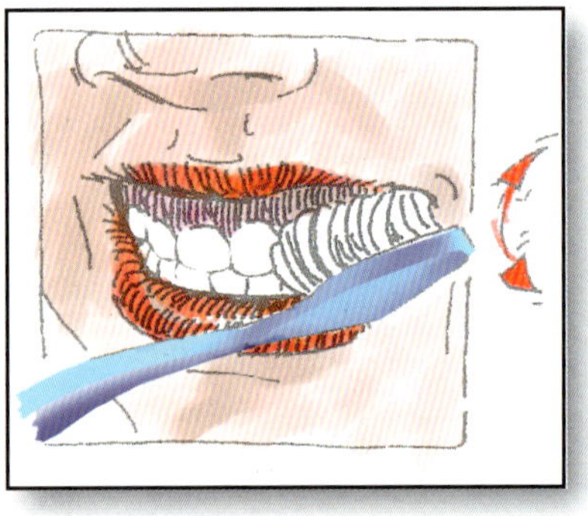

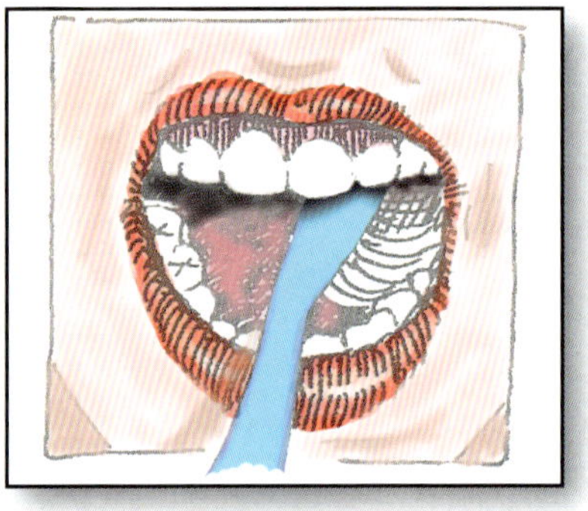

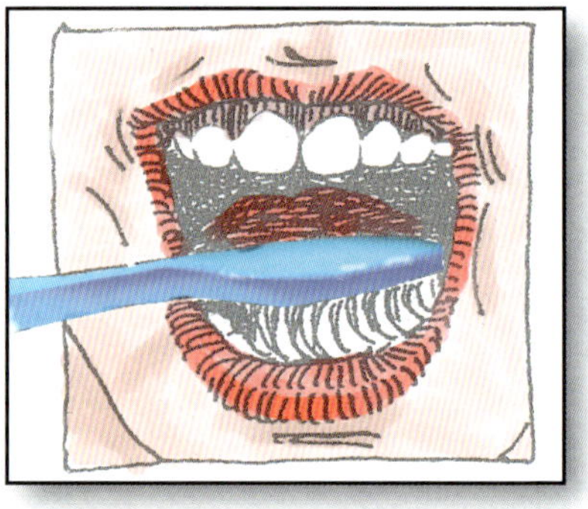

BECAUSE people with diabetes are prone to tooth decay and gum infections, it is important to maintain good oral hygiene.

Healing may also be delayed or decreased so if you suspect any problem exists, seek early diagnosis and treatment. This prevents minor problems from escalating into serious conditions.

Be gentle because brushing too forcefully can damage teeth surfaces and wear away gums.

Remember to tell your dentist you have diabetes.

Where possible choose plain water or milk as a between-meal drink; avoid using sugar in tea or coffee and choose snacks that don't contain sugars or acids.

Use the following tips to maintain a brilliant smile and healthy breath while avoiding serious problems and costly dental repairs.

AT A GLANCE

- **Key factors are daily brushing and flossing, regular consultations with your dentist, and eating the right foods.**
- **At the slightest suspicion of a gum, tooth, denture or mouth problem, see your dental professional.**
- **Eat nutritious snacks that don't contain sugars or acids.**
- **Drink plain water where possible.**

Cleaning

- Use a small, soft toothbrush and replace it regularly.
- Thoroughly clean teeth and gums morning and night; ask your dentist to instruct you in the correct brushing technique.
- Use a pea size amount of fluoride toothpaste at each brushing.

Brushing

It is important to brush teeth and gums thoroughly without causing damage. Here is one method:

- Hold your toothbrush like you would a pencil – this prevents using too harsh pressure.
- Begin on the left side, placing the brush on the outside of the top teeth.
- Place the bristles of the brush on the gum line where teeth meet gum.
- Wiggle the bristles gently back and forward over one or two teeth at a time using a gentle massaging motion.
- Brush from the top left around to the top right.
- Repeat the same steps for the lower teeth.
- Brush the chewing surfaces on both sides of your mouth using backward and forward strokes.
- Finish by gently brushing your tongue and rinsing your mouth with water.
- You can also use a disclosing solution (available from pharmacies) to show up colourless plaque.

Flossing

Flossing cleans food and plaque which may be lodged between your teeth where the brush cannot reach. Floss is a thread available in waxed, unwaxed and mint-flavoured varieties. Choose one that feels most comfortable.

Method

- From the floss dispenser, break off about 30 cm of floss.
- Wrap floss around the middle and/or index finger of each hand leaving a gap of about 10 cm in between.
- Guide the floss between the gaps in the teeth.
- Move floss to the left to curve it around each tooth.
- Keeping the floss in this position, gently slide it up underneath the gum then down a few times.
- Using a new clean section of the floss, place the floss back in the space and repeat the instructions, but for the tooth on the right.
- Always use a clean section of the dispensed piece of floss to prevent transferring bacteria.
- Repeat this procedure between all the teeth in the mouth.

Dentures and plates

People with dentures or removable dental plates are advised to:

- remove dentures and clean them at least once daily
- use a denture brush or soft nail brush kept especially for this purpose
- clean both sides of the denture, ideally over water or a cloth to prevent breakage in case you drop the dentures
- massage gums by brushing with a soft toothbrush to stimulate blood supply
- after eating, remove dentures and brush or rinse them; also rinse your mouth and gently brush your tongue
- remove stains or hard deposits from dentures by soaking them in vinegar for an hour or cleaning with a denture cleaner
- contact your dentist or clinical dental technician if your dentures don't fit well
- have your dentures and mouth checked regularly by a dental professional.

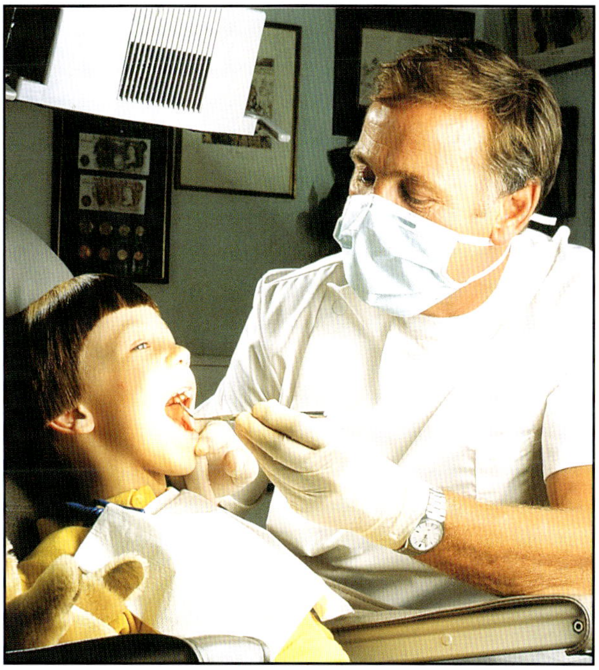

Dry mouth

People with diabetes often get *xerostomia* or dry mouth as a result of their medications.

Hyperglycaemia can lead to an increased amount of urine, depleting the body's extracellular fluids and reducing saliva flow to cause dry mouth.

This decreased saliva flow is not only uncomfortable but can increase the risk of tooth decay and cause:

- bad breath
- difficulty in speech and eating
- cracking and bleeding of lips and tongue
- difficulty in retaining dentures.

If you have a dry mouth, drink water. Other drinks may increase the risk of tooth decay or make you thirsty.

You may find some relief from creams and artificial saliva. Chewing sugarless gum or sucking sugarless and acid-free sweets may stimulate saliva production.

Mouth washes containing alcohol are not recommended as they can further dry the mouth.

Ask your dentist for further advice.

Oral infections

If you suspect any oral problems exist, see your dentist immediately.

Symptoms of infection may include red, sore or swollen gums; white film on gums, cheek or tongue which, when wiped, cause pain, bleeding or redness; lumps; swellings or any unusual conditions in the mouth.

Dental treatment

You are eligible for dental care with the community dental service located in metropolitan and country areas if you hold a:

- Health Care Card
- Health Benefits Card
- Pensioner Concession Card.

**Material developed by the Dental Health Education Unit of the South Australian Dental Service.*

Sexual Problems in Men

◆ By the late Dr Ted Keogh ◆
Revised by Dr Tom Cromer

MEN may have sexual problems at any time of life regardless of whether they have diabetes or not.

As men age, sexual desire (libido) may decrease and the penis may no longer become fully erect, remain erect or become erect at all. This is called erectile dysfunction.

Few studies have been done in Australia but it is estimated that there are more than 25 million men in the USA with erectile dysfunction.

Men with diabetes are more likely to experience some kinds of sexual problems than men without diabetes.

The most common sexual problem is erectile dysfunction, but premature ejaculation, failure to ejaculate and an inability to sustain an erection may also be problems.

Physiology

The penis contains two rods of spongy tissue lying side by side. On the undersurface is a tube – the urethra, which conveys urine from the bladder and semen from the testes and other sex glands. The rods of tissue can become filled with blood. The tiny cavities, called lacunae, expand and compress the veins (which drain blood from the penis) against the rigid outer layer, so blood becomes trapped in the penis. This results in a firm erection.

These events are under nervous and reflex control. When a man contemplates sexual activity, messages travel from the brain down the spinal cord and through nerves that then dilate the arteries. Direct stimulation of the penis will also send signals that eventually dilate the arteries.

If a man becomes anxious while he has an erection, the arteries may narrow. Thus a stressed man, irrespective of the presence of diabetes, may not be able to achieve an erection or maintain an erection.

The onset of erectile problems can be a gradual process, starting with the softening of erections, then a tendency to ejaculate prematurely, inability to sustain erections and, finally, the inability to initiate erections.

This process may be protracted over a decade or occur much more rapidly. Whatever the cause of a man's erectile dysfunction, there is always a psychological component. A good understanding relationship is always helpful, whereas an atmosphere of conflict will only worsen the problem.

Erectile dysfunction may occur in men with signs of other complications from diabetes. On the other hand, it is a common problem in all men as they age and may occur without any other complications connected with diabetes.

Causes of impotence

Up until the mid-1970s most impotence was thought to be psychological. Nowadays we believe that about 70 per cent of impotence is due to a physical cause and about 30 per cent is psychological.

Even when erectile problems have a physical cause, there is nearly always an additional psychological component.

Men with diabetes may suffer from a temporary loss of sexual desire if blood glucose levels are high. This often improves once blood glucose control improves.

A number of drugs can affect erectile function although, in practice, ceasing these medications may not help. Occasionally men may have hormonal abnormalities that can cause a decline in sex drive, but often such men present with impotence.

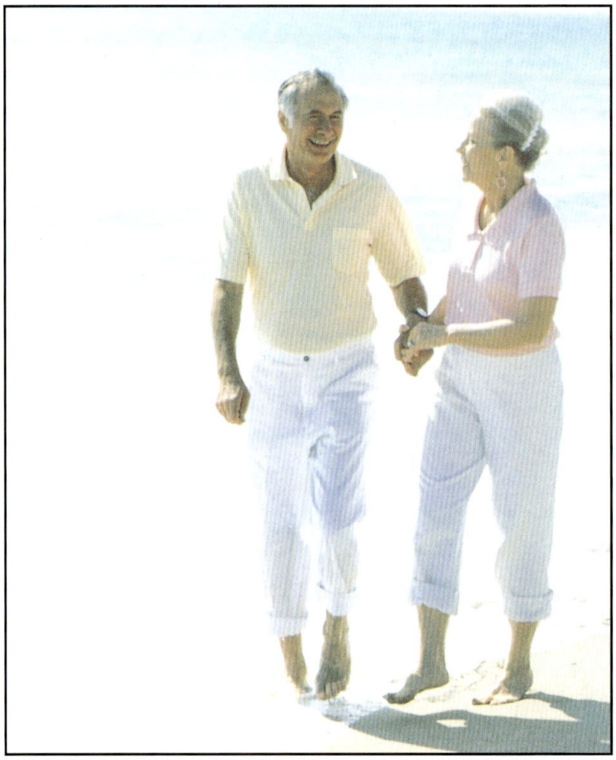

AT A GLANCE

- **Incidence of impotence increases with age and diabetes.**
- **Modern treatment is effective, relatively inexpensive and safe.**
- **About 70 per cent of impotence has a physical cause, the rest is psychological.**
- **The particular cause of the sexual problem determines the treatment.**

Most impotence is caused either by permanent damage to the nerves of the penis or blockage (partial or complete) of the blood vessels supplying the penis.

Definition

A man is impotent when he cannot achieve an erection adequate for intercourse. Penetration and intercourse satisfactory for the man and his partner do not require total erections. Most men can penetrate and have intercourse with erections they rate at about half their normal capacity.

Tests

In most cases the only tests that are needed are a few blood tests and an injection into the shaft of the penis. The blood tests check for hormone levels, HbA1c, cholesterol and liver function.

The main test is a diagnostic injection of a drug, prostaglandin E_1, into the shaft of the penis. This drug opens up the blood vessels in the penis, resulting in its spongy tissue filling with blood – the mechanism of an erection.

Usually after about five to ten minutes the penis becomes erect. This erection lasts about half an hour although, on occasions, it may last two hours and, very rarely, even longer. Occasionally this injection test fails, usually when the arteries supplying the penis are severely blocked.

In rare cases more complicated investigations are necessary, but for the vast majority of men no other investigations are required.

Treatment

Ideally, treatment options will be discussed with both partners.

Not so long ago the only treatments for erectile dysfunction were sex therapy by a sex therapist or insertion of a penile implant. Both treatments are still available but other methods may be more effective, less expensive, and therefore more popular.

Sexual counselling and education are valuable methods of treatment, whether the cause is psychological or not. They are the preferred treatment when psychological issues are suspected as the main cause of erectile problems.

Penile implants are expensive, require complex surgery and are prone to mechanical failure but are still used in certain situations or when other methods have failed.

Implants are available in two types. One is a malleable rod with a metal core surrounded by an inert rubber such as silicone. The penis can be bent down or straightened for intercourse.

The other type of implant is an inflatable device consisting of two sausage-shaped balloons fitted into the shaft of the penis. A reservoir of water is placed in front of the bladder and a pump in the scrotum. The pump is manually worked to fill the balloons with water and cause an erection.

The most popular method of treatment in Australia is intracavernosal injections (injections into the shaft of the penis). Men and/or their partners learn how to inject medication that opens up the blood vessels in the penis (a vasodilating agent, Carerject™ which contains prostaglandin E_1). It sounds difficult and painful but in reality is fairly easy and pain-free. For most men this method of treatment results in satisfactory erections and intercourse.

Injections are not suitable for all men and some are unwilling to learn self-injection therapy. These men can try treatment with a vacuum-assisted device. With this method, the penis is inserted into a rigid perspex cylinder which is pressed firmly against the body. A vacuum created in the cylinder sends blood flow to the penis, causing rigidity. Placing a tight rubber band around the base of the penis traps blood inside causing it to remain rigid. When the rubber band is removed the penis returns to its flaccid state.

Often in the early stages of erectile dysfunction men can achieve an erection but it softens before – or shortly after – intercourse begins. This can often be avoided by placing a rubber ring around the base of the penis during intercourse to trap the blood. However, this method will not work if there is no initial erection.

The future

In April 1998 Pfizer introduced the orally taken drug sildenafil (Viagra™) in the USA for the treatment of erectile dysfunction. Viagra™ was released in Australia in September 1998.

Sildenafil blocks an enzyme found mainly in the penis that breaks down a chemical produced during sexual stimulation. The longer that chemical, called cyclic GMP, remains active, the better chance of an erection. Studies have shown it to be effective in about 70 per cent of men with erectile dysfunction and in about 60 per cent of diabetic men with erectile dysfunction.

It is generally well tolerated but minor side effects have been reported. These include headache, flushing, stuffy nose, diarrhoea and visual changes. Men taking any form of nitroglycerin must not take sildenafil because it can result in a dangerously low blood pressure.

Sildenafil is a great advance in the treatment of erectile dysfunction and no doubt will become the preferred method of treatment for most men with erectile dysfunction.

Diabetes and Women's Health

◆ By Associate Professor Lesley Campbell ◆

ALTHOUGH issues such as contraception and sexuality are very important to women with diabetes, there is little information readily available to them.

This chapter remedies this lack and contains information about the menstrual cycle, contraception and sexuality relevant to women with diabetes.

AT A GLANCE

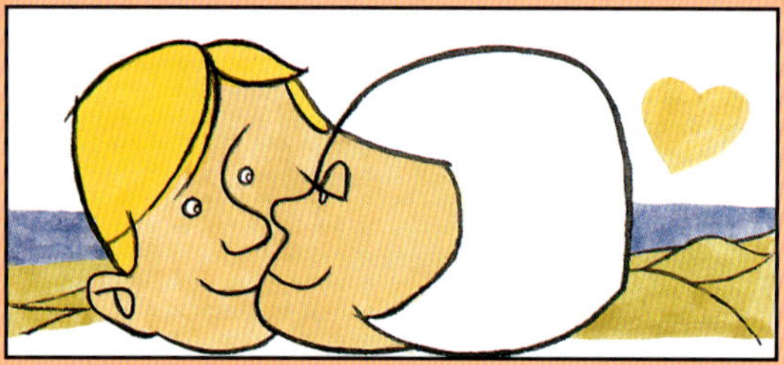

- **There is no evidence to suggest that women with diabetes encounter more sexual difficulties than other women.**
- **Women with diabetes often report a cyclical change in their insulin requirements related to the menstrual cycle.**
- **High blood glucose levels can have a temporarily adverse effect on the sexual aspects of a woman's life.**
- **Diabetes increases the risk of thrush.**
- **Simple and effective treatments exist for most problems encountered.**

The menstrual cycle

The onset of the menstrual cycle in young girls with type 1 diabetes occurs about a year later than in girls who don't have diabetes.

If diabetes is poorly controlled, periods are irregular. During times of very poor blood glucose control, periods temporarily cease.

Women with diabetes often report a cyclical change in their insulin requirements which is related to the menstrual cycle. We don't fully understand this phenomenon but, most commonly before a period, the blood glucose level increases, requiring additional insulin to control the glucose levels.

Once menstruation starts, the need for extra insulin tends to fall. The changes may be directly related to hormonal effects, but probably changes in eating patterns are also involved.

You may have to change your insulin doses for a few days each month to overcome fluctuations. However, there are variations in these patterns and not all women report a major change.

Contraception

Diabetes does not reduce fertility.

To plan a pregnancy and achieve excellent blood glucose control before conception (see page 68 – Diabetes and Pregnancy), women with diabetes must be confident about the effectiveness of their contraception.

While once there was concern about the impact of the contraceptive pill in diabetes, recent research suggests that modern low-dose contraceptive pills have little effect on metabolism in women with diabetes. However, if blood glucose levels change, you will need to adjust your insulin dosage.

As with all oral contraceptives, there is increased risk of vein thrombosis. If you are predisposed to thrombosis, this may rule you out as a contender for the pill. Smoking is an additional hazard for thrombosis. If you have diabetes and are about to start taking the pill, stop smoking.

Blood pressure and blood lipid levels need to be monitored before and during contraceptive therapy, but usually are not affected.

The intra-uterine contraceptive device (IUD) used to be thought less effective in women with diabetes. We know now that it is equally efficient in all women and therefore valid for consideration among all your contraception options.

Barrier contraceptives such as the diaphragm or condom have no side-effects, but may be less reliable than the contraceptive pill in preventing pregnancy.

Sterilisation (of either partner) is an effective means of contraception for older women who have completed their families. It is also a method with no metabolic or blood vessel side-effects.

It is important that each woman with diabetes talks frankly with her doctor about contraceptive options in relation to her medical condition.

You may also need to change the means of contraception as your life situation alters.

Sexuality

While there is much information about the effects of diabetes on various parts of the body, there is still only limited discussion about the impact of diabetes on women's health, particularly in the area of sexuality.

For example, not all women with diabetes know that diabetes increases the risk of infection with monilia (thrush). Monilia is a common yeast (fungus) always present in the body. In women it can cause a vaginal infection with intense itching and a whitish discharge.

This happens more commonly when the blood glucose level is high, or when a course of antibiotics has changed the normal body flora (bacteria), allowing the monilia to flourish. Recurrent monilial infection can cause painful intercourse, creating one form of diabetes-related sexual problem in women.

When there are typical symptoms, the doctor takes a vaginal smear to confirm the diagnosis. Pessaries or creams provide effective treatment. Take the full course of treatment and be careful to reduce the risk of reinfection by maintaining good glycaemic control and keeping the area dry and cool (monilia grows best in moisture and warmth). When infection is recurrent, it may be necessary to treat the woman's partner as well.

The effect of diabetes on women's sexuality is not an easy topic for accurate research. People are often shy about discussing intimate matters and there aren't the simple tests of sexual function in women as there are in men. However, the evidence indicates that there are no reasons why women with diabetes should have more sexual difficulties than other women.

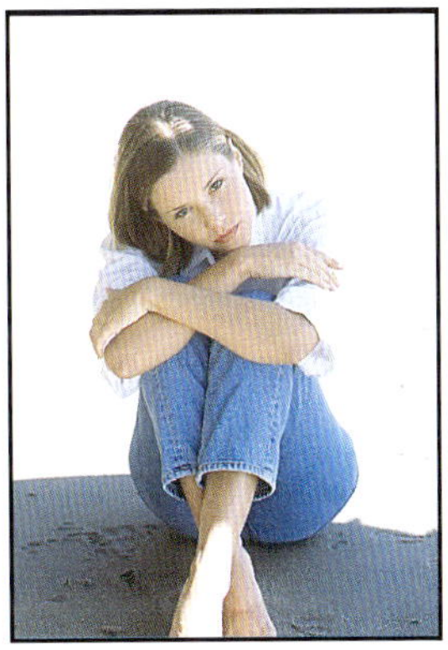

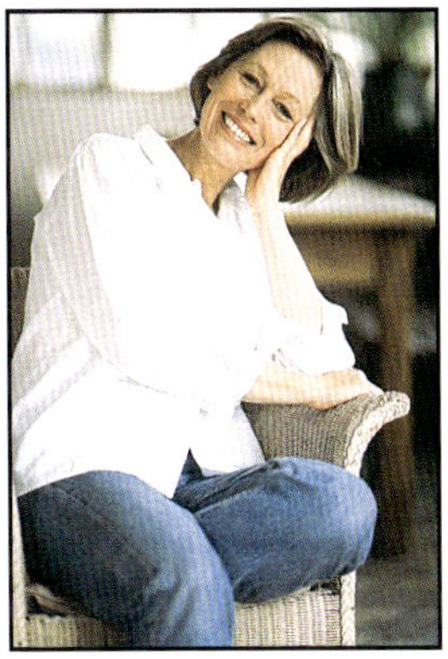

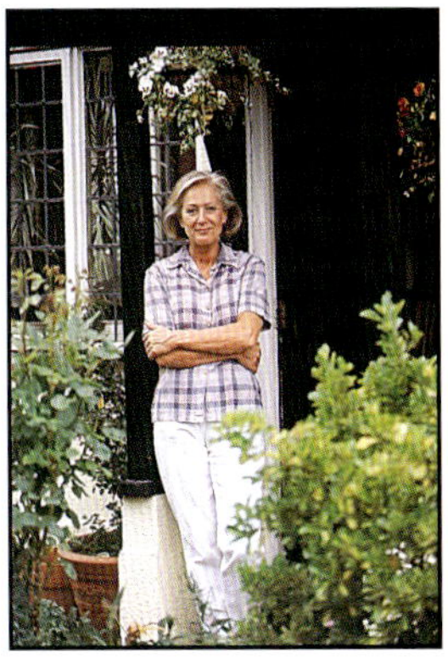

Regardless of whether a woman has diabetes, there are several physical and emotional factors which contribute to a satisfactory sexual life.

Any woman can have difficulties in any step along the sequence of sexual desire, sexual arousal and orgasm. Emotional factors (like depression and marital conflict) and physical factors (like menopause or chronic illness) can all cause some type of sexual dysfunction.

On the emotional side, some studies suggest that late onset diabetes may have a detrimental effect on the marital relationship, including sexual desire and satisfaction. When a woman is diagnosed with type 2 diabetes she may be at a vulnerable time in her life. She may feel less attractive, less healthy and, subsequently, be less sexually responsive.

On the other hand, in couples where diabetes was present before the relationship, the partnership may be stronger because the man has always accepted the implications of his partner's diabetes.

Among the physical effects of diabetes, high blood glucose levels can have a temporarily adverse effect on the sexual aspects of a woman's life. She may feel tired, less interested in sexual activity and less able to enjoy it. These symptoms will respond to a sustained improvement in blood glucose levels, so assess the effect of improved blood glucose control if you have any of these symptoms.

Some men with diabetes who have secondary damage to the nerves or circulation develop impotence, but there is no corresponding sexual difficulty in women with similar complications. There may be some lessening of vaginal lubrication, but that problem is easily treated with a lubricant.

Menopause can also lead to problems such as vaginal dryness or discomfort during intercourse.

Treatment considered a part of normal menopause management may be needed for these problems, otherwise these symptoms may be mistakenly attributed to the diabetes and ignored.

It is uncommon for women – with or without diabetes – to report problems with arousal or achieving orgasm. When they do, often there are several factors responsible including stress, fatigue, ill health, depression or relationship difficulties. It is important for women to be able to discuss these issues and seek help.

If you are worried about some aspect of your sexual relationship, help is available. Ask your doctor or diabetes specialist for advice or a referral to a suitable counsellor for expert confidential treatment.

A happy sex life is one of the most pleasant aspects of a successful relationship and, generally, women with diabetes enjoy a healthy and satisfying sex life.

Diabetes and Pregnancy

◆ By Dr Alison Nankervis and Dr Ian Martin ◆
Revised by Dr Alison Nankervis

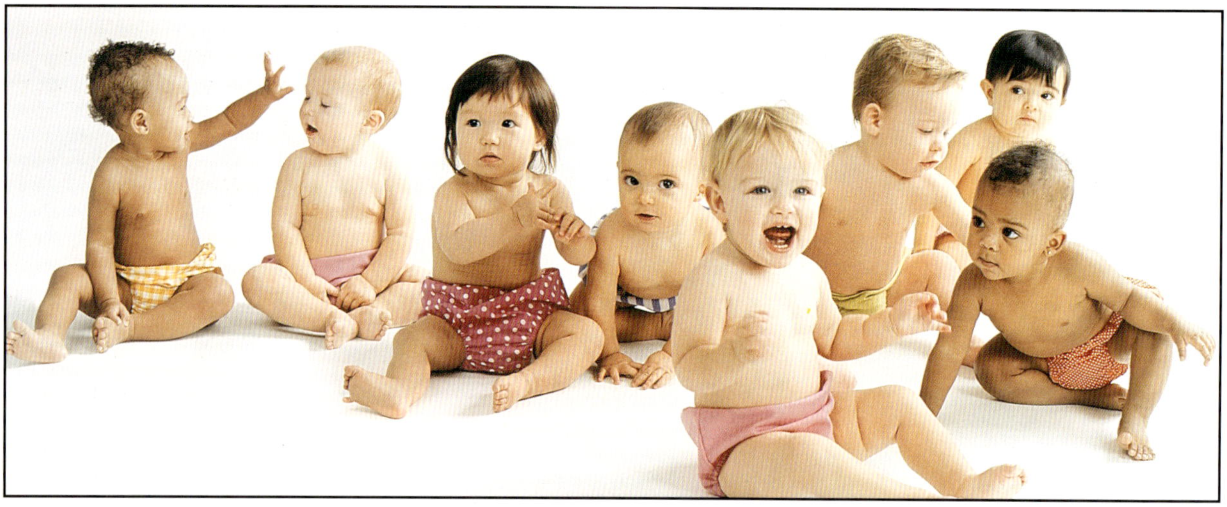

DIABETES in pregnancy and pregnancy in women with diabetes usually result in a normal delivery with no effects on the mother's long-term health.

Thanks to recent advances in the treatment of diabetes, the baby's outlook is also excellent. However, successful outcomes depend on close cooperation between the woman and the medical team caring for her before and during pregnancy.

Metabolic changes during pregnancy

To understand the care required, you need to know the metabolic changes women with diabetes go through during pregnancy.

Sometimes, early in pregnancy, the woman's body becomes more efficient in using glucose so insulin requirements drop slightly. At this time hypoglycaemia can be a problem.

By about the fifth or sixth month, the placenta – the baby's source of nutrition – has increased in size and begins to contribute significantly to the production of hormones which antagonise the effect of insulin. This produces a temporary state of insulin resistance in the second half of pregnancy.

These changes can also cause a deterioration in glucose tolerance in women who are susceptible to diabetes but have not previously had the condition. In these cases a temporary state of diabetes – gestational diabetes – develops, most commonly after the 24th week of pregnancy.

After the baby is born and the placenta delivered, these changes rapidly reverse. In women with type 1 diabetes, the insulin dose falls dramatically. In women with gestational diabetes, the temporary diabetes usually ends.

Pregnancy in women with pre-existing diabetes

Among women with diabetes who become pregnant, the majority will have type 1 diabetes, although some aged 30 plus will have type 2 diabetes.

AT A GLANCE

- **Women with diabetes have healthy pregnancies and healthy babies.**
- **Although there are potential problems, they can generally be averted by taking a disciplined and sensible approach to pregnancy, supported by an experienced medical team.**
- **Pregnancy for a woman with diabetes is usually an enjoyable and rewarding experience.**
- **Seek advice from a dietitian to ensure food intake is adequate for you and the baby.**
- **Excellent diabetes control at the time of conception and during the first eight weeks of pregnancy minimises the risk of birth defects and miscarriage.**
- **Your baby should be monitored carefully in the last four to six weeks before delivery.**
- **Insulin requirements change throughout the pregnancy.**

For these women the best medical care comes from a team experienced in managing diabetes in pregnancy. The most likely team members are an obstetrician, diabetes physician, diabetes nurse educator, dietitian, neonatal paediatrician and ophthalmologist.

It is not always possible to be treated by the entire team, but any pregnant woman with known diabetes requires specialist care and advice.

Pre-pregnancy care

Women with type 1 diabetes have a slightly increased risk of having a baby with a birth defect. Excellent control at the time of conception and during the first eight weeks of pregnancy minimises this risk.

It is therefore extremely important to plan the pregnancy and achieve the best possible blood glucose control before becoming pregnant.

A number of other considerations are important when planning a pregnancy:

- Supplementation with 5 mg folate daily (available over the counter from chemists and health stores) reduces the risk of abnormalities of the spinal cord. Commence folate before conception and continue for at least the first three months of pregnancy.
- Limit the amount of alcohol consumed.
- Do not smoke.

Women with type 2 diabetes who are planning a pregnancy ideally should cease taking tablets and achieve excellent diabetes control on insulin before conception.

Although there is little evidence to suggest that oral hypoglycaemic tablets are harmful to the developing foetus, insulin is used routinely instead of tablets in the treatment of pregnant women with pre-existing type 2 diabetes.

Diabetes management during pregnancy

Throughout the pregnancy the aim is to achieve excellent control of diabetes. There is no absolute rule as to the type of insulin treatment best suited to pregnancy, but it is common practice to start a multiple dose schedule before conception or as soon as you know you are pregnant.

Some women achieve excellent control on twice-daily insulin and do not need to change their management program.

Hypoglycaemia can be a problem in the first three months of pregnancy when nausea may limit carbohydrate intake and there is a tendency to increased insulin sensitivity.

Hypoglycaemia symptoms may also alter at this time and it is important to recognise any change in the ability to recognise low blood glucose. Fortunately, low blood glucose levels do not appear to affect the baby, but severe hypoglycaemia should be avoided.

Later in pregnancy, insulin requirements generally rise, with some women needing as much as twice their usual dose. In the last four to six weeks of pregnancy, insulin requirements may drop slightly.

Careful attention to nutrition is essential, not only for good diabetes control, but to meet the body's increased nutritional requirements during pregnancy.

Exercise is also helpful in maintaining general fitness and good blood glucose control. However, avoid contact sports and overly vigorous exercise, which can raise the body temperature and possibly harm the foetus.

To maintain the best possible diabetes control, meticulously monitor blood glucose levels. Test blood glucose at least four times daily plus occasionally overnight.

Blood glucose levels before breakfast should be less than 5.5 mmol/L and between meals you should ideally achieve levels between 3.5 and 8.0 mmol/L.

The glycated haemoglobin or haemoglobin A1c estimates average blood glucose levels during the preceding six weeks and is very useful to assess overall diabetes control. The HbA1c should be measured on several occasions during the pregnancy and ideally maintained within the normal range.

Urine tests in pregnancy are an inaccurate measure of blood glucose levels so are of little value except to monitor the presence of ketones.

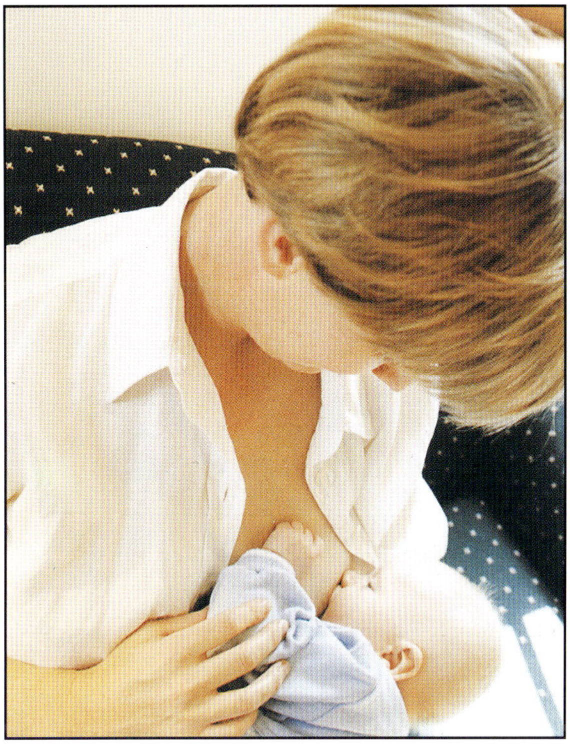

COURTESY NURSING MOTHERS' ASSOCIATION OF AUSTRALIA

Diabetes complications during pregnancy

As well as checks of weight and blood pressure, women with diabetes require regular eye and kidney tests.

Diabetic retinopathy generally does not present a problem during pregnancy. If the pregnancy is planned, the eyes should be checked beforehand and, if treatment is required, have it done before conception.

In most cases there is no significant deterioration in retinopathy during pregnancy but have your eyes examined at least every three months.

Occasionally eye problems develop or worsen during a pregnancy and, if this happens, laser treatment can be carried out during the pregnancy without any ill effects to the baby.

Kidney disease, known as diabetic nephropathy, is of more concern and requires individual assessment. If there is severe kidney disease, the chances of a successful pregnancy are slight. For most women, whether with or without mild nephropathy, pregnancy outcomes are usually excellent.

However, development of pre-eclampsia – a combination of high blood pressure, accumulation of fluid, swelling of the legs and increasing protein in the urine – can be a problem. It occurs particularly in women who have pre-existing high blood pressure or kidney disease but can occur in any woman during pregnancy.

The development of significant pre-eclampsia may require earlier hospitalisation and delivery than otherwise planned.

Urine infections are another potential problem in pregnancy so report any symptoms or unexplained fevers early.

Diabetic nerve problems rarely present problems during pregnancy. Carpal tunnel syndrome – when pressure on one of the nerves at the wrist causes pain, numbness and tingling in the fingers and hand – is common but usually resolves after pregnancy.

Common concerns about the baby

All women are naturally concerned that their baby will be healthy and normal. Often this anxiety is greater in women with diabetes and, in the past, women with diabetes had poorer pregnancy outcomes.

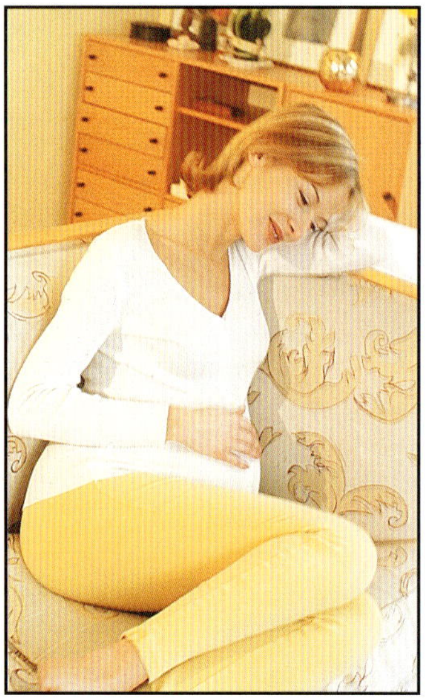

Although it is true that women with diabetes still have a higher than normal risk of birth defects and miscarriages, they minimise this risk by maintaining good control during the early weeks of pregnancy.

Diabetes increases the chance of having a large (macrosomic) baby. Maintaining excellent glycaemic control in the second half of pregnancy is the most effective strategy for preventing macrosomia.

To give a clear idea of the expected delivery date, an ultrasound examination of the baby is usually organised early in the pregnancy.

A second ultrasound is done at 18–20 weeks to check the baby carefully for any abnormalities – particularly of the heart, nervous system and kidneys.

A further ultrasound is usually performed at seven or eight months to estimate the baby's physical growth and development.

Towards the end of pregnancy the baby's health is carefully monitored. The heartbeat is measured by a cardiotogragh (called a CTG, or non-stress test) and if there are any questions about the baby's wellbeing, further ultrasound examinations will be conducted.

After the birth, particularly if the baby is premature, it will be closely monitored in a special nursery for signs of hypoglycaemia, breathing difficulties and jaundice. If these occur they are treated by special staff. Supplemental feeds or intravenous glucose might be required for hypoglycaemia and premature babies sometimes require oxygen until their lungs function normally.

Women are frequently concerned that their babies will have diabetes but there is little chance of this occurring in early life (see chapter 33 – The Genetics of Diabetes).

Obstetric management

Women with diabetes rarely need admission to hospital before delivery time. However, if there is an acute infection or other illness such as pre-eclampsia or major problems with diabetes control, an admission for treatment or stabilisation may be necessary.

Unexpected illness can cause loss of control, dehydration and ketosis more quickly in pregnancy, so contact your physician immediately if you are ill.

For many years it was usual to deliver the woman with type 1 diabetes at 37–38 weeks gestation – about two weeks before term. This was because of an increased risk of stillbirth among babies born to mothers with diabetes.

Better monitoring practices mean that pregnancies often proceed further, sometimes to full term. Continuing careful assessment of mother's and baby's health determines each individual delivery plan. If there is any question about the wellbeing of the baby, the doctor will organise earlier delivery.

Often the woman with diabetes does not go into spontaneous labour. She is usually admitted to hospital on the evening before the planned day of delivery.

The woman is admitted to hospital on the evening before the planned day of delivery and given a dose of Prostin™, a substance which is inserted into the vagina and assists the onset of labour.

If labour hasn't commenced by next morning, the membranes are ruptured, often with the addition of intravenous syntocinon to accelerate labour. Unless there is a problem with the baby or a particular obstetric problem, expect a normal vaginal delivery. A caesarean section is performed if there are obstetric problems, if the baby's health is at risk or labour doesn't proceed normally.

Managing diabetes for either caesarean section or vaginal delivery is not a problem, and is adapted as required. Insulin can be given as frequent small injections or as an intravenous infusion, with or without intravenous glucose to maintain carbohydrate intake.

Have the baby delivered in a hospital where there are full facilities for the care of mother and baby. Following delivery of baby and placenta, insulin requirements fall dramatically for two or three days. The diabetes then gradually readjusts, with insulin requirements returning to near the level before pregnancy.

This stabilisation of diabetes and readjustment of insulin dose is a dynamic process which can last two to three weeks.

Breast-feeding

There is no reason why women with diabetes should not breast-feed. Insulin requirements are generally slightly lower in the breast-feeding mother so take particular care to avoid hypoglycaemia. Insulin does not pass into the breast milk and is not harmful to the baby.

However, oral hypoglycaemic tablets are passed into breast milk, and women on tablets before pregnancy should continue on insulin treatment while breast-feeding.

Gestational diabetes

Among every 100 pregnant women, three to five develop diabetes in pregnancy. Some racial groups such as Indians, Vietnamese, Aborigines and Torres Strait Islanders and Pacific Islanders have a much higher incidence of gestational diabetes.

Gestational diabetes usually develops in the second half of pregnancy and improves after delivery. It is more common in women aged 30 or more who are overweight and have a family history of type 2 diabetes.

Some women are found to have previously unrecognised diabetes when undergoing routine tests in early pregnancy.

The Australian Diabetes Society recommends that all pregnant women are tested for gestational diabetes. The best time is between the 26th and 28th weeks of pregnancy with a blood test for glucose followed by a very sweet glucose drink ahead of further blood glucose tests one and two hours later.

The treatment of gestational diabetes depends on the severity of the diabetes. In many women it is easily controlled and treatment is simply by modifying eating. An appropriate meal plan ensures that energy and nutrition are adequate for mother and baby, although mothers will need low glycaemic index (slowly absorbed) carbohydrate foods, eaten in small quantities, at regular intervals throughout the day.

Management is aimed at careful control of weight gain plus maintenance of normal blood glucose levels.

Most women with gestational diabetes monitor their own blood glucose using either direct reading strips or borrowed blood glucose meters. These help ensure that blood glucose levels are constantly controlled.

If blood glucose levels cannot be controlled by food, insulin treatment will be necessary for the duration of the pregnancy. Usually this starts on an outpatient basis, under instructions from the medical team. Generally, women use a pen injector two to four times daily. Their haemoglobin A1c will be monitored for the remainder of the pregnancy, along with weight, blood pressure and kidney function.

The most common outcome with gestational diabetes is macrosomia (a large baby). If this occurs, greater care is necessary in monitoring the baby and during delivery.

If there are no obstetric problems or concerns for the baby, the pregnancy continues until term and the baby is delivered normally. After delivery, the baby is checked for low blood glucose levels.

Unless the blood glucose levels remain clearly elevated, gestational diabetes usually disappears after delivery, occasionally it persists and requires ongoing treatment. In those women whose diabetes resolves, a follow-up glucose tolerance test is carried out six to eight weeks after delivery. Even if this proves normal, these women have a much higher than normal chance of developing diabetes later in life. Sensible eating, maintenance of normal weight and regular exercise minimise the chances of developing diabetes.

If you have had gestational diabetes, tell your general practitioner and, ideally, have a blood glucose test each year, especially after the age of 40. If you are planning another baby, have a check for diabetes before stopping contraception.

Women with a history of gestational diabetes have a greatly increased chance of developing it again during future pregnancies. Have checks early in the pregnancy.

Diabetes, Menopause and Hormone Replacement Therapy (HRT)

◆ By Dr Mary Parkin ◆

AT A GLANCE

- **Menopause is a normal transition in every woman's life and some women experience no problems or symptoms during this average five-year phase.**
- **Women with diabetes who are approaching menopause and experiencing symptoms are advised to discuss the place of HRT with their doctors and health care professionals.**
- **HRT may be beneficial in reducing the risk of heart disease and osteoporosis.**
- **HRT has side-effects which may be worse than the symptoms of menopause.**
- **It's not yet known whether HRT is as effective in women with diabetes as it is in women without diabetes.**
- **Expect your doctor to monitor your lipid profiles and blood glucose levels before and after you begin HRT.**
- **Menopause management differs with every woman.**
- **Each woman's particular wishes plus family medical history will be taken into account before menopause treatment decisions – if any – are made.**
- **You are entitled to a thorough explanation of the relative risks and benefits of all menopause treatments so that you can make an informed decision.**

EVERY woman will eventually reach the time of change called menopause. Menopause generally occurs between age 45 to 55, although some women experience it before they turn 40.

It is the time when monthly periods cease and with them, a woman's ability to have children.

Among the hormonal changes that accompany menopause is a decreased level of oestrogen.

Lack of oestrogen at menopause may produce various symptoms that can last up to five years, although some women experience no symptoms or problems.

These days women live longer. In Australia their average life expectancy is the early eighties and in the future we will live even longer.

Studies in France predict that more than 50 per cent of female babies born in 1995 will live more than 100 years. This is a vastly increased lifespan compared with 40 years earlier when only 17 per cent of females reached 100.

Because women are living longer, they are at increased risk of developing age-related illnesses plus the longer term problems of oestrogen deficiency – namely osteoporosis (weak bones) – heart disease and dementia.

Complications of menopause

Short term

The most common symptoms of oestrogen deficiency are hot flushes and drenching night sweats. These can disturb sleep, causing tiredness.

Other possible problems are vaginal dryness, causing discomfort during intercourse, diminished sex drive, and urinary frequency, sometimes accompanied by a sense of urgency or loss of control.

Women at this time may also complain of headaches, generalised aches and pains, poor concentration, short-term memory lapses and mood changes. Some describe anxiety and panic attacks or feelings of loss of control and depression.

These symptoms can develop several years before the periods stop. This is the transition stage leading to menopause which is called the peri-menopause.

Whether or not a woman has symptoms – plus how well she copes with them – appears to be influenced by her culture (nationality and traditions), her socio-economic status and individual expectations. These factors also determine whether she'll seek hormone replacement therapy (HRT) or alternative therapies.

Long term

1. Osteoporosis

Osteoporosis means a thinning and weakening of the bones, making them more fragile and susceptible to fractures and breaks. A family history of osteoporosis (such as fractured hips and wrists in elderly relatives) and early onset menopause increase a woman's risk of developing osteoporosis.

Other factors also increase the risk of osteoporosis. These include:

- smoking
- excessive alcohol intake (in women, this is defined as drinking more than two standard drinks a day)
- taking certain medications such as steroids
- excessive thyroxine therapy
- medical conditions including type 1 diabetes, chronic liver and kidney disease, malabsorption of vitamin D, rheumatoid arthritis, hyperthyroidism and hyperparathyroidism.

One in three post-menopausal women develops osteoporosis and half of these will break a bone, most commonly the hip, wrist or back. Common back problems include compression fractures, which lead to pain, deformity (dowager's hump) and a loss of height.

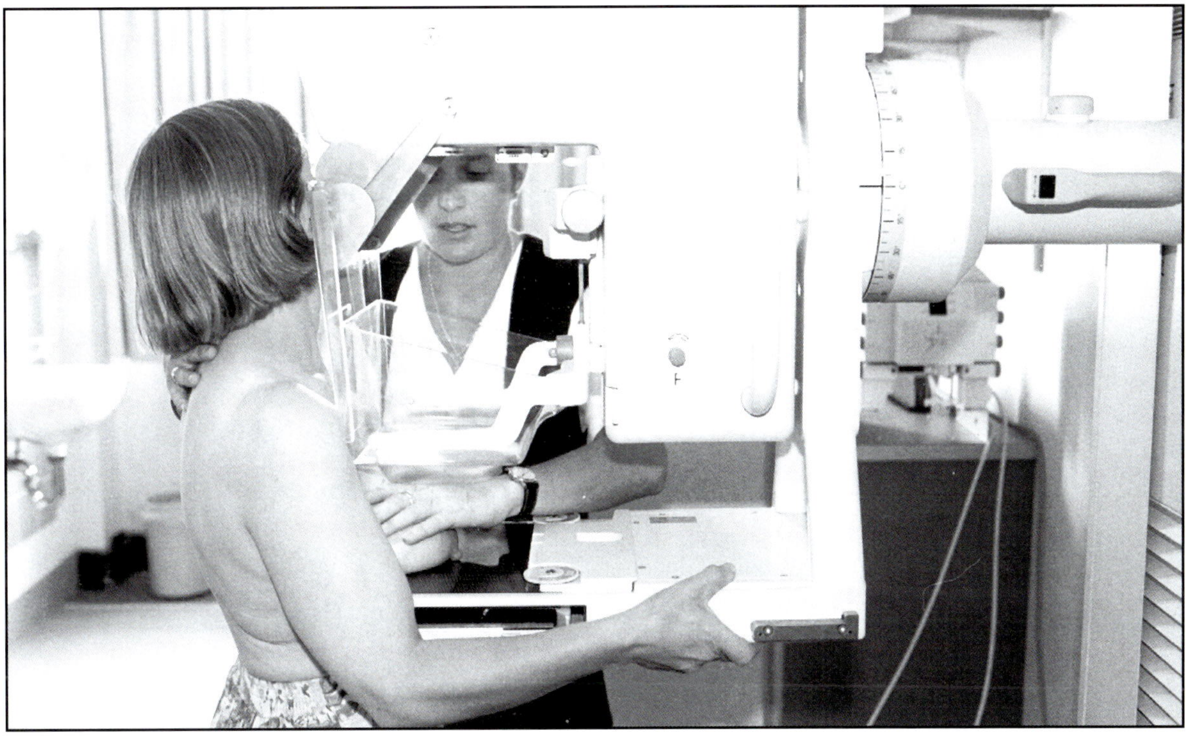

COURTESY NATIONAL BREAST CANCER CENTRE

Bone loss starts during the peri-menopausal phase. Starting HRT at this time will prevent the rapid bone loss common during the first 5 to 10 years after menopause.

Oestrogen helps limit the breakdown of bones. It does not stimulate the formation of new bone. However, once you stop taking the hormones, their protective benefits stop and bone loss continues.

If you haven't done so already, it is important to review your lifestyle at this time of your life.

- Try and stop smoking.
- Moderate your alcohol and caffeine intake.
- Ensure an adequate daily intake of calcium (1000 – 1500 mg of elemental calcium each day).
- Initiate a regular weight bearing exercise program.

2. Cardiovascular disease

Heart disease accounts for more than half the deaths in women, with 50 per cent of these due to coronary artery disease. The likelihood of heart disease increases significantly after menopause and reaches a peak at 75 years old.

Some studies suggest HRT reduces the severity of heart disease.

Oestrogens are believed to have a protective effect on the heart and this is the likely explanation for the very low incidence of heart disease in pre-menopausal women when compared with men of the same age.

Uncontrolled diabetes increases the risk of heart disease in women.

At menopause, women often note changes in their body weight, particularly around the tummy. This apple shape is associated with medical conditions including hypertension, diabetes, dyslipidaemia (frequently high triglyceride levels) and heart disease.

Oestrogens have other beneficial actions on blood vessel walls which increase blood flow. Oestrogens also affect clotting factors and coagulation.

3. Dementia and stroke

Recent studies suggest that oestrogens help prevent dementia and possibly stroke.

More than 40 per cent of women over 80 will develop dementia and the incidence of dementia doubles every four to five years after age 65.

Short-term preliminary studies demonstrate improved mental ability in oestrogen users. However, progestins may reverse some of the benefits seen. (Women with an intact uterus require the addition of a progestin to protect the lining of the womb (endometrium) from developing potentially pre-cancerous changes).

Diabetes

Diabetes leads to reduced life expectancy. This is because people with diabetes develop atherosclerosis or hardening of the arteries at an earlier age than the rest of the population and it progresses more rapidly.

This condition can lead to premature development of heart disease (angina and myocardial infarction) at rates up to six times higher than in people without diabetes.

Strokes, transient ischaemic attacks and peripheral vascular disease – leading to foot ulcers, gangrene and the need for amputation – also occur more frequently.

People with diabetes are also more likely to have other risk factors for cardiovascular disease including high blood pressure, increased abdominal fat, high insulin levels (leading to resistance to insulin and changes in glucose tolerance) and alterations in the chemistry of their blood fat (lipid profile).

Hypertension (high blood pressure) is seen more commonly in post-menopausal women with diabetes than in people without diabetes. However, studies using HRT in hypertensive post-menopausal women did not show increased blood pressure and this was the case regardless of whether the oestrogen was administered by patch or tablet.

For women who had high blood pressure before their periods stopped, HRT is considered safe provided their doctor regularly monitors their progress.

Metabolic effects of diabetes

Diabetes is associated with an abnormal lipid profile. The most common abnormality is an increase in triglyceride levels. LDL (bad) cholesterol levels are increased and HDL (good) cholesterol levels reduced, particularly in those with type 2 diabetes.

Menopause is an additional magnifier of lipid changes in women with diabetes.

Oestrogen tablets may increase the risk of acute pancreatitis because they can increase triglyceride levels. Transdermal oestrogen patches are preferred.

Because of HRT's effects on an individual's lipid profiles, it is vital the doctor checks lipid levels before women with diabetes start HRT. These levels must be continuously monitored.

Alterations in carbohydrate metabolism

HRT may affect metabolic control in women with diabetes. The little information available suggests that changes, if any, are likely to be small.

Any worsening of control may be linked to weight gain but you can't blame this on HRT because women not using hormone therapy also report weight gain.

The effects of HRT on carbohydrate metabolism depend on the type of oestrogen and whether progestins are also used. Transdermal (patch) oestrogens are preferred, but studies show no deterioration in glucose tolerance or change in insulin sensitivity in women taking oestrogen tablets. Progestins appear to have minimal effect.

In women with type 1 or type 2 diabetes on insulin, there is either no change or a slight decrease in insulin requirements.

Menopause management

HRT is a safe and effective treatment of acute oestrogen deficiency symptoms. The risks and benefits of short-term treatment with HRT differ little between women, whether or not they have diabetes.

There are possible side-effects, most commonly breast tenderness, bloating, weight gain, fluid retention and mood change. These symptoms may settle with time but, if they continue, consult your doctor as modifications in dose or changes in the type of oestrogen may help.

Peri-menopausal women or women within two years of menopause will be prescribed cyclical progestins which are taken for 12 to14 days a month.

A withdrawal bleed usually occurs several days after stopping the progestin, although in about a third or more of women the bleeding stops after a few years.

Women whose periods have stopped for more than two years are generally prescribed a combination of continuous oestrogen and progestin (for example, Kliogest™, Menoprem 28™ or Provelle 28™), with which the risk of bleeding is small.

HRT and breast cancer

There is concern about the link between HRT and breast cancer. However, all women have a one in 12 – 14 lifetime risk of developing breast cancer unless their mother and a first degree relative had pre-menopausal breast cancer, in which case the risk is significantly increased.

Short-term HRT (that is, less than five years use) does not increase the incidence of breast cancer when compared in studies to non-users. And five years after stopping HRT there is still no significant increase in risk compared to non-users.

Studies examining longer use of HRT are inconclusive. However, there is a view that continuous use of HRT for more than five to eight years may be associated with a small increase in the risk of breast cancer.

It is important that every woman on HRT undertakes regular self-breast examination plus mammography. If you note any changes, see a doctor immediately for advice.

Natural therapies

Although conventional menopause management centres on the use of HRT, other alternatives are available.

It is important that women eat healthily, exercise regularly and moderate their alcohol and caffeine intake. Smokers should be encouraged to stop.

Natural therapies are increasingly popular, with evening primrose oil, vitamin B6 and remifemin among the most commonly used menopause treatments.

Phytoestrogens are biologically active compounds in plants that produce oestrogenic effects (although anti-oestrogenic effects have also been reported). They are commonly found in cereals, legumes and grasses. The best known phytoestrogens are found in soy beans, soy products and flaxseed (linseed).

Epidemiological studies suggest that in countries where consumption of phytoestrogens is high there is a lower reported incidence of menopausal symptoms and breast cancer.

Phytoestrogens may also provide cardiovascular protection by lowering cholesterol and other mechanisms.

For further reading contact the National Health and Medical Research Council and request their booklet for consumers on HRT.

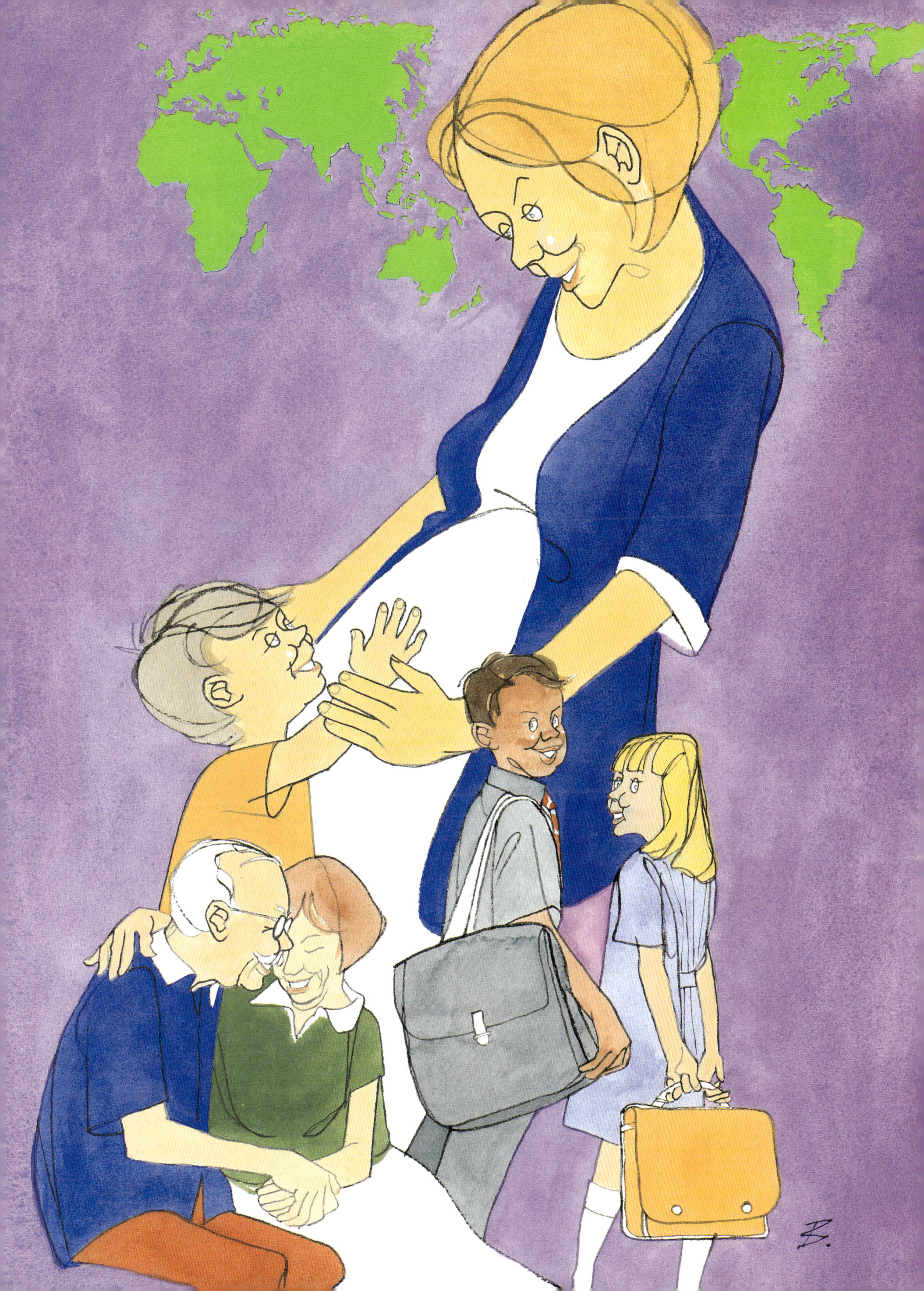

The School Child with Diabetes

◆ By Professor Martin Silink ◆

THE formative early years at school are difficult enough for a child under normal circumstances, let alone with the added burden of diabetes.

The quality of the school experience is important for all children. It helps them develop self-esteem and the ability to interrelate with others, while equipping them with knowledge and problem-solving abilities.

Never underestimate the role of the teacher and parent during these years.

This is not to say that the teacher should consider the child with diabetes as a problem child or poor learner. Diabetes does not decrease a child's ability to succeed academically. In some cases it has the opposite effect.

Expect the same standards of classroom behaviour from a child with diabetes as from any other child.

As with all children, those with diabetes need to be accepted by their peer group. They hate to be considered different. For this reason they should be encouraged to participate in all school activities, including sport.

Diabetes rarely causes significant absenteeism. School attendance is largely unaffected, apart from routine doctor visits every few months. Occasionally, unstable diabetes may lead to hospital admission or increased doctor visits for a while.

Schools are responsible for providing supervision and a safe environment for their students. Having a child with diabetes in class means added responsibility for the teacher.

All school staff should be aware that they have a student with diabetes in their classroom or playground. They should also have a basic understanding of the condition.

Parents can help by providing information about their child's needs. Many schools work with parents or guardians and the child's doctor to develop individual management plans for students who require extra supervision.

Because teachers do not receive specific training on how to cope with a diabetes emergency, many of the larger children's hospitals and Diabetes Australia can arrange for an expert to visit and explain how to do so to teachers and ancillary staff. Parents can also attend these lectures.

These sessions are to be encouraged because it is important that teachers are aware of the physical and psychological challenges facing children with diabetes.

While not treating the child differently from other children, teachers should recognise the warning signs of hypoglycaemia and know what steps to take in an emergency.

Just as they would for other medical conditions such as asthma, teachers should request that the school prominently displays an emergency chart outlining procedures in the staff room and that staff manuals contain policy and procedures to deal with the special needs of students with diabetes.

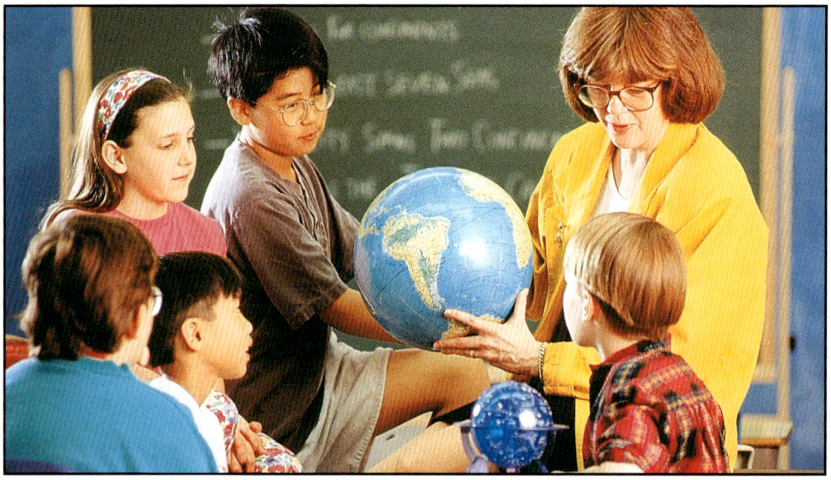

AT A GLANCE

- **Alert all school staff that they have a child with diabetes in their care and offer appropriate information on diabetes management and how to deal with hypoglycaemia.**
- **Having a child with diabetes in class means added responsibility for the teacher(s).**
- **Expect the same standards of classroom behaviour from a child with diabetes as from any other child.**
- **Provide information to the school about the child's diabetes management needs.**
- **Offer school staff expert information on diabetes from professional organisations such as Diabetes Australia.**
- **Encourage communication between teachers, parents and the child with diabetes.**
- **There is a fine line between protecting the child and stifling natural potential.**
- **The child does require certain special treatment but, at the same time, must not feel different from friends and classmates.**

Physical problems

Physically, there are four main areas in which special allowances must be made for children with diabetes.

- They may need to drink and urinate more often than other children. Excessive thirst and urination are often the first clues to the diagnosis of diabetes and may recur whenever the blood glucose level rises for more than a few hours.
- They may need to be allowed to eat – either food, sugar or even sweets – at times different from other students, even in class or at assembly. Check requirements with the parent or doctor. With younger children, meals may need to be quietly and unobtrusively supervised.
- Occasionally a child may need to measure their blood glucose levels or take additional doses of insulin at school. Staff can help by arranging some privacy for children to do these extra tasks.
- They may need to be checked for signs of hypoglycaemia or insulin reaction which, if untreated, may lead to unconsciousness.

Hypoglycaemia – the warning signs

Most people with diabetes experience hypoglycaemia now and then and suffer no long-term ill effects. However, in children, the blood glucose level is generally more erratic than in adults. A child may have a different reaction on different occasions but, if there is an inexplicable change in colour, mood, attention or behaviour in a child with diabetes, suspect hypoglycaemia.

It is important that the teacher is aware that the child with hypoglycaemia is not responsible for his or her actions.

The symptoms to watch for are as follows:

- Headaches. There are no special features of these headaches but, because children rarely get headaches, do not dismiss the symptom lightly.
- Changes in mood. These may range from outbursts of anger or a tendency to cry to unreasonable irritability. If these mood changes are caused by hypoglycaemia, they are beyond the child's control.
- Lack of attention. A child with hypoglycaemia may appear well but seem to be daydreaming. The difference is that children with hypoglycaemia cannot easily be snapped out of their trance.
- Lack of energy; shakiness. These symptoms come on suddenly – in just 5 – 10 minutes.
- Nausea and stomach pains. The pains may be constant or cramping. The nausea will make the child unwilling to eat but sugar must be given.
- Sudden pallor, with or without perspiration. The perspiration is usually visible but fairly subtle, causing the skin to feel clammy. It affects the whole body, not just the face.
- Drowsiness, listlessness, lack of concentration, change of consciousness. This may progress to complete unconsciousness and even to fitting if allowed to go untreated.

After hypoglycaemia, brain function may not return to normal for several hours. The child may not do as well as expected in an examination.

Treatment of hypoglycaemia

The two most important facts about hypoglycaemia are:

- it is usually preventable
- it must be treated quickly.

At the first signs of any of the warning symptoms, the child must be given some form of sugar.

All children with diabetes should be allowed to carry food such as glucose tablets or jellybeans to treat hypoglycaemia. It is a good idea for parents to provide teachers with sweets for any emergencies.

Unlike adults who learn to recognise the warning signs and symptoms of hypoglycaemia and know the best action to take, young children do not. Besides, the symptoms can often come on very quickly, giving them little time to react.

In these cases it is up to the teacher to act quickly and, unless specifically told otherwise by the parent, to give the child something sweet such as two heaped teaspoons of sugar in a little water, half a glass of ordinary lemonade, or four large or seven small jellybeans. Follow with solid food such as a sandwich, biscuit or piece of fruit.

Expect the child to respond within 15 minutes and then be able to resume usual activities.

It is important that the child is left alone (but not unsupervised) during hypoglycaemia and afterwards until completely well. When the hypoglycaemia has passed, the child can rejoin the class with as little fuss as possible.

Inform the parents

The teacher can note for parents the time of the hypoglycaemia, its severity and the treatment given, especially if episodes occur at similar times or during similar activities such as sport. This helps determine if the insulin dose needs adjustment.

If after 15 minutes the child is still unwell, give another dose of sugar followed by solid food. Call the parents or a doctor if there is still no improvement.

Ensure that parents collect the child after a hypoglycaemia episode and never send the child home alone.

Treating severe hypoglycaemia

If the hypoglycaemia progresses rapidly, or if the early warning signs were not detected, the child may become drowsy, fall into a stupor or even have a convulsion.

If the child can swallow, encourage them to take sugar in an easily absorbed form, such as two to four heaped teaspoons of sugar in water or a glass of lemonade.

As soon as the child can eat, give some solid food such as biscuits or sandwiches. If the child cannot take food, give one teaspoon of sugar in water or half a glass of lemonade every half hour until they can eat properly.

Children who have had severe hypoglycaemia may not feel well and could have a bad headache, but they should be given sympathetic but firm encouragement to eat and drink.

Occasionally, the child may be so disoriented that the teacher will need help from an additional person.

If the child loses consciousness, is unable to swallow or simply will not take treatment:

1. Put the child on its side.
2. Clear the airway.
3. Call an ambulance and doctor.
4. Above all, keep calm.

Never give anything by mouth to an unconscious child as the food may be inhaled, causing choking.

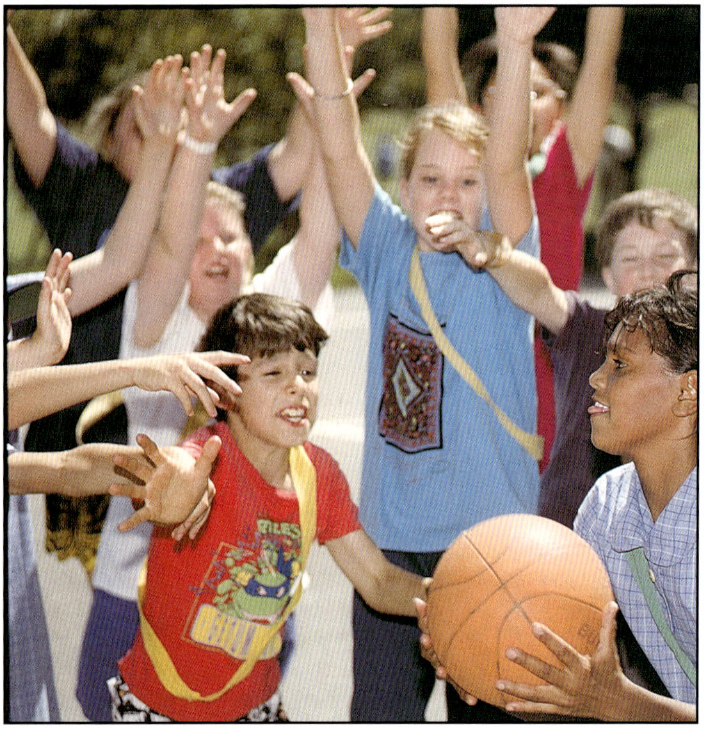

If you can't get a doctor quickly, it's better to call for an ambulance to take the child to the casualty section of the nearest hospital. When calling for an ambulance, it is important to state that there is a diabetic emergency. Some ambulance officers can give glucose or glucagon injections if necessary.

Glucagon is a hormone which makes the liver release stored glucose into the bloodstream. All parents of children with diabetes can learn to give these injections and can discuss the right dosage with the doctor (see chapter 12 – Hypoglycaemia and Hyperglycaemia).

Generally, for children under five, give half the contents of the ampoule (0.5 mg or unit). For others, use the whole ampoule.

Learning to give these injections is an easy skill and one of use to teachers if they take children with diabetes on overnight excursions or school camps.

The effect of the glucagon is temporary and as soon as the child is sufficiently recovered the usual treatment applies – a glass of ordinary lemonade or two heaped teaspoons of sugar in a glass of water, followed by solid food.

Preventing hypoglycaemia

The child with diabetes usually has two insulin injections a day, but many are on three or four daily injections. Once the insulin is injected it lowers blood glucose until the insulin wears off.

The glucose coming from food raises blood glucose. It is important that the child with diabetes eats meals at the same time each day and does not miss meals or snacks.

Because hypoglycaemia occurs most commonly just before meal times or at times of increased or unplanned activity, teachers should keep an unobtrusive eye on the child at these times. If there are any warning signs, give food immediately.

Teachers supervising sport or exercise should be aware of the possibility of hypoglycaemia if there is a child with diabetes in their care.

Exercise causes blood glucose to fall because muscles use more glucose when they are being used actively. Reactions will differ and some children may have hypoglycaemia during exercise, some immediately afterwards, and others not for hours later.

Give extra food before exercise and also during any prolonged activities.

The best type of food is a mixture of rapidly absorbed sugar and a more slowly absorbed form. An ideal mix is a drink of orange juice or sweet lemonade, an orange, or two or three lumps of sugar followed by starchy carbohydrates such as bread or plain sweet biscuits.

A sandwich made with honey or jam is okay, or an energy bar or whatever is advised by your health care team.

Keto-acidosis

Keto-acidosis is a more serious problem for the child with diabetes. It is associated with a high level of glucose in the blood and is a sign of serious inadequacy of insulin.

It usually occurs when the child is unwell with severe colds, influenza or other feverish illnesses when the body requires extra insulin.

Keto-acidosis may also be caused by insulin injections being missed or the dose being too low.

Far less common than hypoglycaemia, keto-acidosis comes on gradually over hours or days and is marked by excessive urination and thirst with subsequent vomiting. It requires prompt medical attention.

Food and diabetes

The young child with diabetes usually brings a specially prepared lunch to school, but as the child grows older and more knowledgeable, can select food from the school canteen.

There is nothing extraordinary about the food. Meals are simply well balanced and low in simple sugars.

However, food must be fairly constant in quality and timing. The teacher is usually asked to ensure that meals are neither skipped nor delayed. It is useful if the canteen stocks low-calorie soft drinks suitable for people with diabetes.

In general, extra food of any kind should only be given before exercise or to stop hypoglycaemia. This means that occasionally the child with diabetes will need to eat between classes or even during examinations.

Psychological problems

The child with diabetes has to contend with many pressures, from daily blood tests and injections to peer group pressure and uncertainty about the future, all of which may cause significant psychological problems.

In turn, this may make the diabetes less stable, adding to the pressure.

To help the school child overcome these problems provide:

- support
- acceptance
- encouragement.

Sports, exercise and excursions

Encourage the child to fully participate in school activities, whether sports, excursions or camps. People with diabetes excel in many fields, including sports.

However, it is important to make certain allowances and take special precautions. For instance, the child with diabetes may require extra time to prepare for sport. They have to eat and clean up afterwards or they may need a blood glucose test – factors to be taken into account by the teacher or sports supervisor.

All students with diabetes need more supervision during exercise and younger ones may also need to have meals supervised, especially before exercise. Keep food or sweets to treat hypoglycaemia where the sport is taking place, not some distance away.

Any sport in which hypoglycaemia would cause risk to either the student or anyone called upon to help can be considered only after careful planning and under strict supervision. Water sports are included in this category because of the dangers of drowning.

Planning is the key to trouble-free excursions. The timing of meals is important and parents or carers need to provide these details. Children with diabetes cannot rely on being able to buy food or snacks when needed and are advised to carry an adequate amount of food such as a sandwich, biscuits or dried fruit.

School camps and travel need additional planning by parents, children and school staff. Parents need adequate information about meal times, planned activities and travel arrangements.

Examinations

Students with diabetes perform best at examinations when their diabetes is under good control.

If the blood glucose level is high, the student will need to urinate more frequently so provide easy access to toilets.

Examinations may pose a special problem if pre-exam nerves stop the child from eating the normal amount of food, if stress and anxiety cause the blood glucose to rise, or if nervous tension burns up more than usual amounts of sugar.

Remember, a child with hypoglycaemia will not be able to think as well as usual. For important senior examinations many school boards make allowances, such as letting students with diabetes eat during exams or leave to go to the toilet.

If hypoglycaemia does occur, ideally give extra time to enable the student to perform to optimum ability. If a more severe episode occurs, especially in the more senior years, encourage the student to file a claim for special consideration due to misadventure.

Camps for children with diabetes

(Also see chapter 22 – Diabetes and Teenagers.)

These camps are a wonderful holiday for children as well as giving parents a break. Camps enhance self-esteem, are fun and promote confidence and independence. The children have a good influence on each other, which can lead to them undertaking responsibilities they previously refused such as self-injecting.

Regular diabetes camps are run in most States and Territories. Check with your local Diabetes Australia branch or the Juvenile Diabetes Foundation Australia.

Some schools and other organisations also conduct camps. In general, children should be able to attend camp when they are reliably independent in the care of their diabetes. This includes the ability to:

- measure insulin doses accurately
- inject reliably
- measure blood glucose levels accurately
- recognise and treat hypoglycaemia early
- understand dietary exchanges of carbohydrates
- understand why meals and snacks need to be on time
- understand the need for extra food before, during and after exercise.

In general, it is best if the child's friends are aware of the diabetes, however, it is essential for all members of staff to be aware. Parents or guardians will need to discuss with organisers well in advance the practical details concerning insulin supplies, storage and injections, testing and meals. If the camp is isolated, then thought should be given to emergency access for help.

With patience, empathy and communication, the school days of a child with diabetes can be just as rewarding and enlightening as for any other child.

Chapter 22

Diabetes and Teenagers

◆ By Gillian Harris and Tony Diment ◆

BEING a teenager is complex enough, but when diabetes is added to the existing mix of physical, emotional and career issues, the individual has specific needs to be considered.

Teenagers are not simply scaled down adults, although they may encounter similar social, cultural, economic and educational problems.

In writing this we were conscious that many older people regard teenagers as wild or uncontrolled. However, teenagers with diabetes do have particular needs and the following is an attempt to help them emerge from these formative years better prepared for a healthier future.

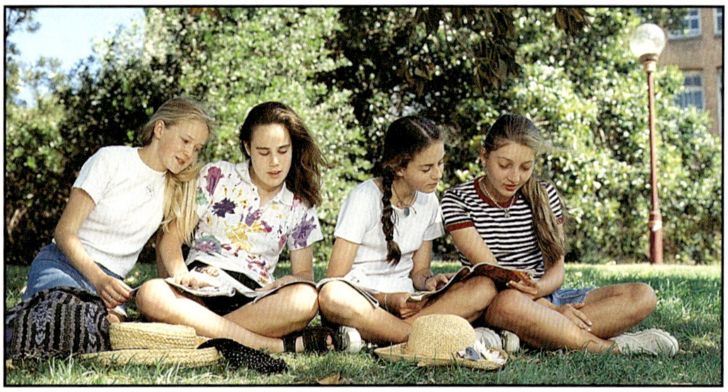

In the average Australian high school of 600–1000 students, there will probably be one or two teenagers with diabetes. These odds have the potential to make the young person feel particularly vulnerable at what is already a challenging time of life.

Because parents want their teenagers to be successful, to achieve and be healthy and happy; it is important that families adapt their lives to include diabetes along with all the hopes and ambitions they hold for the whole family.

AT A GLANCE

- **Teenagers with diabetes may have particular needs but dislike being singled out for special treatment.**
- **Having diabetes need not compromise adolescent life.**
- **Young people with diabetes are often mature beyond their peers.**
- **This is a time for laying the groundwork for a healthy and confident adult life.**
- **Parents and their teenagers benefit from regular contact and discussions with competent doctors and diabetes health professionals.**

Management issues

Adolescence is a period of rapid physical and emotional change. Young people are also less likely to follow a regular routine of physical activity – factors which can make it difficult to achieve diabetes control.

Stress and teenage doubts further complicate the picture.

Doctors and diabetes health care professionals experienced in helping young people can be consulted on a regular basis.

The recent Diabetes Control and Complications Trial means that more teenagers now use insulin three or four times a day. Young people adapt well to this schedule because it gives them more flexibility in their day-to-day life. However, treatment variations depend on the individual and what works well for one may not suit another.

Complications

Early screening for diabetes complications is widespread these days. Regardless of any slight differences in State or Territory practices and health department guidelines, it is an issue doctors will raise with parents.

Following initial diagnosis, there are various health monitoring procedures.

For example, the Australian Paediatric Endocrine Group recommends an annual screen for eye problems after two years of diabetes. Other tests assess kidney and nerve function.

Your health care team will arrange the various procedures after discussing them with you.

Nutrition aspects

Don't let the dinner table become a battleground. Because of young people's rapid changes in growth, their nutrition needs will change. Sensible advice on eating patterns – including parties and take-aways – will benefit everyone in the family.

Regular reviews with a dietitian can help allay concerns about body image and self-esteem, plus offer information on new research of special interest to young people such as sports nutrition and the GI factor (see page 11).

Diabetes health professionals

Further into their teens, young people will take increasing responsibility for their diabetes management. They will take over treatment decisions themselves. There is no set age for this transition and some parents may worry. Be patient and realise that doctors and other health professionals are there to help the young people.

When parents ask teenagers what the doctor, dietitian or diabetes nurse educator said, the usual reply is 'nothing much'. In fact, usually lots was discussed.

Generally, young people prefer to see the doctor by themselves, but it is important that parents understand what is happening. Work out a satisfactory system of communication between you, your teenager and the health professionals. Occasionally, it may be like a three-ring circus but remember, ultimately the ringmaster is the older teenager.

School and friends

(Also see chapter 21 – The School Child with Diabetes.)

Students sitting for senior examinations are advised to apply for the special consideration available. Apply in writing well ahead of the examination date and check your State or Territory's particular procedure with Diabetes Australia or the Juvenile Diabetes Foundation Australia.

During exams, blood glucose control can be erratic and insulin adjustment might be needed.

Teenagers usually find their close friends helpful if they need to treat hypoglycaemia. Encourage them to let their circle of friends know about diabetes and how they can help. Most young people worry about relationships – 'Am I too fat?', 'My pimples are a real turn-off' and diabetes can add to these fears.

As they become more confident, they realise that real friends don't care about their imperfections and diabetes has faded into the background. Nor do they like having to tell other people about diabetes so parents should seek their opinion on what to tell others, especially in front of them. (Also see tips about job interviews in chapter 30 – Diabetes and Discrimination.)

Family issues

Regardless of diabetes this is an interesting time for all concerned. The path towards an independent identity can be a bumpy ride. For teenagers it is a time of rapid change and experimentation. Young people question ideas as they learn spontaneously about the world and new technology; about sexuality and illicit drugs.

For parents or carers this is happening at a time in their lives when middle age is looming (or has arrived!). It is not surprising that there is communication breakdown. Outside help sometimes defuses the situation when diabetes management issues confound the picture.

Having diabetes is not the same as observing it, so the young person's viewpoint (generally focused on the present) is different from the parent's (often looking to the future).

Because of diabetes many teenagers possess maturity beyond that of their peers and accommodate diabetes in their educational, recreational and social lives. As their self-responsibility increases, parental anxiety fades.

Comments from teenagers about living with diabetes:

'Dad can't wait to tell the waiter I have diabetes – I feel like crawling under the table.'

'My brother thinks I'm spoilt because I get more attention.'

And from parents:

'It's a roller coaster ride through life.'

'I get tired thinking all the time about meals – where will I be when he has to eat?'

'I worry about the future consequences.'

'It has brought us even closer as a family in many ways.'

'Am I being too soft – or too strict?'

It helps if the young person with diabetes (and parents) have a good working knowledge of diabetes management. New ideas, facts and technology appear all the time, so it's a good idea to keep up to date.

Educational resources

Support groups: Many hospitals and diabetes centres run support groups for teenagers and/or parents. The groups enable people to learn from others and discuss how to cope in different situations. Highly recommended!

Outdoor educational camps: These help young people develop healthy independence during their teen years. Parents or carers can be confident that the teenagers can look after their diabetes in real life situations. Skills such as management of hypoglycaemia, illness and information concerning development of complications are learned at outdoor educational camps.

Research shows that going to recognised Diabetes Australia camps can change teenagers' attitudes about how they feel about themselves and improve their confidence in handling a variety of common social situations and management predicaments. Camps can do wonders for their self-esteem. The authors feel strongly that attendance at camp is an essential part of the treatment of teenagers with diabetes. Diabetes Australia can put you in touch with camping organisations in your State or Territory by phoning 1800 640 862.

Chapter 23

Diabetes in the Elderly

◆ By Dr Phil Popplewell ◆

AT A GLANCE

- **Early detection and control of diabetes may prevent or delay the onset of complications which otherwise might occur in older people.**
- **Major risk factors for developing diabetes are age, genetic predisposition, being overweight and reduced activity levels.**
- **The effects of diabetes in the aged differ from those in younger people.**
- **Ongoing diabetes education and regular monitoring will minimise the short and long-term impact of diabetes.**

Who are the elderly?

AS a specialist in diseases affecting older people (a geriatrician), one of the most common questions I am asked is 'What do you mean by elderly?'

I don't have a clear answer but, in general terms, people aged 65 years and older are considered elderly.

Each year 56,000 Australians turn 65. Currently this group represents 11 per cent of the population and will increase to 16–18 per cent by 2021. Generally, women outlive men and, increasingly, the older groups of the population are women.

Most older people (90 per cent) live independently in private dwellings, with about 25 per cent – mostly women – living alone. Only 10 per cent live in non-private dwellings such as hostels or nursing homes, but this proportion increases among the very old. The elderly population includes many individuals who are very fit and well, plus others who are very old and frail.

From a geriatrician's perspective, elderly people are divided into the *young old* (65–75 years) and the *old old* (75 years plus). This division has some practical value because, by age 75, a significant number of people will have medical problems and problems with mobility, self-care and memory. This group requires extra care, including assistance from the district nurse, Meals-on-Wheels and domiciliary care services.

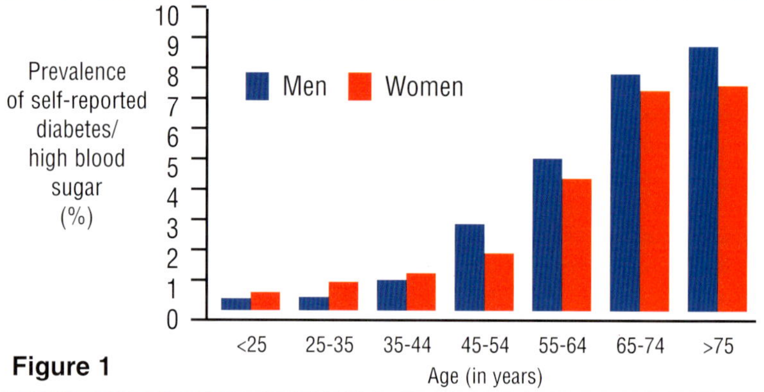

Figure 1

Estimated age-specific prevalence of self-reported diabetes/high blood sugar in Australian men and women: 1989–90 (from Welborn et al, 1995).

The separation of *young* and *old* elderly is helpful in the management of conditions such as diabetes because preventing complications in the younger group often flows into management of existing complications in the older group.

Why do elderly individuals get diabetes?

Diabetes is a common disorder that steadily increases with age (Figure 1). A recent Australian survey of people aged 65 plus found that 11.7 per cent had diabetes (6.4 per cent known and 5.3 per cent previously undiagnosed). A further 11 per cent had glucose intolerance.

There are several reasons why older people are at particular risk of developing diabetes. Major risk factors include age, genetic predisposition, being overweight[1] and reduced activity levels.

Diabetes in older people is different from diabetes in younger people. Diabetes in young people (type 1 diabetes) is associated with progressive loss of beta cells in the pancreas, leading to an absence of insulin.

When diabetes occurs in old age (type 2 diabetes) it is associated with the failure of ageing beta cells to overcome the increasing insulin resistance that occurs with age.

Diagnosis of diabetes

The effects of diabetes in older people also differ from those in younger populations. The classic symptoms of passing large volumes of urine and increasing thirst are less obvious in the elderly. Because the renal threshold for loss of glucose is higher, less glucose is passed in the urine, therefore less water is drawn with it and less urine is produced.

Many older people with diabetes are relatively symptom-free, despite having quite high blood glucose levels. Alternatively, they may have vague symptoms such as tiredness or weakness that are often dismissed by them and their health professionals as 'old age'. Since undiagnosed diabetes is so common (an estimated 5.3 per cent of those aged 65 plus) and the symptoms are so vague and non-specific, testing for diabetes should always be considered, especially in those with a family history of diabetes or those who are overweight[2].

Diabetes treatment

The aim of treating older people with diabetes is to minimise the short and long-term impact of the condition. This is achieved by ongoing diabetes education and regular monitoring.

Regular monitoring includes checking lifestyle issues, blood glucose, blood pressure, blood fats, kidney function and the eyes, plus checking for vascular (heart and blood vessel) problems. There is an ongoing education program covering action plans which address problems you may encounter.

The priorities: healthy eating and healthy lifestyle

Good nutrition, quitting smoking and limiting alcohol consumption are the cornerstones of a healthy lifestyle. Especially important is advice about how to control weight, such as the simple matter of increasing complex carbohydrate while decreasing fat and salt intake. Because older people often have an inadequate intake of calcium and iron, specialist advice by a dietitian might be needed.

Medication for diabetes

Older people with type 2 diabetes may require tablets or insulin and to adopt a healthier lifestyle to control their diabetes. If tablets are prescribed, the sulphonylurea group of diabetes tablets (hypoglycaemic agents) is generally preferred. Treatment will start with the lowest recommended dose – usually half to one tablet a day – and can be increased to a maximum of four tablets a day, usually taken before breakfast and before the evening meal (see chapter 6 – The Use of Tablets).

Because all sulphonylureas work by stimulating insulin secretion and reducing insulin resistance, there is no point in taking more than one kind of sulphonylurea. The risk of low blood glucose levels (hypoglycaemia) occurs when sulphonylurea tablets are taken but some (chlorpromide and glibenclamide) are more likely to cause hypoglycaemia than the newer tablets (gliclazide and glipizide). The older tablets are therefore not often used in elderly people. Tablets are taken with meals to avoid the risk of taking the sulphonylurea but missing the meal.

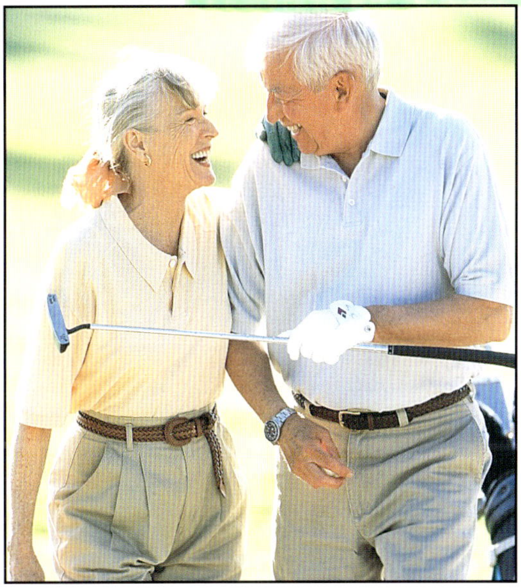

Metformin and Acarbose have different actions from sulphonylureas, directly affecting the way the body uses glucose. Metformin is a useful tablet because it may help overweight people control their weight. Older people with heart, kidney or liver disease are not generally given metformin because of the increased risk of lactic acidosis. Organ damage in older people is often not obvious and not detected by standard tests, so metformin is generally only used for overweight people with normal heart, kidney and liver function.

If symptoms are not controlled or blood glucose targets are not being met, insulin may be needed and should be started as soon as possible. Some older people are afraid of insulin but the doctor or diabetes nurse educator will carefully explain why insulin is necessary. The diabetes team will also explain the risk of hypoglycaemia; how to avoid it and treat it.

Cloudy (intermediate-acting) insulins such as Isophane™ (Humulin NPH™, Protaphane™) generally can be used with safety and are less likely to cause hypoglycaemia than the clear (quick-acting) insulins (Actrapid™, Humulin-R™, Humalog™).

Sometimes tablets and insulin are used together, often using a night-time dose of intermediate or long-acting insulin (Humulin NPH™, Protaphane™, Humulin-UL™, Ultratard™) and day-time sulphonylurea tablets (gliclazide or glipizide) with meals. Relatives and friends may also be involved in diabetes education and taught how to recognise hypoglycaemia and to treat it with glucose lollies, soft drinks or the administration of glucagon by injection.

Blood glucose control

In general, if blood glucose levels can remain between 5 and 10 mmol/L with a HbA1c of approximately 7 per cent, control is satisfactory. Targets can often be met following a modified meal plan and increased exercise.

A suggested checklist for diabetes care in older people is shown in Table 1.

Complications of diabetes in the elderly

Death rates in individuals with type 2 diabetes are about twice those of people without diabetes. More than 20 per cent of older people with newly diagnosed diabetes already have retinopathy and even more have vascular disease affecting the heart (angina or heart attacks), brain (transient ischaemic episodes or strokes) and limbs (claudication).

Although existing diabetic complications are probably irreversible, progression of disease and major problems such as foot ulcers (leading to amputation) and eye damage (leading to blindness) can be prevented. The full diabetes care team is involved: the doctor, to review the medical care; the diabetes nurse educator, to advise on the day-to-day techniques of self-care; the dietitian, to discuss food and activity; the podiatrist, to check on foot care and foot wear plus provide expert treatment if needed.

Early detection and control of diabetes may prevent or delay the onset of complications which otherwise might occur in older people.

The life expectancy for older Australians has increased considerably since the turn of the century. Men aged 65 can expect to live to 80; women aged 65 can expect to see their 85th birthday. Prevention of long-term complications from diabetes is therefore a high priority among the *young old* (65–75), the majority of Australians aged 65 or more. In the *old old* (75 plus) the emphasis is still on preventing complications but also includes management of existing complications and prevention of additional problems such as foot ulcers and falls.

TABLE 1

A check list for diabetes care in older people

1. Diagnosis of diabetes
Annual screening for diabetes by measuring random venous plasma glucose.
If venous plasma glucose equals or exceeds 11.1 mmol/L, confirm diabetes with a fasting venous plasma value equal to or exceeding 7.8 mmol/L.
Review the patient with newly diagnosed diabetes for cardiovascular, vascular, renal and ocular disease.

2. Glycaemic control
Remain aware of the risk and ill effects of hypoglycaemia in older people.
Emphasise the importance of diet, exercise and healthy body weight.
In general targets for fasting and preprandial venous plasma glucose values are below 7.8 mmol/L. Maintain two-hour postprandial plasma glucose values under 11.1 mmol/L in patients on diet or oral hypoglycaemic agents or under 15 mmol/L in patients receiving insulin.
Patients and staff should perform regular blood glucose monitoring and be taught to use and maintain equipment and carry out quality control.

3. Education
Older people with diabetes should have access to community-based diabetes programs designed for this age group. Preventive strategies for home safety should be emphasised. Institutions housing older people with diabetes should have professional diabetes education for staff.

4. Nutrition and lifestyle
Identify vascular risk factors such as hypertension, dyslipidaemia, smoking and overweight. Ensure regular individual or institutional review, ideally by a dietitian.
Structure diet around the recommended dietary intake to achieve and maintain a body mass index of 20-25 if possible; to maintain 50% carbohydrate, 30% fat and 20% protein; and to ensure an adequate calcium and iron intake.
Encourage regular aerobic exercises in fit older people, and exercise to maintain mobility and circulation in those who are less fit.
Encourage cessation of smoking and limitation of alcohol to 40 grams per day for men and 20 grams per day for women.

5. Medication
Exclude secondary causes and give nutrition and lifestyle modification an adequate trial.
Consider individual factors that might affect medication choice and make hypoglycaemia a special risk.
Give preference to shorter acting sulphonylureas.
Do not delay insulin treatment if glycaemic targets are not met with oral medication.
Quick acting insulins are rarely necessary in older people with type 2 diabetes.
Ensure relatives can recognise and treat hypoglycaemia.

6. Monitoring complications
Eyes. Arrange regular review by an ophthalmologist.
Foot care. Examine the feet of older people with diabetes at least annually. Ensure nursing staff in institutions review older people with at-risk feet at frequent intervals (sometimes daily)
Kidneys. Monitor renal function at least annually by measurement of plasma creatinine with urinalysis to exclude urinary tract infections.
Preventive care. Examine patients every 3-4 months and regularly review risk factors and indicators of complications, and update vaccination status for tetanus, influenza and pneumoccal disease.
Note: This table is adapted from the NH&MRC Series on Diabetes No 3 Diabetes in older people. Popplewell P, Phillips P, Burston R, Lowther B, Shearn M. Canberra: Australia Government Publishing Service 1992. Commonwealth of Australia copyright reproduced by permission.

Common conditions that co-exist with diabetes in older people

Management of diabetes can be further complicated by additional medical problems and medications.

Diabetes, high blood pressure and kidney damage are a dangerous trio which can accelerate the rate of kidney damage and raise blood pressure, increasing the risk of heart attack or stroke.

Medications used to treat one condition (such as fluid tablets – diuretics – for high blood pressure) may affect the control of another, for example, by increasing blood glucose levels. This can become a two-edged sword, where potential benefit from the medication comes with an increased risk of an unwanted side-effect. For example, ACE inhibitors used to treat high blood pressure may protect the kidneys in some circumstances but, in others, such as vascular disease, may reduce kidney function.

Other medications used to treat high blood pressure and angina (beta-blockers) are very useful but may increase blood glucose levels, mask the signs of hypoglycaemia and worsen symptoms of vascular disease affecting the legs (claudication).

Monitoring complications

Eyes

An eye specialist will review all older people with diabetes at the time of diagnosis and regularly afterwards, as appropriate. Blindness can be prevented by modern eye care and regular eye reviews are part of the follow-up routine. Laser treatment can prevent damage to the back of the eye and lens implants can improve visual function in people with cataracts.

Foot care

People in their seventies who have diabetes are 50 times more likely to develop gangrene because of associated vascular disease, nerve damage and increased risk of infection. Regular review by a podiatrist is recommended and foot examination, including blood supply, sensation and reflexes, should be undertaken by the general practitioner once a year.

Kidneys

In Australia, diabetes is the most common condition requiring ongoing renal dialysis. It is recommended that blood tests of kidney function are performed annually to pick up problems early. Urinary tract infections are common in the elderly and more common in people with diabetes. However, early detection, treatment and prevention can reduce the frequency and severity of urinary tract infections.

Blood pressure and blood fats

High blood pressure and blood fats are likely to

accelerate the course of cardiovascular, kidney and eye diseases and foot problems. Blood pressure and blood fats should be monitored carefully and treated if levels are above target values.

Other preventive care

Because people with diabetes are more prone to infections if blood glucose levels are high, regular influenza, pneumonia and tetanus vaccinations are essential. Aspirin is beneficial in preventing heart attacks and strokes and may be given to any person with diabetes at risk of vascular disease. Most people with diabetes who are aged 50 or more will be advised to take aspirin. Just as for people without diabetes, regular cancer screening is also important.

A member of the health care team may assess the very old and frail to determine how they are coping at home and provide any necessary assistance and support.

Footnotes

1. As a general rule someone's ideal weight (kg) equals their height (cm) minus 100, for example, a 1.8 m tall man should weigh (180 – 100 = 80) approximately 80 kg.
2. Older people should be tested annually during routine visits to their general practitioner. The diagnosis is made by a simple blood test which measures the blood glucose level. Once the diagnosis has been made, the doctor will examine the person and review any medications the person is taking as some medications can affect the body's ability to handle glucose.

Chapter 24

Diabetes in Aboriginal People

◆ By Professor Kerin O'Dea ◆

THERE is no evidence that diabetes or other lifestyle diseases such as obesity, cardiovascular disease or hypertension occurred among Aboriginal people when they lived traditionally.

Today most Aboriginal people live a westernised lifestyle, eating western foods and leading sedentary, physically inactive lives.

Under these circumstances many become overweight and develop type 2 diabetes.

Although diabetes is common among non-Aboriginal Australians, with 3.4 per cent contracting the condition, in most urbanised Aboriginal communities the prevalence is much greater, ranging from 5 per cent in the least westernised communities, to 24 per cent in the most westernised, overweight communities.

In many Aboriginal communities more than half of the over 40 year olds have either diabetes or impaired glucose tolerance. They also have a greater risk of cardiovascular disease, hypertension, hyperlipidemia, ECG abnormalities and high insulin levels consistent with insulin resistance.

The public health implications of these high rates of diabetes are enormous. People with diabetes are at higher risk of coronary heart disease, stroke, peripheral vascular disease, gangrene, skin infections, renal failure and peripheral neuropathy.

However, the implications are even more serious when you consider many Aboriginal people contract diabetes in their early twenties and thirties. The younger they are, the greater the risk of complications occurring at a young age.

Apart from the soaring financial costs of treating these conditions, there are personal costs in terms of lost quality of life.

For cultural, historic and economic reasons, diabetes in Aboriginal people has not responded to conventional therapies. New and different strategies are essential if we are to control the epidemic.

AT A GLANCE

- **It can be argued that humans are genetically programmed for a hunter-gatherer lifestyle.**
- **It makes sense to return to that lifestyle in our search for solutions to some current health programs.**
- **If successful, these solutions may have wider application than simply preventing and treating type 2 diabetes.**
- **Any aspect of a person's lifestyle which could worsen insulin resistance may act as a trigger to bring on diabetes.**
- **Diabetes is not only potentially reversible in Aborigines, but potentially preventable if people initiate major lifestyle changes.**

Why Aboriginal people are vulnerable to diabetes

Type 2 diabetes – the same form predominant among non-Aboriginal Australians – is common among Aboriginal people.

Type 2 diabetes develops when genetic or inherited susceptibility is triggered by certain lifestyle factors.

The precise nature of the genetic susceptibility is not well understood, but we believe that resistance to the action of insulin may be the main factor. Therefore, any aspect of a person's lifestyle which could worsen insulin resistance may act as a trigger to bring on the disease.

We also know that lack of exercise, obesity and eating energy-dense foods (that is, rich in fat and sugar but low in fibre) worsen insulin resistance and are also risk factors for type 2 diabetes.

It is likely that Aboriginal people's traditional hunter-gatherer lifestyle protected them against type 2 diabetes by maximising their insulin sensitivity.

They were nomadic, lean and fit, eating meals derived from wild animals, fish, and vegetables – bulky, low energy-dense foods. The traditional diet had all the qualities important in treating and preventing type 2 diabetes – high fibre and low fat plus slowly digested and absorbed carbohydrate.

Wild animals and fish are low in fat. Uncultivated vegetables contain slowly digested carbohydrate and are high in fibre, vitamins and essential trace elements.

Eating these foods while being lean and physically active maximises insulin sensitivity.

When they adopted a western lifestyle, Aboriginal people's physical activity declined dramatically and eating styles changed radically. Out went the fibre, in came an increased energy intake of sugar, fat and alcohol.

Aboriginal people's efficient metabolism of hunted and gathered foods – once a survival mechanism – now promotes overweight, diabetes and the associated conditions of hypertension and cardiovascular disease.

It is possible that all these conditions share a common pathway – insulin resistance provoked by lifestyle change.

Reversing the process

If lifestyle change causes diabetes in Aboriginal people, can it be treated by reversing the process?

This was the idea behind a study in 1982, when 14 Aboriginal people from a remote community in Western Australia – 10 with diabetes and 4 without – participated in a study during which they adopted the traditional lifestyle.

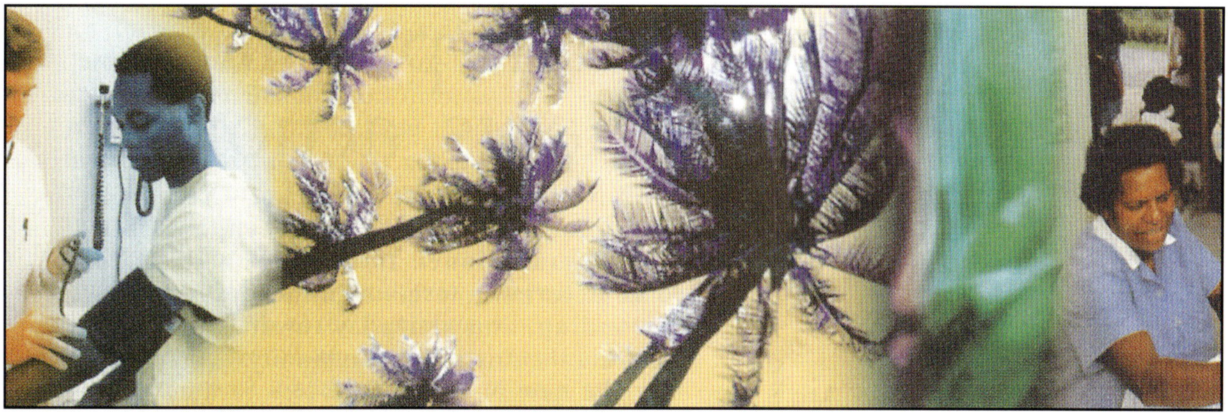

Metabolic tests were conducted before and after seven weeks of living off the land.

The results were striking, with marked improvement in all the metabolic abnormalities of diabetes, plus a reduction in several risk factors for cardiovascular disease.

Some of these diabetes-related abnormalities – such as high plasma triglycerides – were completely normalised. Others – such as fasting glucose, glucose tolerance and insulin secretion – were not, although they improved greatly.

Had the study continued longer, these abnormalities may have been corrected. As it was, seven weeks of traditional lifestyle were enough to substantially reverse a disease that took years to develop in the urban environment.

The public health implications are enormous. Not only is diabetes potentially reversible in Aboriginal people, but potentially preventable as well.

The results of the study are a dramatic illustration of the relationship between lifestyle and health.

The three major traditional lifestyle components which contributed to participants' improved metabolic control were regular physical activity, a low-fat, high fibre meal plan, and weight loss.

These are a natural part of the hunter-gatherer lifestyle, but each needs to be addressed separately in an urban context.

Increased physical activity

Ideally, incorporate in the daily routine by walking rather than driving; carrying out manual labour or taking part in sport. Ironically, the traditional hunter-gatherer would have minimised unnecessary energy output in the interests of efficiency.

Low-fat, high-fibre eating

A key component for many communities is their local general store where short-term profit rather than health is the major factor determining types of food sold. There are a few financially profitable stores in Aboriginal communities which stock high quality food and promote the consumption of fruit, vegetables, wholegrain cereals, lean meats and low-fat dairy products. However, these success stories depend on intensive input from public health professionals such as nutritionists.

Weight loss in the overweight

By adopting the first two components – increasing physical activity and eating low-fat, high- fibre foods – you will automatically lose weight.

Because of the epidemic of lifestyle diseases such as diabetes in Aboriginal communities, community-wide treatment and prevention programs are essential.

Prevention is better than cure and the cluster of lifestyle diseases such as obesity, diabetes and hyperlipidemias will all respond to changes in eating and exercise.

The challenge for Aboriginal people is to design, implement and own appropriate strategies to encourage health-promoting change in their communities.

The success of the back-to-the-bush study was due in part to its Aboriginality. The benefits went far beyond the physical health of the participants; their self-esteem also increased enormously. People who were considered failures in town – such as alcoholics – turned out to be capable and successful hunters in the bush.

The strong links Aboriginal people have with their land and the renewal evident when they return to it, highlights the important relationship between land rights and health.

Probably the most important implication to be drawn from the association between diabetes and the westernisation of Aboriginal people is the clear potential for preventing type 2 diabetes.

This is particularly relevant for the children and other close relatives of people with diabetes.

One of the best predictors of susceptibility to type 2 diabetes is a family history of the disease. The stronger the family history, the greater the risk.

However, this genetic susceptibility need not be taken as a foregone conclusion. Aboriginal people did not get diabetes when they lived traditionally and the principles of that lifestyle could be applied to protect the offspring of people with diabetes.

As all people with diabetes are only too aware, prevention is preferable to treatment and, theoretically, is possible in most cases.

Unfortunately, by the time many people are diagnosed as having type 2 diabetes, the condition is well established and intervention to reverse the process is more difficult.

Implications for non-Aboriginal people with type 2 diabetes

The same principles inherent in the hunter-gatherer lifestyle can be applied to the treatment of type 2 diabetes generally.

Regular physical activity, low-fat, high-fibre meals and weight loss remain essential therapies for the vast majority of people with type 2 diabetes. Each is independently effective in improving metabolic control in type 2 diabetes, with the underlying mechanism of effectiveness apparently related to improved sensitivity to insulin.

As also demonstrated in the bush study, these lifestyle changes have numerous other beneficial health consequences, including improved self-confidence. This arises when people with diabetes take control of their own treatment.

Since type 2 diabetes is a condition brought on by lifestyle factors, it stands to reason that the most rational approach to its treatment is through lifestyle modification.

However, this approach does not work for all people with type 2 diabetes.

It is particularly appropriate for those with insulin resistance. In cases of type 2 diabetes where insulin resistance is not a major feature, diabetic control may not be improved greatly by lifestyle modification.

Different from type 1 diabetes, type 2 diabetes is symptomless in its early stages, which can last for years. Frequently, the condition is picked up only by chance or when complications develop.

Treatment by lifestyle modification has the best chance of success during the early stages of type 2 diabetes, when major metabolic abnormalities appear to be reversible.

Chapter 25

Diabetes – A Problem in Any Language

◆ By Bernadette Lowther ◆

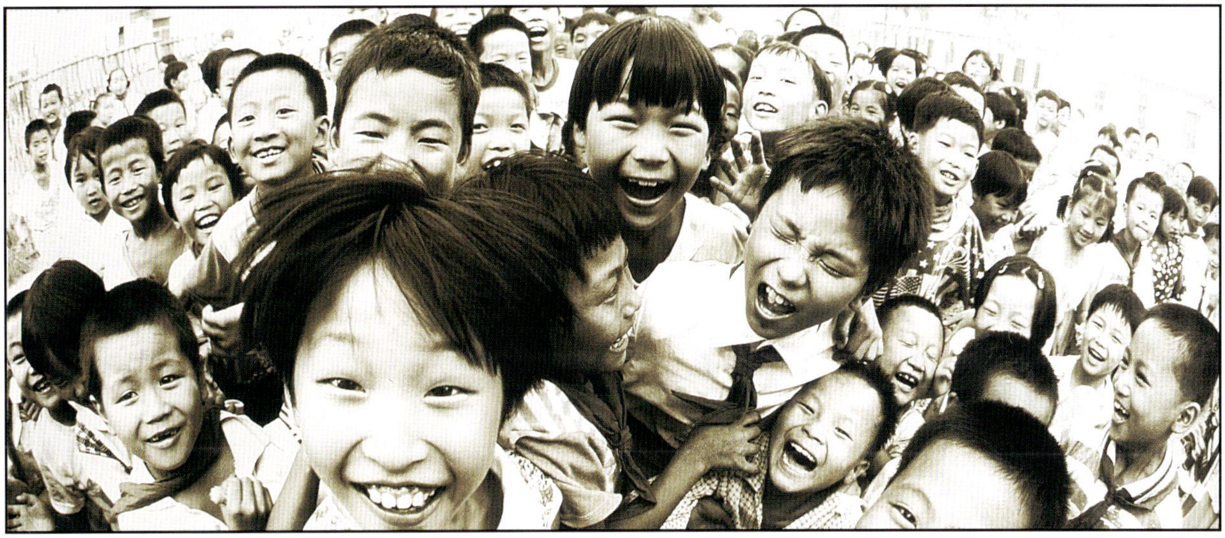

Diabetes, who has it?

DIABETES is a much more common problem among people who migrate to Australia than for the Australian-born population. This is especially so for Asian Indians, Chinese, people from the Middle East, Southern Europeans and Pacific Islanders (see chapter 34 – Around the World with Diabetes).

Why are some races more prone than others?

Researchers believe that there are many reasons for this, some of them to do with the new environment and different lifestyle in a new country; some related to inherited genes.

For similar reasons, diabetes is also more common in Australian Aboriginal people who, since European settlement, have changed their traditional way of living for a western lifestyle (see chapter 24 – Diabetes in Aboriginal People).

Diabetes in pregnancy

Diabetes may first appear during pregnancy and all pregnant women should be tested for diabetes between the 26th and 28th week of pregnancy.

Diabetes during pregnancy is called gestational diabetes. It is more prevalent among more recently arrived migrant groups such as Vietnamese, Africans, Filipinos, mainland Chinese, Sri Lankans and Pacific Islanders.

Women from these backgrounds are at risk of developing gestational diabetes and their doctors should check them for diabetes during the pregnancy. If the condition develops, it needs appropriate management to help ensure delivery of a healthy baby (see page 68 – Diabetes and Pregnancy).

AT A GLANCE

- **Certain migrant groups are more prone to type 2 diabetes.**
- **Australian residents are entitled to free health care through the public health service.**
- **Women from South East Asia, Africa, People's Republic of China, the Middle East and the Pacific Islands are more prone to develop gestational diabetes.**
- **For people with diabetes who are not confident in English, it is imperative that a professional interpreter is present during health care discussions.**
- **The Federal Government subsidises the cost of syringes and test strips. Contact Diabetes Australia to register for the subsidy.**

Women who develop diabetes during pregnancy are at risk of developing diabetes in later life. They will need to be tested annually for the rest of their lives and to eat properly. Food should be low in fat and high in fibre, with only moderate amounts of sugar. These women can also help prevent diabetes from developing by incorporating regular exercise into their lives.

Access to education

Learning about diabetes management is difficult for people who can't speak or read English, and especially challenging for those with reading difficulties in their own language. However, it is important they know what health services are available and what they need to do to keep their diabetes under control.

Health professionals in migrant communities are generally conscientious about informing those with diabetes where their support services are, how they work and how they can be accessed.

Foreign language pamphlets or newspaper items are one way to advise people about health care services. Others are ethnic radio broadcasts and video presentations in community health centres.

Health professionals are always looking for new and effective ways to reach different migrant communities.

However, health care workers can become frustrated if they are unable to get their message across. They may confuse a lack of comprehension with unwillingness to follow instruction. It helps if both parties recognise this risk and have the means at hand to prevent further misunderstanding, such as an appropriately trained interpreter.

Special considerations

People from non-English-speaking backgrounds are all different. While there are problems they all share, there are many cultural differences that need to be considered.

Religion, racial customs and traditions plus issues relating to gender, seniority and who is the best or most appropriate person to provide health messages must be considered.

Cultural differences

It is important that health professionals recognise the differing cultural requirements of people with diabetes or other health conditions. It may be totally unsuitable to expect one family member to pass information on to another, especially if it is a young person passing information to an older one. The age of the person may be especially significant when making decisions about how to provide education and who should be involved. In some cultures it may not be appropriate for a woman to try to educate a man, or it may not be reasonable to expect a woman to make decisions about changing traditional cooking methods for her own benefit without first consulting her husband.

The part played by food in different societies may be especially relevant – food may be linked to social status, or excess weight may be associated with good health or prosperity.

Some ethnic groups may shrink from the idea of taking blood from the body to test blood glucose levels. In a multicultural society the issues are many and varied, so education must be tailored to suit the needs of individuals in the context of their particular cultural background.

Interpreters

Just because someone is of a certain age or has lived here for years doesn't mean that they'll necessarily understand how to manage their diabetes.

People from Southern Europe and Asia who have been here a long time often remain unable to communicate in English and many people from these groups develop diabetes. Some people who speak enough English for everyday survival have diminished understanding when they are under stress and trying to understand educational messages about their diabetes. For these people an interpreter will deliver the messages in their native language.

Too often family members are used as interpreters.

It is essential that non-English-speakers have a professional interpreter present when they are consulting a health professional.

In most States and Territories a Government Interpreter Service or Migrant Health Unit can assist. However, it is important that the health worker knows in advance that an interpreter will be needed so they can arrange one. In an emergency, a telephone interpreter service is usually available to translate information from the health professional to the patient.

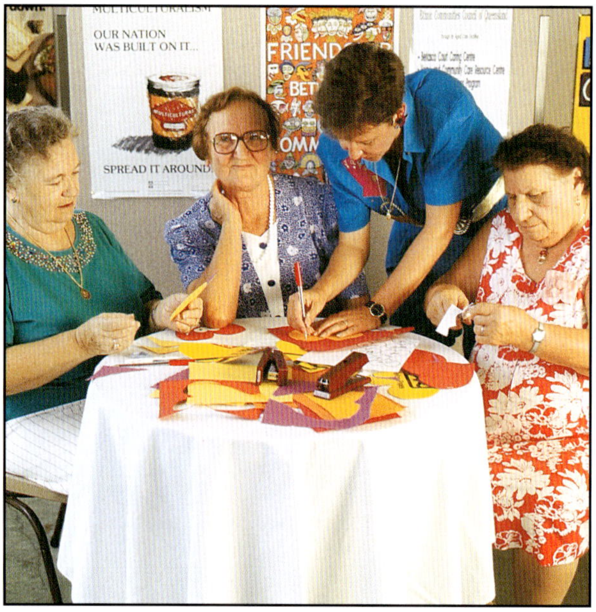

Health care in Australia

In Australia, all permanent residents have the right to health care. People with diabetes are entitled to education and medical treatment to help them manage their diabetes and remain healthy.

Resources

Many resources exist to assist people to manage their diabetes. Most large hospitals or community centres have diabetes education and support services available to all. The general practitioner is the best person to ask about services such as a relevant specialist physician, dietitian, diabetes educator, podiatrist, eye specialist or psychologist.

It is important that people learn how to perform their own tests so they can assess their success at diabetes control. The doctor or a diabetes nurse educator can advise about the best method for each person to test their blood glucose levels.

Written, audio and video-taped information is also available in several languages. Ask Diabetes Australia or your local Diabetes Education Centre to help you find it.

Diabetes Australia

Diabetes Australia exists solely to help people with diabetes. The organisation has a branch in each State and Territory and telephone numbers for Diabetes Australia offices are in this book (see chapter 32 – Further Resources) and in your telephone directory.

National Diabetic Services Scheme (NDSS)

The cost of blood and urine test strips and syringes is heavily subsidised by the Federal Government through the NDSS. To qualify for the subsidy you must be a permanent resident of Australia and register at a Diabetes Australia office. There is no charge for registration.

For further information, see chapter 32 – Further Resources.

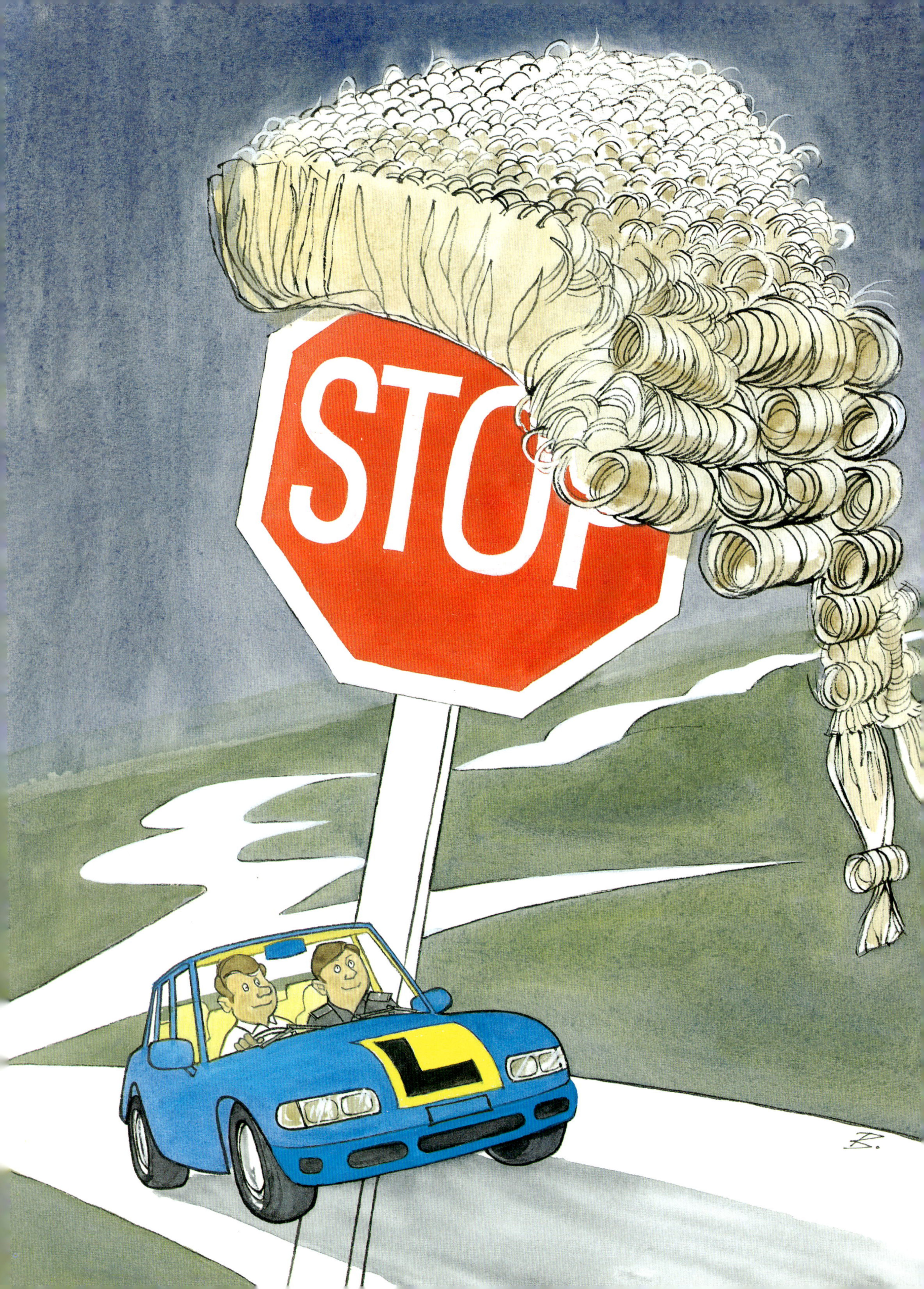
STOP

Chapter 26

How to Work with Your Health Care Team

◆ By Dr Pat Phillips and Dr June Raine ◆
Revised by Maureen Unsworth

The team approach

YOU live with diabetes 24 hours a day, 365 days a year with no holidays, balancing food, exercise and medication, trying to keep in control. Fortunately, you do not have to face it alone.

In Australia there are a range of health professionals to help you handle your diabetes. They usually work as a team, each bringing special skills and knowledge to your total health care plan.

The team leader and most important member of the group is *you*. It is easy for your doctor, diabetes nurse educator or dietitian to lose track of your total health status. Often, you are the only one who knows the whole picture – what has been done, what needs doing and any on-going challenges.

AT A GLANCE

- **Maintain your ideal body weight.**
- **Be active every day.**
- **Set achievable goals.**
- **Take your medication correctly.**
- **Monitor you blood glucose levels regularly.**
- **Look after your feet.**
- **See your doctor regularly.**
- **Have annual checks with key specialists.**
- **Join Diabetes Australia to receive a variety of services to help you.**

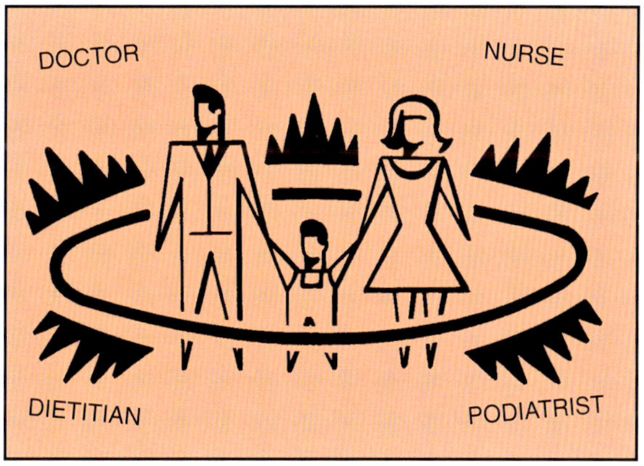

Your responsibilities in day-to-day care

Maintain a healthy ideal body weight. Extra weight makes it difficult for you to control your diabetes. Weight is a major reason body cells become resistant to insulin. In addition, extra weight can make it hard for you to control blood fats.

Develop a regular exercise pattern. Exercise has many advantages, in particular it helps to:

- control blood glucose
- reduce or maintain your weight
- increase the effect of insulin, thus helping control your diabetes
- keep blood fats normal
- reduce stress levels
- reduce the risk of long-term problems associated with diabetes and much more.

The following will help you to become more active:

- Deciding on an activity that fits well with your lifestyle. Think of a variety of personally enjoyable activities to keep you motivated.
- Choosing an exercise you like such as walking, cycling, tennis, golf, aerobics, swimming, jogging, gardening, dancing or some other form of exercise.
- Starting at a low level and gradually building up.
- Making activity a part of the day, for example, use the stairs instead of the lift, walk an extra bus stop or two, exercise in your lunch break, walk rather than drive short distances.
- Exercising with a friend may be more fun than doing it alone and you can motivate each other.

Take your medication/insulin correctly. Many people with diabetes require tablets to help control their diabetes. There are certain important steps to follow if you are taking oral medications:

- Take your tablets with meals at the same time each day.
- Never miss or delay a meal.
- Do not take more than your doctor prescribes.
- Never stop taking your tablets without first discussing this with your doctor.
- Get to know the name and dose of your tablets.
- Contact your doctor or your diabetes nurse educator if you are unwell or not sure what to do.
- Store your tablets in original, accurately labelled airtight containers, away from direct sunlight.

Some other medications can react with diabetes tablets, for example, medication for blood pressure, arthritis and asthma. You may want to discuss possible reactions with your doctor.

If you are prescribed insulin injections, your diabetes nurse educator will tell you how to purchase supplies and inject insulin (see chapter 9 – Injections and Injectors).

Wash and inspect your feet daily. Proper daily care of your feet and regular foot checks by your doctor or podiatrist can prevent serious foot problems (see chapter 17 – Foot Care and Foot Wear).

Visit your doctor regularly. Your doctor will want to check your:

- medication/insulin schedule
- overall diabetes control
- blood pressure

- ability to manage your exercise program and healthy eating pattern
- results, so that anything abnormal can be followed up. This may include blood tests for cholesterol and other blood fats; your average three-monthly blood glucose result; and any elevated blood pressure or long-term complications.

Your doctor is also responsible for referring you to a suitable education program or other health professional, such as a dietitian or podiatrist.

Year-to-year care

In addition to day-to-day responsibilities, there are also annual tasks for people with diabetes:

- an annual medical check-up is essential for all people with diabetes
- arrange an annual consultation with your eye specialist.

There are many record cards that can remind you and your doctor of all the areas you need to have checked annually. An example is displayed on page 95.

Have you considered the following:

- Joining Diabetes Australia, so you can keep up to date with new developments and know about relevant meetings, support groups and resources? This is all information to help you better manage your diabetes (see chapter 32 – Further Resources).
- Buying a Medical Alert bracelet? All people on insulin are advised to wear a bracelet or necklace or to carry a card in case of emergency.
- Joining an ambulance scheme? Subscriptions are not expensive and can help you avoid an enormous bill.
- Informing the relevant State or Territory motor vehicle department – such as the Roads and Traffic Authority – and insurance companies that you have diabetes? In some States it is illegal not to inform the relevant authority. Ask your Diabetes Australia branch about your State or Territory requirements.

To keep track of these issues, set a date each year (perhaps your birthday or other significant date) to check through your responsibilities.

Your doctor's responsibilities

The role of your doctor involves:

- diagnosis of diabetes
- initial and ongoing treatment
- coordination of care and referral to other members of the health care team such as diabetes nurse educator, dietitian, podiatrist, eye specialist and diabetes specialist for regular follow-up
- annual medical check-ups
- regular review of your tablets and insulin routines.

Your doctor is a key member of your health care team whose role is to help you access all the services you need to support your diabetes management.

Discuss regular follow-ups with your doctor and arrange a mutually convenient schedule.

There are areas your doctor will need to follow up regularly.

- **Your home blood glucose monitoring results**. The Diabetes Control and Complications Trial and UK Prospective Diabetes Trial demonstrated that people with above-normal blood glucose levels have a higher risk of developing the long-term complications associated with diabetes. Recommended blood glucose levels are tabled below:

Your control	Before meals	Two hours after meals
Ideal	Less than 6 mmol/L	Less than 8 mmol/L
Satisfactory	6–7 mmol/L	8–11 mmol/L
Unacceptable	Greater than 7 mmol/L	Greater than 11 mmol/L

- **Your blood pressure**. People with diabetes often have high blood pressure, which puts an extra strain on blood vessels. Imagine the effects of pounding the delicate tissues 100,000 times a day. That's the number of times your heart beats daily. As the heart contracts and pumps out blood, the pressure in the blood vessels rises to a peak (systolic blood pressure). The empty heart then fills up with blood and the pressure falls to a trough (diastolic blood pressure). In general, the lower the blood pressure the better. Your aim is to get values under 140 systolic and 90 diastolic. (Blood pressure is recorded like this: 140/90.) Your doctor will want to check your blood pressure at regular intervals.
- **Your overall diabetes control**. This entails measuring your long-term diabetes control by checking your haemoglobin A1c or glycated haemoglobin. This test measures your average blood glucose over approximately two months. This can be measured by calculating the percentage of glucose attached to the red blood cells. If you use insulin, your doctor will perform this test three-to-six-monthly. If you don't, the test will be 6-to-12-monthly.
  Glucose in the blood attaches to blood proteins. The part with glucose attached is said to be *glycated* (glycos = glucose). If blood glucose levels are often high, more glucose attaches to the haemoglobin protein. Since haemoglobin stays in the body for some time, this measurement reflects all the highs and lows of blood glucose levels during the past weeks and months. The higher the average blood glucose, the higher the glycated haemoglobin. Targets vary from person to person, but recent trials suggest values of 6–8 per cent were ideal. Discuss your target with your doctor.
- **Your weight**. Your doctor will measure your height and weight. Usually weight is measured at your initial assessment and then every three months. If you are trying to lose weight, your doctor may measure your weight more often.
- **Your medication**. Your doctor is responsible for ensuring you are on the right medication and the right dosages for your needs. Everyone's requirements change over time. Some people need a higher or lower dose or the type of medication may need to be changed. Your doctor will regularly ask

questions about your medication. On average, medication assessments are done at three-monthly intervals.

- **Your healthy lifestyle**. Your doctor shares your aims to keep healthy. He or she will provide ongoing support for:
  - maintaining a healthy eating pattern
  - maintaining an active lifestyle
  - drinking alcohol in moderation
  - giving up smoking.

On an annual basis:

- **Your eyes**. You need to have your eyes examined annually. Your doctor will organise for you to see an eye specialist. The tests performed include visual acuity (how well you focus). This is recorded as a fraction: 6/6 means when you are six metres away you can read a chart designed to be read at six metres. 6/9 or 6/12 would mean at six metres away you can't read the six-metre chart and can only read the one designed to be read at nine or 12 metres.

  KEEP YOUR OWN RECORD OF YOUR VISUAL ACUITY

  Other conditions the eye specialist will test for are cataracts, retinopathy and glaucoma.
- **Your kidneys**. Early signs of kidney damage can be detected by testing for small (micro) amounts of protein in your urine. This test is called microalbuminuria and should be performed at diagnosis and then every 12 months for people with type 2 diabetes. For people with type 1 diabetes, the test should be conducted five years after diagnosis, then every 12 months.

  Other checks performed on kidney function are for infection. Your doctor may also do a blood test to check the level of waste products in your blood (creatinine and urea levels).
- **Your feet**. If you are not able to care for your feet, see a podiatrist regularly. Your doctor is interested in checking your pulses for blood circulation and will also check your sensation to determine what your feet feel so that you can prevent potential damage.
- **Your injection sites (for insulin users)**. You are responsible for giving the injections properly (preferably in the abdominal area) and for making sure you rotate the injection site to avoid hitting the same spots. Your doctor will check for lumps or hollows which could affect the absorption of insulin. An annual check is adequate.

Keeping track of your care

Because you may see your doctor several times a year, it's easy for you both to lose track of what has and has not been done. Many people keep a log book to record their monitoring procedures.

Your vital input

Remember, you are the most important member of your health care team. You lead the team approach to diabetes care.

DATE	FEB	JUNE	OCT	FEB	JUNE	OCT	FEB	JUNE	OCT
GENERAL Weight									
Blood Pressure									
Glycated haemoglobin									
EYES Visual acuity									
Ophthalmologist due in									
KIDNEYS Microalbuminuria									
Dipstick									
Creatinine									
FEET Arteries									
Nerves									
INJECTION SITE									
VACCINATIONS									
Due in									

Record card for annual check up.

Rights and Responsibilities

◆ By David Nathan ◆
Revised by Maureen Unsworth

PEOPLE with diabetes are no different from other members of the community in that they have rights and responsibilities.

They have the right of access to treatment, education and support services to enable them to best control their diabetes.

They have the responsibility for themselves, taking charge of their own treatment to ensure successful management of their condition.

AT A GLANCE

• It is your responsibility to manage your diabetes and your right to access the resources you need.

• Among your rights is access to a professional health service and treatment plus confidentiality of your personal health care records.

• You are entitled to access to health information, support and supplies.

• Your other rights include a career of your choice, life and health insurance cover, appropriate job training and most civil licences and permits.

• Among your responsibilities is to declare your diabetes when applying for insurance, licences and permits.

• Failure to declare your diabetes to an employer may render you ineligible for workers' compensation.

Your rights

Like anyone else you have rights. If you wish, you are entitled to the following:

- *Access to a professional health service and treatment*. You need a medical practitioner to prescribe correct treatment plus review your medical management and refer you to other health services. Other health services you will need are a specialist physician; eye specialist; dietitian and other specialists as necessary. You may also need specialist care when you are in hospital for other conditions. You are entitled to a second medical opinion if you are not totally satisfied with a medical diagnosis or treatment.
- *Access to information.* You are entitled to a clear and understandable explanation about your condition plus a sympathetic hearing and discussion with health professionals who will provide any necessary treatment, referral or investigations. If necessary, you can request and receive interpreter services.

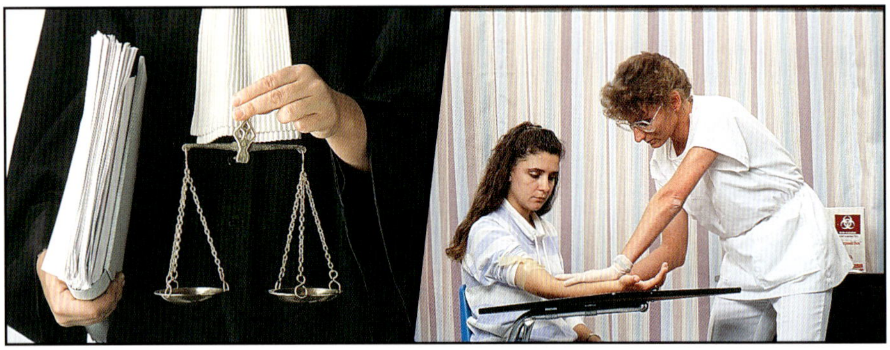

- *Access to support and supplies.* The National Diabetic Services Scheme is available through Diabetes Australia branches in each State and Territory. This scheme is federally funded and gives you access to blood glucose testing strips, syringes and pen tips at minimal cost. All you have to do is register with your State or Territory branch of Diabetes Australia (for contacts see chapter 32 – Further Resources). Diabetes Australia branches provide several services to people with diabetes including support groups, counselling services and other initiatives providing ongoing help. A variety of products and equipment is available through State or Territory branches to assist you in managing diabetes.
- *Access to blood glucose monitoring equipment and supplies* for giving your own insulin.
- *Confidentiality of your personal health information.* As a general rule, no information concerning your health records is released to another person without your consent. Sharing your personal health record can only occur if:
  - the court releases a subpoena for the record at a court proceeding

  or
  - if you are endangering lives and it is in the public's best interest to disclose confidential information (done only in serious situations)

  or
  - if there is a statutory obligation that states certain confidential information must be

reported to a specific government body

or

– if you are in a life-threatening health situation or crisis, information can be shared for the purpose of providing emergency treatment.

- *A career of your choice, life and health insurance cover, appropriate job training, civil licences and permits.* (see chapter 30 – Diabetes and Discrimination). There should be no discrimination against a person with diabetes in the workforce. However, in specific areas there are restrictions that preclude you from lines of work that may place you or your colleagues in danger. These include frontline combat in the armed forces; working in fire brigades or off-shore rigs; pilots in commercial airlines; bus drivers and fieldwork in remote areas. You can incur an increase in premiums for life and travel insurance or, in some cases, be denied insurance cover because you have diabetes. If this occurs, contact your Diabetes Australia branch for advice about insurance companies which do not disadvantage people with diabetes.

  Most civil licences and permits are accessible to people with diabetes. State and Territory requirements differ, for example:
  - in some States and Territories you must declare you have diabetes to obtain a driver's licence
  - for a driver's licence other than class A or B, you may require a letter from your specialist for licence and renewal (commercial bus drivers and commercial pilot's licence may be refused)
  - a special medical and training program is required for issue of a Certified Scuba Diver's licence.

In all cases of seeking insurance, licences or permits, it is advisable to declare you have diabetes. Failure to do so may cause your insurance company to reject your claim. In a work environment, failure to declare your diabetes may make you ineligible for workers' compensation.

Remember, you have the right to the last say.

What you need to know

Never forget that the responsibility for control of your diabetes ultimately rests with you. You will be advised and monitored by your doctor but regular daily procedures such as meal planning, blood testing, exercising, taking medications, foot care and coping with high or low blood sugars are up to you.

In some instances the responsibility must be shared or delegated. In the case of a young child, the aged, infirmed or mentally handicapped, relatives or other carers will have to step in and take charge.

However, in the majority of cases, reasonable standards of care and delegation of responsibilities are achieved by the people with diabetes themselves.

Diabetes is never mild

Even those with control by an eating plan alone can develop complications. Prolonged poor control increases the chances of damage to eyesight, kidneys, sexual potency, blood flow to the heart, brains and legs. Whether or not your body has some damage, there is much you can do to prevent further problems.

Some of the steps to better control of diabetes

There are eight steps to better control of diabetes:

1. Become as fully informed as possible about your diabetes management. Contact your State or Territory branch of Diabetes Australia for extra information. Seek out and attend diabetes education courses which may be at your local hospital, health centre or diabetes education centre. Learn all the skills you need. Ask to see a diabetes nurse educator.
2. Ask your GP to refer you to a dietitian if you haven't seen one recently for a meal plan. All people with diabetes need this advice at diagnosis and at regular intervals thereafter.
3. Discuss with your doctor the need for assessment by a specialist experienced in diabetes care. If you are on insulin injections, your GP will seek an assessment by a specialist. If you are planning to become pregnant, it is advisable to see a diabetes specialist before stopping contraception. If you are already pregnant, discuss this with your doctor or obstetrician as you will need referral to a specialist experienced in diabetes care. If you are on a meal plan alone or a meal plan and tablets, your GP may send you to a specialist physician if you're having problems with your diabetes. Ask questions, follow the specialist's advice and improve your knowledge of diabetes.
4. Identify any factors that alter your diabetes control. Stop smoking, cut down on your alcohol intake, take regular exercise (after checking with your doctor), start losing excess weight. See a dietitian about eating healthy food. This will include reducing the fat in your whole family's diet plus increasing the intake of vegetables, fruits and cereals.
5. Test your blood glucose levels regularly and record the results so that you have the information to make correct decisions about your medication and food plan.
6. Learn what to expect when you visit your GP or specialist physician.
7. Become interested in the pathology tests ordered by your doctor. Common ones are:
   - **glycated (or glycosylated) haemoglobin**
     This valuable test is usually done three times a year and shows your average blood glucose control for the previous few months.
   - **cholesterol, triglycerides and high density lipoprotein**
     These are important blood fats the doctor usually measures each year.
     High cholesterol is an important cause of heart attacks (coronary artery disease) and circulation problems. Meal plans – with or without certain medications – can reduce high cholesterol levels.

- **microalbuminuria**
  This is another test on your urine sample conducted to detect early kidney damage due to diabetes.
- **creatinine and urinary protein**
  These are tests of your kidney function and are usually done once a year.

8. Remember it is your responsibility to manage your diabetes control using the advice and help given to you.

What the doctor wants to check

Your eyes

If you are under 30, see a medical eye specialist after five years of diabetes and at intervals after that, as advised.

If you are over 30, see a medical eye specialist at the diagnosis of diabetes and at intervals after that, as advised.

Remember, serious eye damage (retinopathy) can be developing even though your eyesight is still excellent. Early detection means early treatment and preventing blindness (see chapter 16 – Diabetes and Eyes).

Your blood pressure

High blood pressure (hypertension) may worsen any damage caused by diabetes to your kidney, heart and circulation and eyes. Treatment of high blood pressure can prevent this damage.

This is why it is important your doctor checks your blood pressure at every visit and puts you on treatment if it is necessary.

Your feet

Diabetes can damage the circulation and sensation in your feet, making them susceptible to damage. If this happens, foot care is even more important.

This is why your doctor regularly checks the skin, pulses and sensation in your feet and may refer you to a podiatrist. Remember to dress appropriately because your doctor needs to be able to examine your feet easily (see chapter 17 – Foot Care and Foot Wear).

Your weight and height

Being overweight by itself makes diabetes control difficult because it contributes to poor blood sugar control, elevated cholesterol, high blood pressure and heart disease.

This is why your doctor weighs you regularly to assess your progress. If you are still growing, he will also measure your height because growth may be reduced by poor glucose control.

Your insulin injection sites

Your doctor needs to examine these because problems at these sites can hinder your diabetes control.

It is your right to access the resources that you need and it is your responsibility to manage your diabetes.

Chapter 28

Diabetes in General Practice

◆ By Dr Chris Holmwood ◆

FOR most of us, when we are ill, the general practitioner (GP) is the first port of call.

Australia is fortunate in having a well-trained, affordable and accessible workforce of GPs. Because diabetes is such a common condition, the average GP probably has 30 or 40 people with diabetes attending the practice and is the most likely person to diagnose your diabetes.

GPs help people with diabetes manage the problems associated with the condition, including helping them navigate and benefit from an increasingly complex health care system.

They also deal with people's other health concerns in the context of the individual's ongoing diabetes management.

Some GPs have established clinics for people with diabetes. This means that people can access specialised care in an environment that may be preferable to a hospital setting.

GPs are a convenient means by which people with diabetes can access other health professionals and utilise the hospital system, specialist private practitioners, local community health centres and general practice service divisions.

Diabetes is a multifaceted condition and aspects of care involve many different areas of practice.

For example, a GP might see a woman aged 54, with type 2 diabetes, who is going through menopause and feeling depressed.

The GP can assist with the management of her diabetes; offer the option of hormone replacement therapy; conduct routine cervical smears, breast checks and mammograms; counsel her about possible depression and provide specific therapy where necessary.

Not only is such composite care convenient for the patient, it is also cheaper and less likely to become disjointed.

Although the GP does not have the depth of knowledge of a specialist in each area, it is highly likely that the GP has built up a good relationship with the patient. This helps in management of most problems, although there may be the occasional referral for specialist help when needed.

GPs deal with people's most common and frequent problems. In most cases these are issues that do not need specialist input.

Choosing a general practitioner

One of the great features of the Australian health care system is the degree of choice people have about health care.

There are many theories about what makes a good GP and evidence suggests that people have better health outcomes if they attend GPs who listen and try to see the world from their perspective.

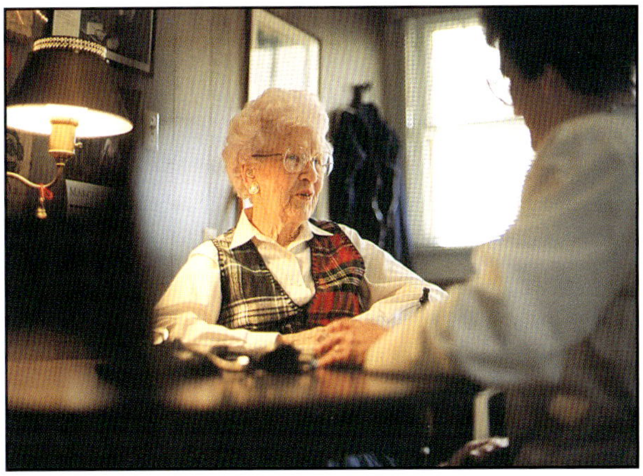

AT A GLANCE

- **Find a GP who is respectful and with whom you feel comfortable.**
- **Optimum diabetes care requires regularly scheduled GP consultations for adequate review and management.**
- **Look for a GP who is experienced in diabetes care and who has an organised approach.**
- **Use your GP as a health care resource to refer you on when you need specialist help.**
- **Don't be afraid to seek a second opinion.**

These are GPs who are genuinely interested in each person who consults them and who involve them in decisions affecting their health care.

Good general practice is based on providing the best care and access to resources for all who seek help and advice. The GP is the person's advocate when negotiating the health care system.

People seeking advice from GPs may not always agree with them and GPs may challenge the views of those seeking advice.

What the GP believes is the best course of action may not be the easiest course of action for the person with diabetes.

The best advice for people with diabetes is to keep well informed.

You are on the right track if you can develop a professional relationship with your GP based on trust and cooperation. Ideally, you will be in control of your own care, liaising regularly with the GP who manages the broad picture of your diabetes while providing you with access to a broad range of services.

How to get the best care from your general practitioner

Diabetes care is complex. Many people only see their GP when they are feeling unwell or when they need a prescription or referral.

If neither of you has an opportunity to look at the diabetes in a strategic way, you may miss the big picture.

For optimum diabetes care, see your GP every three to four months about your diabetes and have an extended consultation every 6 to 12 months.

If your GP coordinates your diabetes care, ensure that once a year you have a full management review. During this process your GP will:

- review your blood glucose levels
- rule out complications and other cardiovascular risk factors
- discuss future management.

When to get specialist help

The depth and range of skills of each practitioner (whether specialist or general) varies greatly.

Some general practitioners have expertise and skills in special interest areas.

Others have limited skills in some areas but they will refer you to appropriate specialists as required.

Some larger practices cross-refer people with diabetes to other GPs in the practice who have a special interest in diabetes. This means that there is some flexibility surrounding which professional to see for specific concerns.

Arrangements can be different in country areas where there may be a lack of specialist care. Often GPs develop skills to fill gaps where specialists are not available.

Because of the importance of self-management of diabetes, it is a condition requiring good communication between people with the condition and their health professionals. The more candid the communication, the better the care.

Chapter 29

Travelling with Diabetes

◆ By Dr Paul Moffitt ◆

THESE days there is virtually no limit to where people with diabetes can travel, yet as recently as the 1980s they faced difficulties, whether travelling overseas or through remote parts of Australia.

These days, no matter how old you are, the type of diabetes you have, your destination or mode of transport, your preparation and travelling routine will be similar.

Preparation is vital before any trip but even more so if you have diabetes. The key is to make lists of things to do and take well ahead of departure.

Essential preliminary preparations

On the first list write essential matters which cannot be left until the last minute. Include contacts for health problems in the countries to be visited (and emergency contacts back home); list your vaccinations, passport renewal details (in case of loss), plus the names and addresses of diabetes services available at your destination.

This early preparation should also include vital phrases in the language of your destination. Approach your local high school or relevant foreign consulate requesting a written translation of essential sentences such as 'I have diabetes' and 'Please quickly give me some sugar or something to eat'.

It is important that you carry some form of identification – a bracelet, locket or, less desirably, a card stating the carrier has diabetes and requires certain medications. This is vital when travelling and should be obtained long before departure – ask Diabetes Australia or your local Diabetes Education Centre.

Insurance

Medicare is not responsible for health expenses incurred overseas, which can be very expensive. In a worst case scenario, imagine your passport, tickets, travellers' cheques, credit cards or luggage are stolen. What will you do?

The answer is to take out travel insurance before departure. It is cheap and covers your health and your possessions. Ask your travel agent or Diabetes Australia for details.

AT A GLANCE

- **Plan ahead by making lists.**
- **Carry a letter from your doctor saying you have diabetes and describing your medication requirements.**
- **Pack a *traveller's survival kit* which contains:**
  - **quick-acting carbohydrate (for example, glucose)**
  - **slow-acting carbohydrate snack (for example, dried fruits)**
  - **glucagon and syringes**
  - **quick-acting insulin (neutral, clear)**
  - **blood testing equipment**
  - **Medical Alert bracelet**
  - **basic first aid requirements**
  - **key contacts details at home and abroad**
  - **useful and relevant phrases in the language of your destination.**

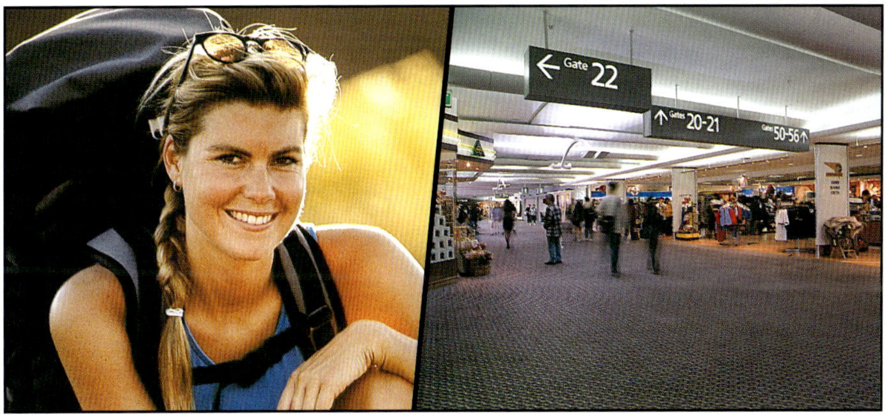

Your itinerary

Have your travel agent prepare an accurate itinerary of your trip, not only with departure and arrival times plus duration of flight sections, but also with stopovers and approximate meal or snack times (see Table 1 – page 106).

People on insulin need this information as it is essential for the safe and intelligent administration of their medication. For this reason, do not accept the excuse that such information is not available. This is also a good time to notify the airline of any special needs you or your child with diabetes may have during the flight.

Personal documents

A list of personal documents is another list to prepare ahead of time. It includes Australian and foreign currency, travellers' cheques, passport, air tickets, health certificate, international credit card, addresses of contacts, letter from your doctor and itinerary details.

Carry copies (include serial numbers of original documents) and store separately from the original to ensure that, in case of loss, you still have a record of details to enable you to get replacements quickly.

Hand luggage

No matter what the mode of transport, whether in Australia or overseas, you will require hand luggage. Prepare a list of what this should contain ahead of departure. Take twice the quantity of medications you will require and divide equally between your hand luggage and that of your travelling companion. If you are travelling alone, have two full sets of your medications, for example, one in your hand luggage and the other in your stowed luggage.

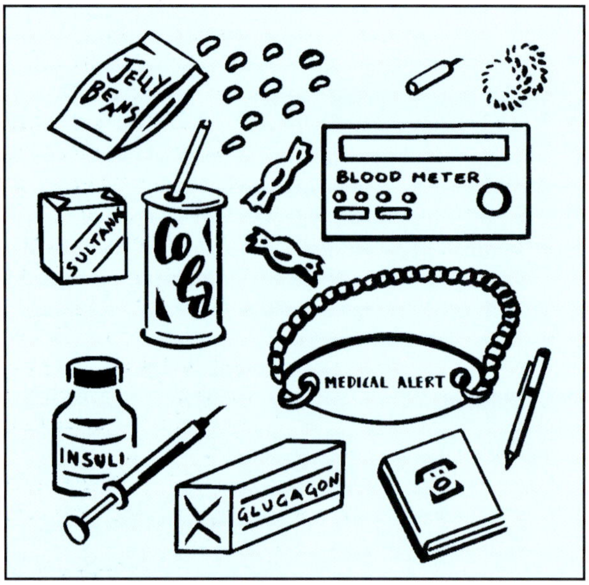

Food and drink en route

International flights usually offer an abundance of food, but this does not mean meals or snacks will be available when you require them. It is essential to carry extra carbohydrate in your hand luggage no matter what the mode of transport.

As any traveller will tell you, no matter what form of transport you take, delays are a fact of life. Be prepared – carry food with you on and off planes, buses or cars.

This is equally important for people with type 2 diabetes on diabetes tablets because tablets can produce hypoglycaemia and unconsciousness if a meal is missed.

Notify the airline at least 48 hours ahead of departure that you have diabetes and will need appropriately prepared meals. Not only will this ensure that you have the correct food, but also that the cabin crew will be aware of your diabetes.

Your specially requested meals may be served ahead of the other passengers' food, although this is of no real advantage unless you need to eat sooner and have specifically asked to be served first. An alternative is to eat the usual food served and to request extra bread.

Don't expect the airline to roll out the red carpet just because you have diabetes. Don't ask for unnecessary services such as meals outside the scheduled times. However, a request for extra carbohydrate between meals would be rarely refused, particularly if you're carrying a letter from your doctor (see the example of the doctor's letter below).

Drinking adequate fluid is also important. Travellers tend to become dehydrated, especially if they drink alcohol, so remember to drink lots of fluid (and not too much alcohol!)

Example of doctor's letter:

To Whom It May Concern:

Re: Mr/Ms S. Smith of 4 Brown Street, Smithtown, Victoria.

Mr/Ms Smith has type 1 diabetes. He/She is therefore carrying insulin, glucagon, syringes and equipment for testing the blood and urine for the presence of sugar. He/She also has other medications incuding Oroxine (thyroxine).

His/Her insulin dosage is Actrapid (Novo Nordisk) 8-12 units before each meal with Humulin UL (Eli Lilly) 42 units at 10.00pm.

He/She is knowledgeable about the management of diabetes and it is unlikely he/she will have any medical problems while travelling. However, any requests for food or non-alcoholic drinks should be immediately granted.

I would appreciate any assistance you can give my patient.

Yours sincerely

DR C.M. THROUGH

Upon arrival

One of the joys of travelling is to eat the local food but in some countries this must be done with discretion. The scenery might be a delight, but the diarrhoea which comes after indiscreet eating or drinking is not. Avoid drinking water, milk or other liquid from unsealed bottles; plus eating uncooked vegetables, salads and peeled fruit.

Mineral water bottled by reputable firms is available in most countries. However, in spite of the utmost diligence, you can expect one of your party – maybe you – to develop traveller's diarrhoea, so be prepared.

Insulin

As already stated, carry your medication in your hand luggage and in your travelling companion's hand luggage. If you are travelling alone, keep the second set of medications in your stowed luggage, with one exception.

Be aware if stowing insulin in the baggage compartment that baggage in some aircraft occasionally reaches freezing point, thus destroying insulin.

It is highly unlikely that this will occur on a large, international airline, but it is possible with some older or smaller aircraft on long flights. Insulin which has frozen and thawed looks no different so there is no way of determining its status.

To reduce the likelihood of insulin being frozen, pack it in a polystyrene container and further insulate by wrapping in clothing and placing it in the centre of your suitcase.

Heat also destroys insulin so, apart from carrying it in a polystyrene container, don't leave it in glove boxes, trunks or roof racks of motor vehicles; nor in outside pockets of back packs, or near heat sources such as engines.

Insulin is *not* affected by airport baggage scanning x-ray equipment.

All insulin used in Australia and New Zealand is 100 units/ml. This is also available in the UK, the USA and many other countries, although in some areas such as parts of Europe only more dilute insulins may be available.

If forced to buy these more dilute insulins – 40 units/ml or 80 units/ml, buy the correct syringe at the same time and use your own dosage with that syringe.

Do *not* purchase a syringe without a marking to identify it as being designed for U40 or U80 insulin.

If in doubt, use your own U100 syringes and adjust the dosage accordingly. U40 insulin used in your U100 syringe requires two-and-a-half times as much fluid as your U100 strength insulin. For example, a dosage of 30 units of U40 needs 30 x 2½ = the equivalent of 75 units in your U100 syringe.

Using U80 insulin in your U100 syringe requires 1¼ times the usual dose and therefore 30 x 1¼ = the equivalent of 37½ units in your U10 syringe.

The insulin used in an insulin pen in Australia is also U100 and can be used in an ordinary U100 syringe if the pen is broken, lost or stolen. Remember you don't need to put air in first if taking insulin out of a penfill. Remember to take a few additional syringes as well as your pen.

Insulin dosage

Insulin dosage should not be of concern during travel unless there is or will be a marked change in your exercise or eating routine. A rapid change in time zone as you travel will also have an effect. Any change in meal plan should have been anticipated and prepared for through consultation with your doctor or dietitian. If you have access to appropriate recipe books or restaurants, you may wish to experiment with anticipated dishes before you leave.

Major changes in exercise are covered in chapter 7 – Diabetes and Exercise – and are unlikely except with those people experienced in such changes. The basic rule is that if you expect to engage in prolonged exercise, either increase your carbohydrate intake before, during and after exercise and/or reduce your insulin dosage before the exercise. This will be a matter of judgment based on experience.

Airline flights towards the north or south do not create significant time changes and won't interfere with insulin dosage. However, eastward and westward flights, depending on their duration, may cause substantial changes which need to be considered when adjusting your insulin dosage.

The problem is that flying east is going in the opposite direction to the passage of the sun, which shortens the day. In other words, if you had stayed in Sydney you would have eaten your evening meal at 6pm knowing the next day's pre-breakfast insulin was 13 hours away.

However, if you had flown to, say, Los Angeles, the time there would be midnight, not 6pm as in Sydney, and the next day's pre-breakfast insulin would be only seven hours away, six hours earlier than it would be had you stayed in Sydney.

Conversely, flying in a westerly direction means travelling with the sun, extending the day and making the time between pre-breakfast insulins longer than if you had stayed at home. This means that you need to change your insulin schedule to make up for the change in the length of the day you are travelling.

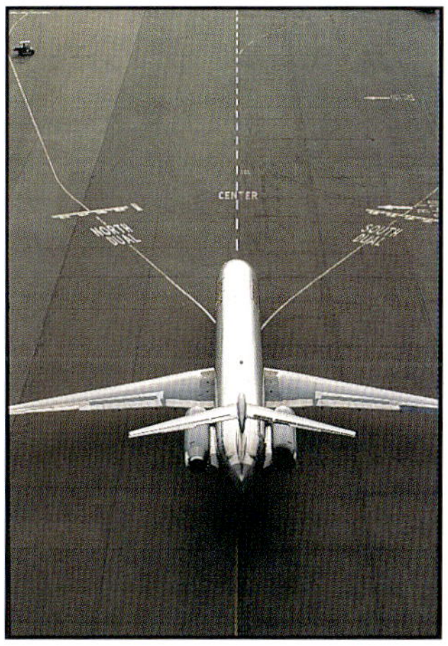

This won't be of great importance if your travel time between the Australian departure point and destination is less than four hours.

No one on insulin should undertake a long air flight without some basic information upon which to make intelligent decisions about insulin dosage.

That is why it is imperative to demand information from your travel agent well ahead of departure that will allow you to compile a chart similar to Table 1 (page 106). Information required for each leg of the flight is:

- departure time
- duration of flight
- local time of arrival at each stop and time spent there before next take-off
- the approximate delay after each take-off before meals or snacks are served.

Don't be put off if your travel agent seems reluctant. The information is available so do not accept excuses. After all, why should some uninterested or uninformed person jeopardise your health?

Whether you are flying north, south, east or west, keep your watch on your home time and use this as a guide to when your insulin should be taken.

The dosage may require some adjustment in size or timing, depending on other factors during the flight.

Armed with the knowledge of the times of meals during the flight, you should be able to predict increases or decreases in dosage. However, in all cases, these decisions are easily verified by testing your blood sugar every two or three hours throughout the flight. You may also wish to test for the presence of ketones in the urine if the blood glucose is high.

Regardless of the direction or duration of your

flight, you are unlikely to experience any great difficulties if you use an insulin pump or basal long-acting insulin once daily, with small dosages of a short-acting insulin ahead of your three main meals.

If you are on once or twice-daily single or combined insulins you'll require changes, the complexity of which will differ depending on your normal daily dosage.

If you strike a single blood glucose estimation above normal, it is no cause for alarm unless it is associated with moderate or heavy ketones – an unlikely event but one which requires immediate short-acting insulin.

A second or third moderately raised blood glucose level without ketones in the urine is also no cause for alarm if the routine insulin injection is due shortly. If not, consider an extra injection of short-acting insulin.

When considering whether or not to take extra short-acting insulin, be aware that mid-flight hypoglycaemia is not recommended. Safety is the key to success in the air – not perfect control of your diabetes. Therefore, design your adjustments to insulin or meals to avoid hypoglycaemia.

Hyperglycaemia and/or keto-acidosis is unlikely but hypoglycaemia is a possibility if you make, or are advised to make, poorly considered dosage changes.

If you don't own a glucose meter, get a prescription from your doctor or see Diabetes Australia for blood glucose test strips which compare the colour on the strip with those on the strip container. These strips are easy to read, but practise using them before your trip.

If you want to learn the procedure, ask your Diabetes Australia branch for your nearest Diabetes Education Centre.

If you plan to travel with your own blood monitor, don't forget to take spare batteries.

If your flight is in an easterly direction, you'll experience a shorter day and require less insulin. If your flight is in a westerly direction, you'll experience a longer day and require more insulin.

People flying east with a shortened day should reduce their morning, intermediate or long-acting insulin by 20–30 per cent unless they also receive an intermediate or long-acting insulin before the evening meal, in which case reduce this insulin.

There will be occasions when the normal evening short-acting insulin dosage might also have to be reduced or even omitted, such as when you reach your destination around midnight, local time, before the normal evening insulin was due. The same could apply if you were still en route eastward without any prospect of a meal within the next six hours.

Westward flights lasting less than four hours rarely require insulin dosage adjustment. Flights longer than four hours extend the day and therefore the amount of food taken, meaning an increase in insulin requirements.

This is best achieved by giving an extra small dosage of short-acting insulin, or you could use intermediate-acting insulin – the key being in each case the maximum effect of the insulin must not occur when you are asleep.

Insulin should never be taken until the meal is in front of you or within sight. Arrival at your destination does not mean that you can relax as either hypoglycaemia or hyperglycaemia could occur then or the following day. You may require extra short-acting insulin at unusual times throughout the day or night after arrival or, alternatively, snacks to prevent hypoglycaemia brought on by unexpected delays in customs or elsewhere.

Jet lag

Jet lag is caused by a number of factors, particularly because the body's natural daily rhythm cannot change fast enough to keep pace with rapid changes from one time zone to another. The effects of jet lag are aggravated by lack of sleep, excessive alcohol and lack of exercise. You can accomplish a degree of exercise by walking up and down the aisle of the plane and walking – rather than sitting – in transit lounges during stopovers.

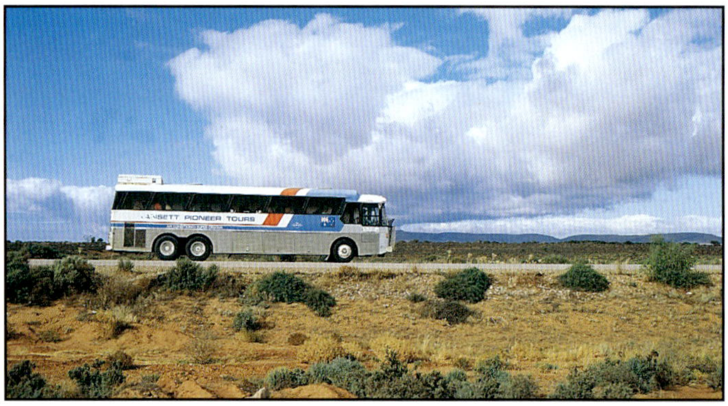

Even a few hours sleep is beneficial and may be easier if you use earplugs (obtainable from any pharmacy) and a short-acting sedative. Using a sedative for the first few nights after arrival may speed up your body's adjustment to the new time zone.

What to do if you get sick

Chapter 14 – Sick Days – Feeling Unwell? – contains the essential elements you'll need to care for yourself during an acute illness away from home.

Soft drinks and biscuits are usually easily purchased and dried packet soups are neither heavy nor bulky and may be just the thing when you're too ill to eat anything else. You can buy a small electric coil to heat broth, coffee or tea at most electrical stores.

If you use insulin and are ill, remember to test your urine for ketones. The presence of moderate or heavy ketones is an ominous sign and demands an urgent medical consultation. The casualty department of a hospital is usually the source of the quickest and best treatment.

Blood and urine testing

Chapter 10 – Self-monitoring of Blood Glucose – explains that urine testing has only a minor role for people on insulin but a greater role for those whose diabetes is controlled by food alone or food and tablets.

Non-insulin users should test more frequently than usual while travelling because a different food and exercise schedule may either markedly improve or worsen their diabetic control.

If you don't use insulin, ask your doctor before departure what to do if there is a sudden and persistent increase or decrease in the amount of glucose in your urine.

If you use a blood glucose meter, remember that it may malfunction or be stolen on your travels so practise strip reading for a few weeks before departure. In case readout is not possible with the meter, carry an emergency supply of visually read strips.

Medications

As explained, you'll travel with two sets of medications plus carry a letter from your doctor explaining your medications, with both trade and generic names. The generic (or real) name will be useful in places where trade names differ from those used in Australia.

If you use insulin, carry one or more ampoules of glucagon when travelling in remote areas of Australia or overseas. If you are unconscious through hypoglycaemia, you'll regain consciousness within 15 minutes of receiving an intramuscular glucagon injection.

Drill your travelling companion in the practice of giving a glucagon injection. If you are prone to hypoglycaemia and travelling alone, instruct another person such as a flight attendant.

Additional points for safe travelling

- Most States and Territories have travel centres listed in the phone book. Staff at these centres are experts and will advise on all aspects of travel.
- You may need medication prescriptions from your doctor.
- Travel with effective sunscreen lotion and insect repellent in hot climates.
- Take mosquito repellents into malarial areas. Malaria is common in some countries and some forms may be fatal. Drugs used to treat or prevent malaria are effective but may cause side-effects. Discuss treatment with a medical practitioner or obtain advice from the Department of Health. Information is contained in *Malaria Guidelines for Medical Practitioners*, produced by the National Health and Medical Research Council of Australia.
- Carry soluble painkiller for infants and an antibiotic ointment or a paint to treat cuts, blisters or minor injuries.

Diarrhoea and travelling

Traveller's diarrhoea has been around so long it has been given quaint names like Bali Belly and Montezuma's Revenge. These names suggest that the condition is short-lived and harmless, which it generally is but not always. Some cases cannot be self-treated, such as when there is blood in the bowel motion and a raised temperature. In these cases the patient requires medical attention.

However, the majority of travellers with diarrhoea can treat themselves, a procedure requiring two stages. The first stage is to try to stop the diarrhoea.

Use drugs such as Imodium™ or Lomotil™ to suppress the contractions of the bowel and stop the diarrhoea. These drugs cannot be used for children under the age of 12 and an alternative is Kaomagma. Imodium and Lomotil should not be continued if there is a prolonged fever or blood in the bowel motions. In these cases seek medical advice immediately.

If the diarrhoea lasts longer than 48 hours, you can use drugs to kill the organism responsible for the diarrhoea. This is the second stage.

Bactrim™, Resprim™ and Septrim™ are trade names for a combination of two drugs used to treat a number of medical conditions, including the organism responsible for traveller's diarrhoea. People of all ages can take these drugs.

Another effective treatment is tetracycline or doxycyline, which cannot be used for children or during pregnancy or breast-feeding. Probably the best drug for the treatment of traveller's diarrhoea is norfloxacin.

Don't use any of these drugs for longer than five days and be aware that they do not kill all the organisms responsible for diarrhoea, for example, cholera.

If you're visiting a country where doxycyline is the drug of choice for the prevention of malaria, you are fortunate in that doxycycline also gives some protection against traveller's diarrhoea.

If you know from experience that you will develop traveller's diarrhoea every time you visit a certain country, you may wish to take low doses of these drugs throughout your visit, providing it is no longer than two or three weeks. The daily dosage for an adult is 100 mg of tetracycline or doxycyline or one double-strength tablet of Bactrim™, Resprim™ or Septrim™.

All medications for traveller's diarrhoea can have serious side-effects so always seek medical advice before using them.

The fluid lost in the diarrhoea is an essential component of the human body and must be replaced or dehydration will occur, which can lead to death in the very young or old. It is essential if you have diarrhoea that you drink adequate replacement fluid in the form of broths or other sterile, non-alcoholic beverages.

Travelling with chronic illness

If you have a medical condition which may flare up while you're overseas, anticipate the worst. Take all the medications you would need if the problem arose. For example, if you have colitis, carry prednisone and salazopyrin and be aware how to use them.

If you get in a bind you can generally phone your general practitioner or specialist, no matter where you are. Lots of my patients have phoned me from overseas with concerns about their insulin dosage during times of illness. Let's face it, the price of the phone call is preferable to seeking, finding and paying for medical advice in the overseas country. Besides, advice from your own practitioner will always be preferable to that given by somebody who does not know you or your history and may speak a different language.

Motion sickness (sea sickness)

People with a past history of motion or sea sickness can reduce these symptoms by using Avomine™ (promethazine), Dramamine™ or Travacalm™ (diphenhydramine). Don't use these drugs if you are pregnant. Don't drive or operate machinery if you use these drugs as they may impair your judgment, especially when combined with alcohol.

Table 1 Frank Harris

	Am	Pm
Humulin R©	14	6
Humulin NPH©	36	16

HOME TIME	AIRPORT	LOCAL TIME ARR.	LOCAL TIME DEP.	DURATION	FROM DEPATURE TO MEAL	FROM DEPATURE TO SNACK	INSULIN	OTHER*
1545	SYDNEY		1545	9½ hrs				
1700							Humulin R© 4	Blood Test
1800					2 hrs		Humulin NPH© 12	
1900								
2000								Blood Test
2100								
2200								
2300								
2400								
0100	BANGKOK	1015						Blood Test
0200	BANGKOK			1¼ hrs	At Bangkok Airport			Walk around
0300	BANGKOK		1130					
0400				12 hr 25 min		¾ hr		
0500								Blood Test
0600								
0700								
0800							Humulin R© 6-10	Blood Test
0900								
1000								
1100								
1200								Blood Test
1300								
1400					11hrs		Humulin R© 6	
1500							Humulin NPH© 36	
1600	LONDON	0555						Blood Test

* After arrival in London take additional Humulin R© between 1100 and 1400 hours, if necessary, then normal evening dosage. Blood glucose levels under 7 mmol/L require extra food. Meals and snacks listed are those provided by the airline.

Chapter 30

Diabetes and Discrimination

◆ By Dr Aidan McElduff ◆

DISCRIMINATION occurs when someone is treated unfairly or less fairly than someone else in the same situation and – for the purposes of this chapter – due to that person having diabetes.

Protection against discrimination is important to Australians and there are various laws, tribunals and commissions to prevent or correct discrimination against various groups.

Although there are no specific laws relating to diabetes, discrimination based on the condition would be covered by the *Human Rights and Equal Opportunity Commission Act 1986*, the *Disability Discrimination Act 1992* and possibly others.

In practice, most problems relate to work or employment. Other areas of concern relate to sport and recreation, insurance, superannuation and driving.

AT A GLANCE

- **It is illegal to use diabetes as a reason not to employ a person unless there is good evidence that diabetes would prevent the person from adequately performing the genuine and reasonable requirements of the position.**
- **There are no specific discrimination laws relating to diabetes.**
- **Discrimination based on the condition is covered by the *Human Rights and Equal Opportunity Commission Act 1986*, the *Disability Discrimination Act 1992* and others.**
- **Most problems relate to work or employment.**
- **Contact Diabetes Australia if you believe you have been discriminated against because of your diabetes.**
- **There is an official policy on driving and diabetes (phone 02 6289 1430 for information).**

Diabetes Australia and discrimination

Diabetes Australia is your consumer representative group. In the absence of a formal policy from the organisation, here is this author's summarised interpretation of Diabetes Australia's approach to discrimination. Diabetes Australia ...

- opposes discrimination in situations where the fact that a person has diabetes is of no relevance
- emphasises the need for fairness in the treatment of people with diabetes in situations where diabetes is an issue
- recommends individual consideration in difficult areas rather than applying blanket laws.

Where the individualisation of policy comes into consideration is when there is a clash between an individual's rights and responsibilities and the rights and responsibilities of society at large. This clash has been outlined in the National Health and Medical Research Council's (NHMRC) policy on diabetes and driving.

Diabetes and driving

The NHMRC, in conjunction with the Australian Diabetes Society (the medical and scientific section of Diabetes Australia), has formalised Australian policy on driving and diabetes (phone 02 6289 1430, 24 hrs for information).

The introduction of this policy stresses the need to balance the usual rights and responsibilities of persons with diabetes to hold a driving licence against the need to protect the person with diabetes, and the public at large, against the consequences of hypoglycaemia while driving.

The policy was greatly influenced by the growing evidence that diabetes – including type 1 diabetes – was not a significant contributor to accidents.

The policy emphasises the need to balance the individual's rights against the need to protect both individual and public. The policy reinforces an approach which:

- individualises decision-making
- uses evidence as it becomes available
- emphasises the responsibilities which come with accessing one's rights.

Your responsibilities

As a person with diabetes, you have a responsibility to handle your diabetes appropriately to avoid increasing the risk of adverse outcomes. For example, while driving you need to actively follow strategies which will lessen the likelihood of having hypoglycaemia.

Diabetes and insurance

Dr John Carter discusses Insurance and Diabetes in chapter 31. The chapter acknowledges insurance is an area where people with diabetes may be treated differently. A person with diabetes seeking life insurance will receive a loading on their premium. Diabetes Australia argues that this loading must be fairly determined; and must take into account up-to-date statistical data on the risk involved, plus an appreciation of modern treatment approaches. It is worth noting that the Disability Discrimination Act does not cover superannuation or insurance when decisions are made on actuarial or other reasonable information.

Diabetes and work

Getting the job

Fear and/or misunderstanding of diabetes is still common in our community and among employers. They believe that people with diabetes will 'black out' all the time, or have frequent sick days.

During the job interview or on the application form, you may be asked to identify health problems. You only have to state you have diabetes *if it is relevant to the position*. You should be prepared to answer questions as to how diabetes may affect your work. For example, stating how you would adjust your insulin/tablets/eating routine to accommodate the work shifts involved, or mentioning the need for occasional short breaks to have a snack or test your blood to prevent problems.

If required, you should be able to convince the interviewer that you are knowledgeable and have the ability to cope with your diabetes.

You should stress the positive aspects of having diabetes, such as following a healthy lifestyle, having yearly medical checks, following routines and, above all, having a responsible attitude towards your health, which rubs off on to other life attitudes, including your work.

It is illegal to use diabetes as a reason not to employ a person unless there is good evidence that diabetes would prevent the person from adequately performing the genuine and reasonable requirements of the position.

Unfortunately, some jobs are not suitable for people with diabetes. These jobs include working in dangerous situations; or jobs in which there may be sudden, unpredictable and unavoidable calls to continue working, preventing you having a snack, which would put you at increased risk of hypoglycaemia and place you and others at risk.

You can therefore understand why a commercial pilot cannot have diabetes requiring medication. Other similar occupations might include steeplejack or commercial diver.

Remember to ask your endocrinologist for a letter of support discussing your health and knowledge of diabetes. Ask to deal particularly with any difficult aspects of the job for which you have applied.

Colleagues

It is probably wise to give workmates a simple explanation about diabetes so that they understand what is happening if you suddenly need to eat. Be sure that they know what to do in the event of an unexpected hypoglycaemic episode.

Responsibilities

It is important that you do not expect to use diabetes to gain special treatment, and if your diabetes does cause a problem, you take steps to correct this problem.

Summary of hints for work

Looking for work

- Apply for jobs for which you are suited and qualified.
- Mention diabetes on your application form or at interview if necessary or if requested.
- Discuss your diabetes in an interview only in relation to the work you will be doing.
- Stress the positive aspects of diabetes where possible.

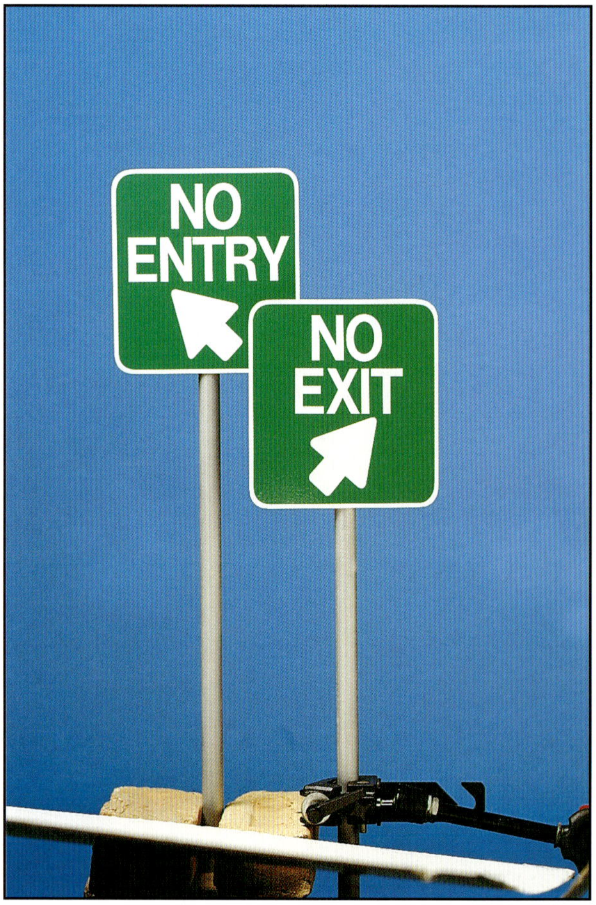

What to do if problems arise

- Take steps to solve the problem yourself.
- Discuss the problem with your supervisor.
- Discuss the problem with the occupational health staff.
- Contact your diabetes doctor, diabetes nurse educator or another member of your health support team.
- Contact your union representative.
- Contact Diabetes Australia.

Diabetes and society

Just as you have responsibilities that accompany your rights, so does society. Should society make decisions which disadvantage people with diabetes, then society has a responsibility to those people.

This is an evolving area influenced by political thinking. However, examples of this responsibility are:

- The community rating system for health insurance. A person with diabetes does not have to pay more for health insurance.
- The National Diabetic Services Scheme which allows cheaper purchase of glucose monitoring strips, insulin syringes and needles.

As our society evolves in the current user-pays environment, the principle of society's responsibility to the individual must be a consideration in future decision/policy-making. One basic premise in the Australian health care system is the goal of universal coverage and equitable access to health care.

This principle needs to be guarded, particularly by groups with chronic diseases such as diabetes which require long-term care.

Complications

I have avoided discussing specific complications of diabetes. However, the rules outlined apply equally to those with specific complications. The need for individualisation of assessment would remain important.

Be aware that some complications may be covered by other interest groups. For example, those with visual impairment could be advised and assisted, if required, by the Royal Blind Society.

Summary

Diabetes Australia's position appears to be that people with diabetes can be treated differently from other people without diabetes but such treatment should be based fairly on the best evidence available and individually determined.

The rights of an individual can clash with the rights of the community and this clash must be reconciled. People with diabetes have a responsibility to minimise potential risks.

What to do if you are discriminated against

Discuss the problem with your doctor, health care team and/or Diabetes Australia before thinking of a legal approach. Diabetes Australia has a great deal of experience with discrimination and can help. Many battles, which never receive any publicity, are won on behalf of people with diabetes.

Insurance and Diabetes

◆ By Dr John Carter ◆

FOR most people, life insurance is a case of picking up the telephone and choosing the lowest premium. Not so for people with diabetes.

For many years the diabetes community has been concerned about the expense and hassles associated with obtaining life insurance.

Not always easy to obtain, when a life insurance policy is granted, the premium is considerably higher than for people without diabetes.

To a certain degree you can understand this. However, many of us believe statistics used by the insurance industry to justify these increased premiums are outdated and fail to acknowledge the benefits of modern diabetes management.

AT A GLANCE

- **People with diabetes traditionally faced problems when seeking to take out insurance or obtain a driver's licence. However, improved life expectancy figures and consumer pressure are having an effect.**
- **Insurance policy prices are coming down due not only to improved health outcomes but to market competition and lobbying by Diabetes Australia.**
- **People with diabetes will benefit from adequate informed preparation before applying to an insurance company for cover.**
- **If you encounter any setbacks when seeking insurance, employment packages or specialised licences, contact your local Diabetes Australia office for advice.**

Good news

There is no question that regular breakthroughs in diabetes treatment have improved quality of life and increased life span, yet some people are still denied insurance while others are charged annual premiums they regard as unfair.

The good news is that improved life expectancy figures and consumer pressure are having an effect and many Australian companies are changing their outlook, albeit more slowly than in other countries.

In Denmark, for instance, extensive studies documented during the past 50 years show improved quality of life and increased life span among people with diabetes. For example, the figures show that people with type 1 diabetes now live 15 to 30 years longer.

The findings have been accepted by the Danish insurance industry and the savings passed on to policyholders with diabetes.

The attitude of the Australian insurance industry is not so enlightened, although some progress is being made.

The company view

Offering insurance to people with diabetes does present difficulties for the underwriter.

This is because diabetes is not a single disorder but covers a cluster of possible conditions which are all related to disturbed metabolism of glucose. And just as there is no fixed definition of diabetes, there is no fixed rule when it comes to insurance.

For this reason it is unusual for pure life insurance – that is, insurance with the sum being payable on death or on survival to a specified date – to be turned down solely because of the proposer's diabetes.

Usually cover will be offered on some grounds.

Information required

Before final assessment of the proposal, the insurance company will require comprehensive medical information consisting of:

- a diabetes questionnaire regarding history and management of the condition
- a detailed report from the person's doctor, including the date of diagnosis, type of diabetes, nature of treatment and response to treatment
- a report on a current medical examination.

For larger policies, the company will require more comprehensive medical information.

The underwriter would take particular note if the medical information showed:

- childhood onset diabetes
- duration of diabetes of less than a year since diagnosis
- poor control of the condition
- poor self-management of the condition
- any existing diabetes-related complications
- additional medical or lifestyle risks
- inadequate documentation of medical history.

The assessment rating would become even more severe, perhaps even resulting in the proposal being turned down, if there were further complicating factors such as:

- evidence of kidney disease, particularly if large amounts of protein were detected in the urine
- evidence of diabetic retinopathy
- high blood pressure
- heart disease
- excessive alcohol intake
- smoking
- being overweight
- evidence of peripheral neuropathy
- unfavourable family history, particularly relating to early deaths from heart and kidney disease.

For adults with diabetes, the best terms are offered if diabetes is of short duration, such as less than 10 years, as long as there are none of the unfavourable factors listed above.

Generally speaking, the later the age of onset, the more favourably the company will look at the proposal.

Insurance premiums generally increase with age, plus advancing age often means other medical complications which may further limit availability of insurance. Because of this it is important to purchase insurance early.

The official policy

According to the Life Insurance Federation of Australia, the terms offered to people with diabetes – as with everyone else – are based on available statistical evidence supplemented by the considered judgment of medical experts, underwriters and actuaries.

Each proposal is treated strictly on its merits and in accordance with the underwriting policy of the company concerned, after consideration of evidence gathered at the time.

Each company could differ in some degree in its ratings, although the assessment criteria generally does not vary.

One company states: 'It needs to be borne in mind that it takes some time for both favourable and unfavourable developments in treatment, diagnosis, survival rates etc to be reflected in the terms offered.'

In addition, it should be emphasised that underwriting rules represent only part of the underwriting process and the differences in policy and competitive factors will often result in different offers from different insurance companies on proposals for the same person with diabetes.

Taking all this into consideration, insurance cover for people with diabetes is generally available in Australia, although the terms offered vary according to several criteria.

An otherwise healthy person with well-controlled diabetes can expect to be insured, although it may be with significantly increased premiums.

Influencing factors

There are some factors influencing premiums over which people with diabetes do have significant control. These include:

- excessive alcohol intake
- smoking
- control of blood pressure
- being overweight
- conscientious management of diabetes
- the presence of any additional medical or lifestyle risks.

Because insurance companies place such importance on good diabetic control and freedom from complications, be sure that your doctor understands the significance that will be placed on his or her medical report. Poorly presented medical evidence will undoubtedly result in a higher premium.

Advice on insurance

Advances in treatment continually occur in Australia and Diabetes Australia actively lobbies insurance companies, keeping them informed of the latest data relating to improvements in quality of life and life span.

Because of increased competition in the marketplace, Diabetes Australia supplies up-to-date advice on insurance policies available.

People with diabetes or at risk of contracting diabetes are urged to take out insurance as soon as possible. Those with diabetes can investigate the possibility of employment packages which include group insurance or join groups which may give them more favourable consideration.

If in doubt about life assurance, sickness, accident or travel insurance, ask Diabetes Australia for advice.

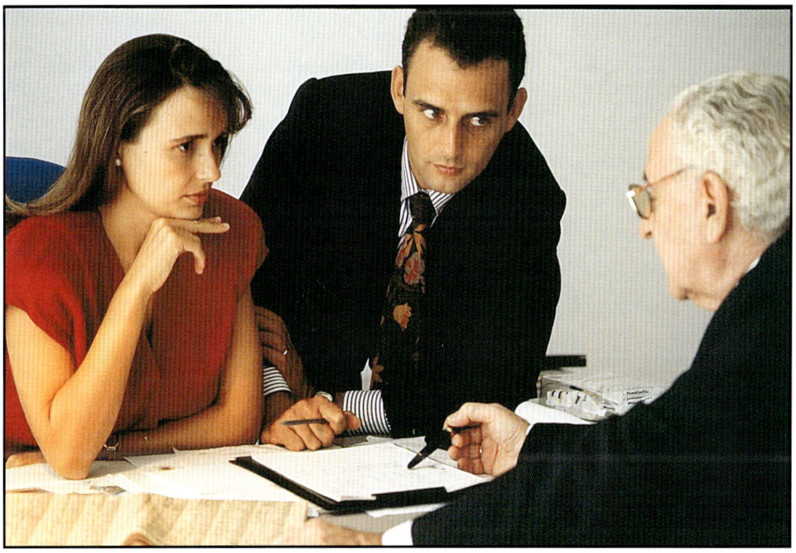

Superannuation

Superannuation can be regarded as an investment whereby a lump sum or pension, or combination of the two, will be paid to you when you retire. People who retire early, say, for medical reasons, receive a lower benefit.

This investment component is not specifically affected by the presence of diabetes, but many superannuation policies also include life insurance and/or disability insurance. The factors outlined earlier influence this type of policy.

Some workplaces have automatic superannuation/life insurance/disability insurance cover. This may be advantageous for a person with diabetes because the regular superannuation contributions would include the insurance premiums – without any loading.

Take superannuation into account and carefully study the fine print when you consider a new job.

Diabetes and driving

Traditionally, people with diabetes found it slightly more difficult to obtain a driver's licence than did those without diabetes. The main concern of the licensing authorities was the possibility of hypoglycaemia while driving and/or diabetes complications – especially eye problems – affecting the ability to drive safely.

These are understandable concerns when you consider the potential for danger – not just to the driver but to other people.

However, recent research suggests that the risks are not as great as first feared and, following intense lobbying from the Australian Diabetes Society (the medical and scientific section of Diabetes Australia), the National Health and Medical Research Council (NHMRC) endorsed Diabetes Australia's guidelines and most Australian States and Territories have either changed their regulations or are in the process of changing to comply with NHMRC guidelines.

In general, the guidelines for drivers with diabetes can be summarised as follows.

1. **Licences for driving cars and motorcycles:**
   (a) Diet control – no medical examination necessary.
   (b) Tablet treatment – medical examination every five years unless more frequent examinations are required by your doctor or a licence issuing officer.
   (c) Insulin-treated persons – two-yearly medical examinations but more frequent examinations will be necessary if required by your doctor or a licence issuing officer.
2. **Licences for buses, taxi trucks, articulated vehicles and dangerous goods vehicles:**
   (a) Diet controlled – annual medical examination (by a consultant physician) but more frequent examinations may be required at the discretion of the examiner or licensing authority.
   (b) Insulin-treated persons – ordinarily, these persons should not be eligible for this type of licence but a mechanism is available for the granting of the licence at the discretion of the Roads and Traffic Authority on the recommendation of a consultant physician. If the licence is granted, there should be annual review by a consultant physician.

Diabetes Australia feels strongly that there should be a balance between ensuring safety for all concerned when driving and minimisation of any unfair discrimination by licensing authorities against people with diabetes.

If you feel that you have been hard done by, please contact your local Diabetes Australia office for assistance.

Chapter 32

Further Resources

◆ Diabetes Australia by Shirley Murray ◆

AT A GLANCE

- **Each State and Territory has a Diabetes Australia office. Join for information, assistance, savings and advice.**
- **Reference literature and guidance on the latest and most up-to-date diabetes literature is available through Diabetes Australia.**
- **Information is also available from your health care team and, if they don't know the answers, they will refer you to others who do.**

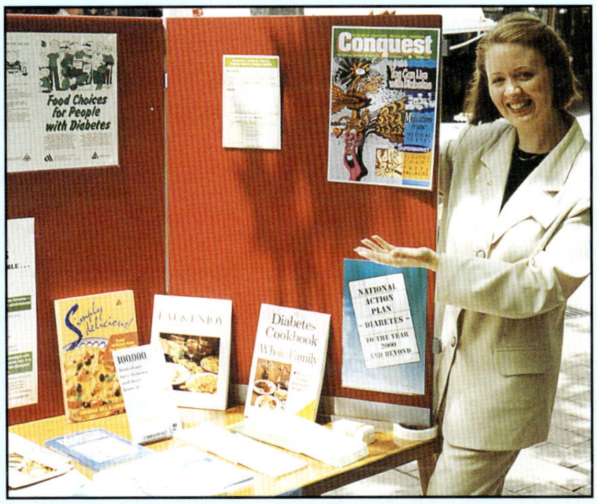

THE quest for sourcing additional resources to help with diabetes management continues through life. This book, *Diabetes & You – The essential guide*, is an excellent reference tool you can use to help your diabetes management.

However, eventually the desire to find out what is happening in areas such as research, the latest treatment techniques or where to go for specialised care may lead the person with diabetes to seek more information about these subjects.

A call to your State or Territory branch of Diabetes Australia will set you on the right track. Diabetes Australia is a national organisation representing people with diabetes. It is made up of eight State and Territory member bodies, plus scientific and educational arms.

Each capital city has a Diabetes Australia office.

Diabetes Australia is a member of the International Diabetes Federation. Apart from supporting and promoting research in Australia, it is also linked to worldwide diabetes information which it disperses to its members.

Most of the eight State and Territory organisations have branches or regional networks which provide services to rural areas.

The branches can provide assistance on a wide range of topics or refer you to specific services for specialised help.

Diabetes Australia provides the following information:

- Up-to-date reference material – videos, books, journals and reports. Many of the State and Territory organisations have established lending libraries for members' access.
- Details on the National Diabetic Services Scheme – a government initiative supplying products such as syringes and testing strips to people with diabetes at a reduced cost. This service is operated by Diabetes Australia.
- Information on health care for those travelling overseas, plus contact information about other member organisations abroad.
- Advice on life and sickness insurance.

  Diabetes Australia can:
  - provide access or referral to a range of other professional services, including diabetes education, nutrition and podiatry services
  - arrange an introduction to groups or self-help meetings where those with diabetes can share their experiences and feelings. The majority of State and Territory organisations conduct camps for children and young adults. Some also conduct family camps. Just ask your local branch office
  - provide details on national and local activities.

Membership of Diabetes Australia is easy. Contact your nearest State or Territory office or ask your doctor or diabetes nurse educator for an application form. All States and Territories charge a small fee. There is a discount for seniors. Membership ensures that you are swiftly notified of new publications, breakthroughs in diabetes management and activities in your area.

All members of Diabetes Australia receive a copy of *Conquest*, the national magazine, plus a copy of their local branch newsletter. Members are offered a discount on products and services provided by their State or Territory organisation.

Doctors and other health professionals

Specialists in diabetes care – usually endocrinologists – can provide you with a range of resource and educational material. Many hospital clinic paediatricians are also specialists in diabetes care. They can assist families who have a child with diabetes by sourcing educational materials and supplies or referring them on to other health professionals.

Most general practitioners carry information on diabetes and know where people can find further information and relevant services.

Diabetes nurse educators can be located at hospital clinics, Diabetes Australia or through the telephone book.

Some dietitians and podiatrists specialise in diabetes and these, too, can be contacted through hospital clinics, Diabetes Australia or the telephone book.

Your local pharmacy or community health centre may also be a source of information.

State and Territory libraries and/or bookshops often carry references of particular interest to people with diabetes, such as cookbooks. However, the management of diabetes is a rapidly developing health care area with new technology and scientific updates occurring regularly. Books can date quickly. Check with your doctor or diabetes nurse educator before you buy.

The development of new technologies plus new means of communication such as the internet and/or video telemetry are broadening the amount of information available from local and international sources.

Enquire at Diabetes Australia if this service is available in your area.

Phone 1800 640 862 for your nearest Diabetes Australia branch office or visit DA's website: www.diabetesaustralia.com.au

◆ Juvenile Diabetes Foundation Australia by Karen Barfoot ◆

AT A GLANCE

- **The Juvenile Diabetes Foundation Australia helps families of children, teens and young adults with diabetes.**
- **The foundation puts families of children with diabetes in touch with each other so that they can share experiences and provide mutual support.**
- **The foundation is an excellent and inexpensive source of diabetes information and literature, specially designed for children and young people with diabetes, their families and friends.**

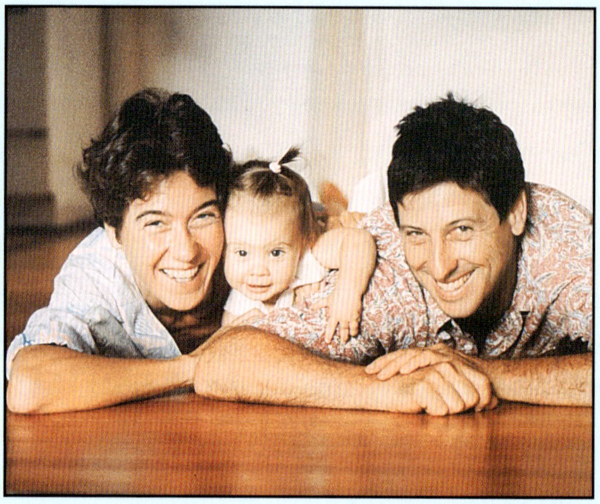

THE Juvenile Diabetes Foundation Australia (JDFA) is a non-profit health organisation dedicated to discovering a cure for diabetes and ways of preventing its complications through funding of basic and applied medical research.

Nationally, JDFA is represented in six State offices and specialises in type 1 diabetes, particularly in children.

Most of JDFA's members are families of children, teens and young adults with diabetes.

The foundation helps put parents of children with diabetes in touch with other parents so that families can establish a support network. This gives them the opportunity to share experiences and offer mutual advice and support.

JDFA is part of the Juvenile Diabetes Foundation International (JDFI), which supports the world's best diabetes research. This connection gives JDFA members access to international information, in particular the JDFI quarterly magazine, *Countdown*, the leading lay magazine on diabetes research, and JDFA's quarterly newsletter, *Update*.

JDFA offices keep a constant supply of literature written specifically for people with type 1 diabetes and their families. Some of the resources available from JDFA offices include:

- *Kids With Diabetes* video and brochure
- *In Control*, a book for teenagers with diabetes
- *Your Friend Has Diabetes*
- *Babysitting an infant or young child with diabetes*
- *Diabetic Complications*
- *Look on the Bright Side*, for teenagers
- Camp/school diabetes information sheet.

For a small annual subscription you can become a member of JDFA and take advantage of the information and resources plus JDFA's education and support services. Educational materials are usually provided either free to members or at a substantial discount.

An estimated 700,000 to 800,000 Australians have diabetes. This is an alarming figure, placing Australia in the category of one of the highest rates of diabetes incidence in the world. Yet those who do not have a family member with diabetes seem to know little about the condition. As a result, the insidious nature of diabetes is underestimated, reducing the sense of urgency in the Australian community to fund research to find a cure.

For this reason, the Juvenile Diabetes Foundation Australia acts as an advocate for the needs of children, teenagers and young adults with diabetes and their families. JDFA's aim is for national recognition of diabetes as a serious health issue. The organisation lobbies State and Territory Governments and the Federal Government on matters of significance to families of children with diabetes.

Increasingly, there is hope that diabetes and its complications can be cured. Significant progress has been made and JDFA funding has been involved in the following areas:

- causes of diabetes
- genetic factors in diabetes
- the immune system
- the auto-immune process
- understanding the basic mechanism of insulin-producing cells
- proteins, peptides, enzymes and other substances involved in diabetes
- the metabolic process and signals sent and received by cells
- transplantation and related procedures involving beta-cell replacement
- prevention – to prevent the disease from occurring and to prevent the disease from recurring after beta-cell replacement therapy
- complications – retinopathy (eyes), neuropathy (nerves), nephropathy (kidneys), vasculature (heart and stroke) and hypoglycaemia/labile.

JDFA funds such research through programs such as the Walk for the Cure and The Only Remedy is a Cure campaign.

Phone 1300 363 126 for your nearest JDFA branch office or visit JDFA's website: www.jdfa.org.au

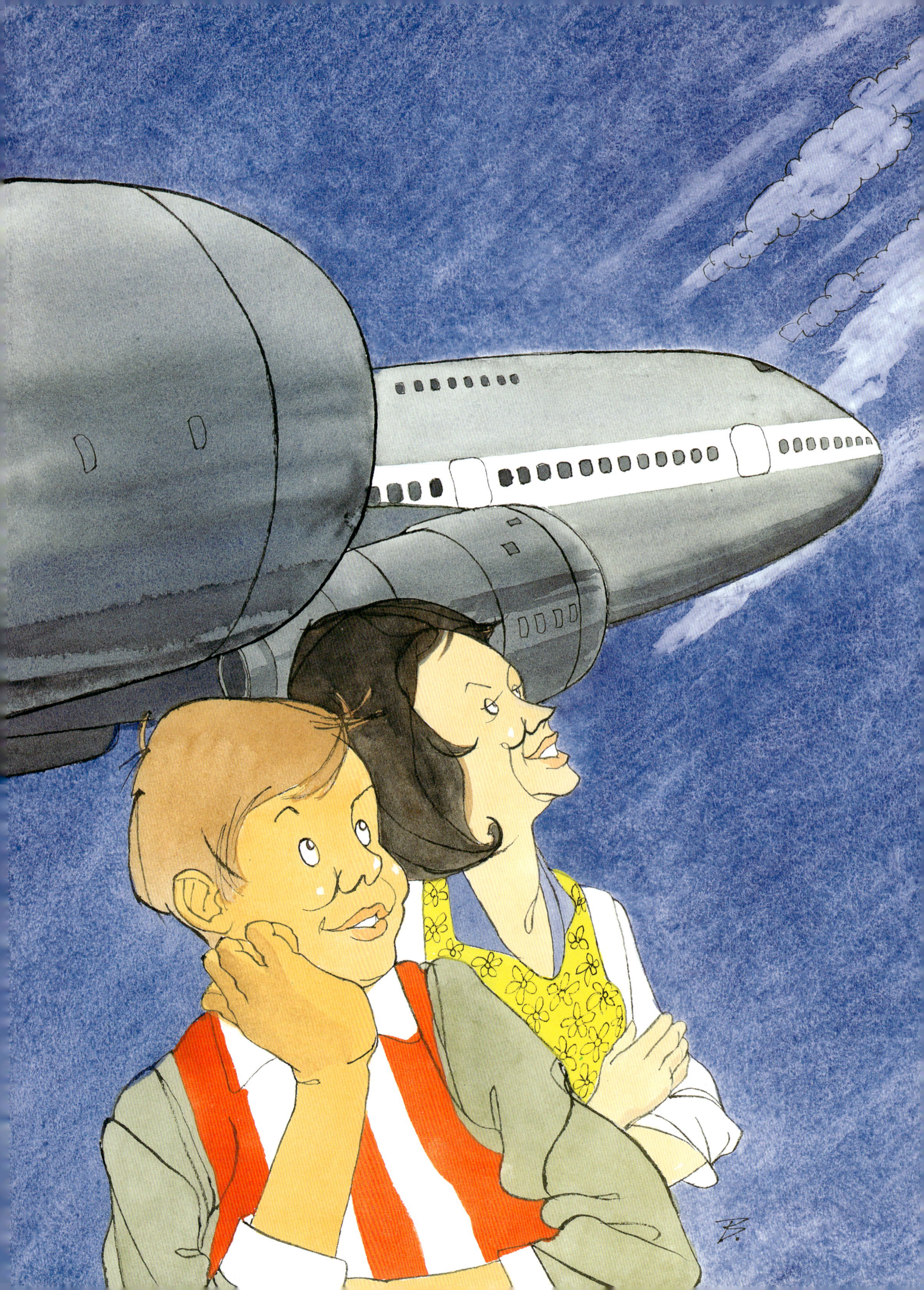

Chapter 33

The Genetics of Diabetes

◆ By Professor Susan Serjeantson ◆

IT is only to be expected that people with diabetes fear that their children will also develop the condition. Just as common and understandable is the fear of parents who have one child with diabetes that their other children will acquire the disorder.

However, type 1 and type 2 diabetes are distinct conditions and in each the causes of high blood glucose are different.

Type 1 diabetes results from a process that destroys the insulin-producing cells of the pancreas.

In type 2 diabetes there is insulin, but the body is in some way resistant to its action.

Each type of diabetes is caused by different genes and the importance of genetic factors has been demonstrated by studies of identical twins.

If an identical twin develops type 1 diabetes, the chance of the other twin getting diabetes is 1 in 3, compared with about 4 per 1,000 in the general population.

However, just because there is diabetes in the family does not mean that people genetically at risk automatically contract diabetes. In fact, two out of three identical twins do not get diabetes.

Additional factors such as viruses trigger the disease in people who have the genes for type 1 diabetes.

If an identical twin develops type 2 diabetes, it is likely that the other twin will also get the condition. In fact, the lifetime risk to the other twin is greater than 90 per cent. In other words, in type 2 diabetes, genetic factors are more important than in type 1 diabetes.

Because each form of diabetes is a distinctly different clinical and genetic disorder, each must be considered separately.

AT A GLANCE

- **Just because there is diabetes in the family does not mean that people genetically at risk will automatically contract diabetes.**
- **Genetic factors influence both types of diabetes, although each is a distinctly different clinical and genetic disorder.**
- **The majority of people with high risk antigens for type 1 diabetes never develop the condition.**
- **The overall chance of developing type 1 diabetes for a brother or sister of someone with the condition is 6 per cent, or about 1 in 20.**
- **Even though a person may have inherited a tendency to develop type 2 diabetes, food and exercise may postpone the onset of the condition or prevent it from developing.**
- **Relatives of people with type 2 diabetes are at risk of developing the condition.**

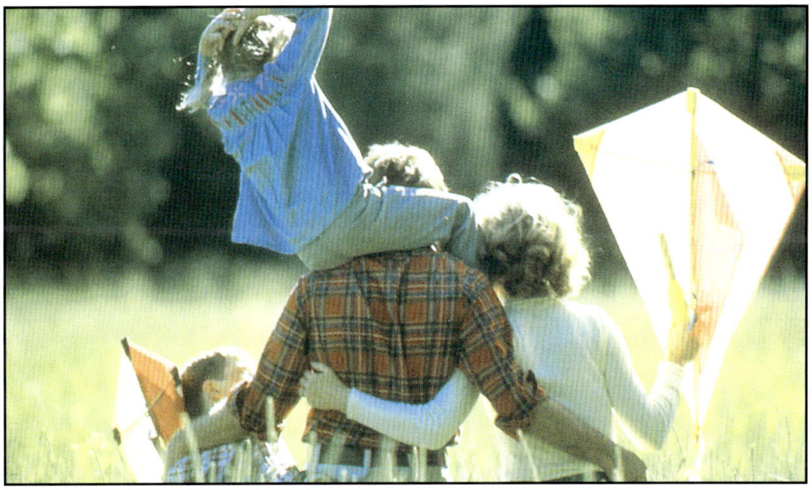

Type 1 diabetes

In the mid-1970s it was discovered that people with certain Human Leucocyte Antigens (HLAs) were more likely to develop type 1 diabetes than others.

HLAs are blood groups on white cells. Antigens are substances which, when injected into animal tissue, will stimulate production of antibodies. In the same way that red cells have antigens – such as the ABO system – white cells also have antigen systems.

The important antigen systems in type 1 diabetes are called HLA-DR and HLA-DQ. In the ABO system, people can be blood group A, B, O or AB. A person who has the AB blood group has inherited the A gene from one parent and the B gene from the other. In the same way, HLA genes are passed from one generation to the next, with each parent contributing one set of HLA genes to the child.

If a child inherits HLA-DR3 from one parent and HLA-DR4 from the other, its HLA type is DR3, DR4 and this combination gives the highest risk for diabetes.

If a child inherits HLA-DR2 from one parent and HLA-DR5 from the other, its HLA type is DR2, DR5 giving almost no chance of developing type 1 diabetes.

The high-risk antigens for diabetes are HLA-DR3 and HLA-DR4 yet, in spite of this, the majority of people with these HLA types never develop type 1 diabetes.

A recent study lead by Dr Glenys Thomson, an Australian working at the University of California, analysed statistics from several families with type 1 diabetes from Australia, Europe and the USA.

The study covered about 1,800 people with type 1 diabetes whose family members had been tested for HLA types. As the largest set of data compiled on type 1 diabetes, the study provided an answer to the common question: 'Will my other children get diabetes?'

The overall chance for a brother or sister of a type 1 diabetes patient developing type 1 diabetes is 6 per cent, or about 1 in 20. However, this overall figure masks the fact that some siblings have a low risk (1 in 75) while some have a much higher risk (1 in 5). This is because the actual risk for diabetes depends on the HLA types of the patient and that of the sibling.

If the patient has the HLA type DR3, DR4, while the sister or brother is also DR3, DR4, then the sibling has a risk for diabetes of 1 in 5 (19 per cent).

If the patient's sibling inherits neither DR3 nor DR4 from his or her parent, then the risk for diabetes is only 1 in 50 (2 per cent).

If the sibling inherits one of the high-risk HLA genes, then he or she also has a low (4 per cent) risk for diabetes.

The diagram at right shows how HLA-DR types are inherited and how brothers and sisters of a person with diabetes can have different risks for type 1 diabetes.

The precise risks for siblings of people with diabetes depend on HLA types of the person with diabetes and their sibling.

On average, if the person with diabetes and their sibling have identical HLA types, the risk for the sibling is 13 per cent. If the sibling shares one HLA antigen with the parent who has diabetes, the risk is 5 per cent. If the sibling has no HLA antigens in common with the parent who has diabetes, the risk is 2 per cent.

In one case in four, an unaffected brother or sister has HLA types identical with the person with diabetes. This means that in a family of five children, where one has type 1 diabetes, one sibling will, on average, have a higher risk for diabetes (13 per cent) while the others will have a lower risk (2–5 per cent).

These figures are reassuring to families where one child has type 1 diabetes. If healthy parents of an affected child are considering another pregnancy, they can be assured the risk for type 1 diabetes in a subsequent child is about 1 in 20 (6 per cent).

The risks given here are lifetime risks, calculated at birth. Clearly, the older the child, the less the risk for type 1 diabetes.

And so to the other most asked question: 'Will my children get diabetes?'

Adults with type 1 diabetes are often concerned with the possibility of passing on the disease to future offspring.

The risk for children of a father with type 1 diabetes is about 1 in 20 (6 per cent) and there is a lower risk for children of a mother with diabetes. In one study, this risk was only 1 in 100 (1 per cent).

Several studies have shown that children with a type 1 affected mother may have some immunity to developing diabetes, but we don't yet understand how this works.

When the father has diabetes, the risks for his children are once again dependent on the children's HLA types. There are low risks in some categories such as, for example, when the mother transmits the resistant DR2 type to the children.

The highest risk is for DR3, DR4 children, where the chance of diabetes exceeds 1 in 5.

Intending parents will make the ultimate decisions but, because individual cases vary, they may wish to obtain skilled advice from genetic counsellors.

Counsellors will present the facts to the best of their ability, taking into account family history, HLA types and so on.

The parents can then consider the facts and decide whether to have children, or whether to have more children if one has type 1 diabetes. Counsellors only provide the facts; the decision is made by the parents.

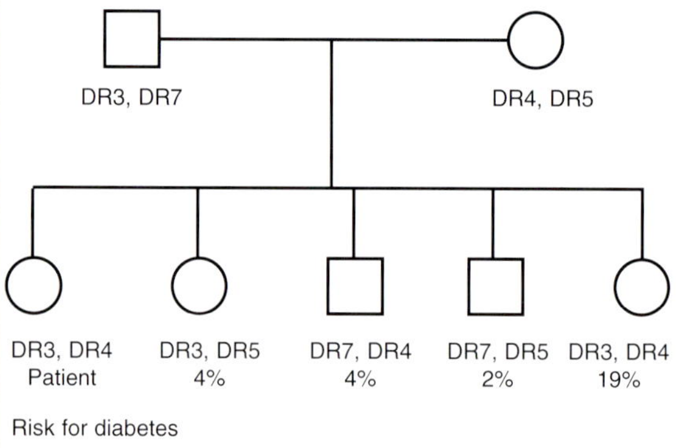

Inheritance of HLA-DR types. Siblings of a type 1 diabetes patient have different risks for disease, depending on their HLA-DR types.

Type 2 diabetes

The mechanics which cause type 2 diabetes are unknown.

This is because diabetes causes so many disorders in bodies' sugar and fat metabolism, that it is difficult to pinpoint the primary defect among many secondary problems.

Research is now focused at genetics to try and define the basic inherited defects of the condition.

Candidate genes – including the insulin gene and the gene for the insulin receptor – have been examined in great detail at the molecular level.

There are rare instances when defects in these genes cause diabetes but usually, in type 2 diabetes, these genes are normal.

Research attention is now on other genes encoded with insulin receptor pathways. So far no specific genetic defects have been identified, but it appears that many different genetic changes can result in type 2 diabetes.

We do know that there is a risk to relatives of people with type 2 diabetes.

There is a very high rate of concordance of diabetes in identical twins. If one twin develops type 2 diabetes, the other has a greater than 60 per cent chance of developing the condition.

However, for type 2 diabetes, even though a person may have inherited a tendency to develop diabetes, food and exercise may postpone the onset of the condition or diabetes may not develop at all.

There seems to be a gene dosage effect in type 2 diabetes. When one parent has type 2 diabetes, the chance of offspring developing diabetes is about 1 in 10, but if both parents have type 2 diabetes, the chance of offspring developing diabetes is about 1 in 5. Likewise, the condition may develop earlier in people who have inherited two 'diabetic' genes.

Type 2 diabetes is a mature onset disease and the increased prevalence of type 2 diabetes in some populations may reflect an increase in life expectancy.

In Caucasian populations, disease onset is often at 60 years or older. In contrast, in high diabetes prevalence groups such as Pacific Islanders, disease onset is often at 40 years or older, with onset in 30–40 year olds not uncommon.

In some women with a tendency to diabetes, pregnancy can cause the condition to develop earlier than would otherwise be the case. In other women, blood glucose levels rise during pregnancy but return to normal after the child is born (gestational diabetes). These women have a tendency toward diabetes later in life.

Women who have had gestational diabetes should adopt a healthy lifestyle to keep diabetes at bay, or at least under control.

Type 1 and type 2 diabetes

There is, by chance, the occasional family with cases of both type 1 and type 2 diabetes.

The conditions are, however, clinically and genetically distinct, with no interaction between genes involved.

Thus a family with cases of type 2 diabetes has the same risks for type 1 diabetes as the general population, while relatives of a person with type 1 diabetes have the same risk for type 2 diabetes as the general population.

Therefore, parents with a family history of type 2 diabetes need not be concerned about passing type 1 diabetes to their children.

Chapter 34

Around the World with Diabetes

◆ By Margaret McGill ◆

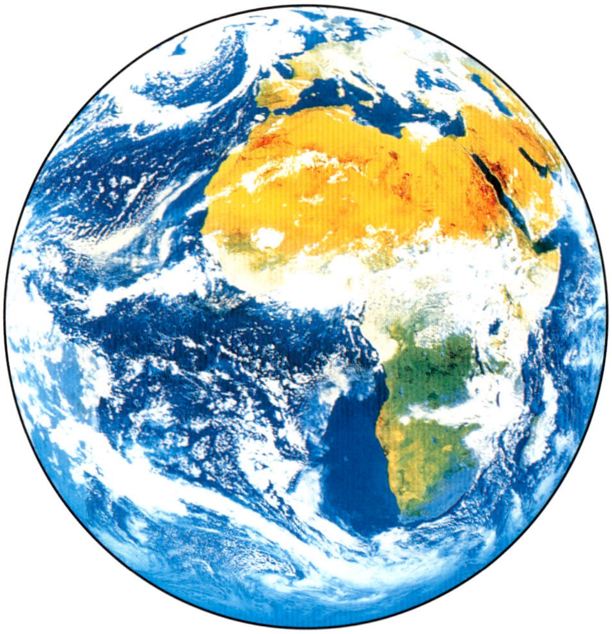

AT A GLANCE

- Travelling in countries unfamiliar with type 1 diabetes presents special risks if you become ill or need surgery, as insulin must never be omitted.
- Lifestyle changes from strenuous rural existence to sedentary city life are linked to an ongoing and dramatic increase in type 2 diabetes.
- Because of countries' different approaches to health services, the International Diabetes Federation works at several levels to improve people's access to medication and care.
- Regardless of where they live, people with diabetes and their families face similar issues and problems, but the solutions need to be culturally specific.

The worldwide distribution of diabetes
Diabetes is a growing threat to the world's health.

ONCE considered a disease of wealthy Caucasians with only rare occurrences among people in Asian and African countries, diabetes is now a serious problem for developing countries as well. This is due to changes in culture and lifestyle, especially the move from the rigours of rural life to relatively easy urban existence, plus the fact that we live longer.

Diabetes is found in almost all populations throughout the world. However, the distribution and occurrence of the two main types of diabetes – type 1 and type 2 – show major differences between countries and ethnic groups.

The rate of type 1 diabetes is up to 60 times greater among children from high-risk countries such as Finland than in those from low-risk areas in Asia, where type 1 diabetes is still relatively uncommon. Why this is so is still not fully understood.

The increasing rate of type 2 diabetes has reached almost epidemic proportions in many developing countries. What is even more alarming is the increase in type 2 diabetes in adolescence seen particularly in Asia and the Western Pacific. Lifestyle changes, such as moving from physically strenuous rural life to more sedentary city living; the change from traditional foods to fast foods (as has occurred in newly industrialised and developing countries), create dramatic increases in type 2 diabetes.

It also appears that many non-Caucasian populations such as our Pacific neighbours and the American Indians, are even more susceptible to developing type 2 diabetes.

This suggests that people with type 2 diabetes may exceed one hundred million by 2000 and a substantial proportion of these will live in developing countries.

How will you be affected by this different distribution of diabetes?

While it is interesting to look at the distribution of the different types of diabetes, there is a practical point to the exercise.

If you have type 1 diabetes and are travelling or visiting a country where it is a rare condition, be aware that many local health professionals will not understand the special characteristics of type 1 diabetes.

If you get sick in these countries, be careful that your attending doctor knows your insulin must be continued, even before surgery, when you are sick and not eating.

It is likely that local medicos won't be familiar with treating keto-acidosis or using glucagon for hypoglycaemia.

We are fortunate in Australia to have access to the highest international standard of diabetes care. This does not make living with diabetes easy, but it does help reduce worries about the level of care you receive. Unfortunately, this is not typical elsewhere in the world, where the level of care experienced by people with diabetes varies enormously.

The role of the International Diabetes Federation

The steady and widespread increase in diabetes creates major international issues to be addressed. This is part of the objective of the International Diabetes Federation (IDF).

The IDF, with its head office in Brussels, Belgium, is the only international diabetes body. It divides its activities between seven regions: North America, South America, Mediterranean, Western Pacific, Asia, Africa and Europe. Australia is a member of the Western Pacific region, which has a membership of 13 countries from South East Asia and the Pacific. To qualify for membership, a country must have a diabetes organisation servicing the nation's people with diabetes.

Diabetes Australia is our link with the IDF. To identify the needs of people living with diabetes and to try to improve worldwide standards of diabetes care, the IDF has established various task forces and consultative sections.

Meanwhile, in developed countries, the availability of technology has increased the burden on people with diabetes because expectations are so great for them to manage their condition and achieve good control. This often unrealistic expectation by health professionals may add to the already heavy load carried by people with diabetes.

Children with diabetes

In 1996 the IDF's consultative section on childhood and adolescent diabetes held a Leadership Needs Assessment Workshop for the Western Pacific region. Its objective was to establish a model for use by representatives from the 14 countries which attended. The model would establish the needs of young people with diabetes and those of their families.

Interestingly, despite the great cultural diversity of participants, the barriers to family acceptance of diabetes and the issues for young people were the same throughout the region.

The cost of diabetes

Probably the most significant international diabetes issue is its cost to governments and to individuals with diabetes and their families.

In many countries health care is not free. Furthermore, insulin – classified as a lifesaving drug – is not readily affordable or accessible in many developing countries. This means that the cost of a vial of insulin is much higher than in the developed countries of Europe and North America. For example, the difference might be US$12 versus US$2.50. The IDF's insulin task force works hard to encourage governments to abolish taxes on insulin and make it accessible and affordable for the people who need it. Lobbying governments is the only solution to this problem.

People with diabetes from poorer countries also have difficulty affording monitoring equipment, medications and appropriate food. Diabetes education facilities are often minimal and services that screen and treat the long-term complications of diabetes are almost non-existent.

The western view of treating type 2 diabetes – improving lifestyle, appropriate and early use of medication, reducing fat intake and regular exercise – implies that members of the community have the choice to do so. In many countries, life is a struggle for survival and treatment for diabetes is not an option. Only those family members who are healthy survive.

We may take for granted our access to services that screen for and treat the long-term complications of diabetes. In many countries, screening for eye disease, for example, is not performed, because even if diagnosed, there is no available treatment, such as laser therapy.

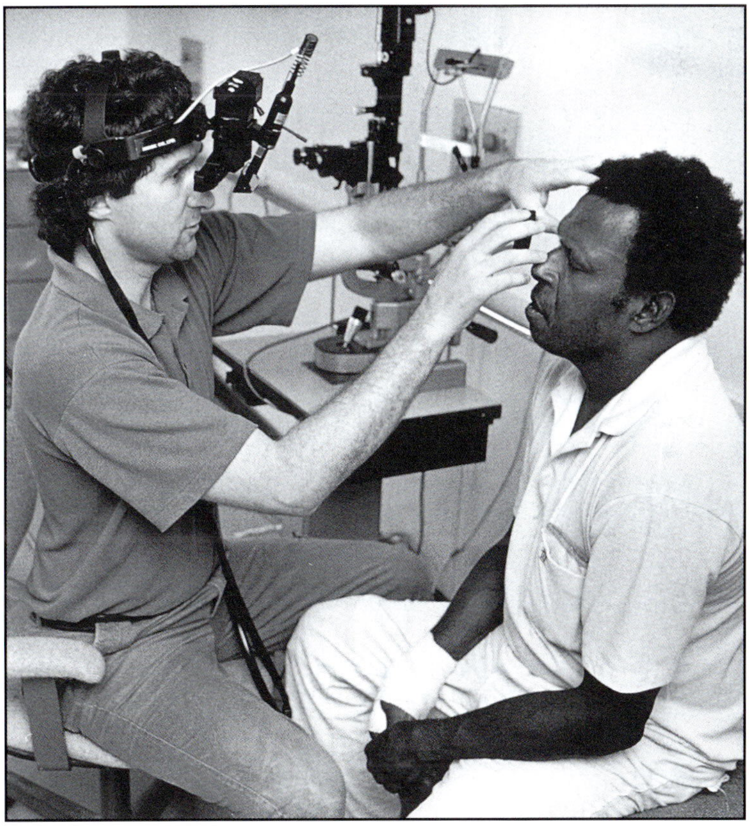

PHOTO: MICHAEL AMENDOLIA. COURTESY THE FRED HOLLOWS FOUNDATION.

Critical issues for the region include:

1. Lack of awareness about the special needs of young people with diabetes. This was particularly the case for health professionals, the general public, employers and the government.
2. Lack of multidisciplinary teams – doctors, diabetes nurse educators, dietitians and specifically trained paediatric social workers. Although diabetes services were available, many were adult-focused and did not meet the medical and psychological needs of young people.
3. Lack of protocols and guidelines for care.
4. Social discrimination: predominantly this referred

to a young person's marriageability. This is an important issue in countries where arranged marriage remains an integral part of the culture. In some countries, young people with diabetes cannot attend the top universities, in spite of their academic achievement, simply because they have diabetes.

The workshop reinforced the perception that, no matter where children with diabetes live in the world, the issues and problems for them and their families are similar. However, the solutions may need to be culturally specific. The same philosophy applies to people with type 2 diabetes.

The use of traditional medicine

In many countries diabetes is considered a modern disease. However, for many centuries a local medicine man looked after the community's health and wellbeing. In China, traditional medicine is so respected that it is incorporated into the medical degree.

It is therefore essential to acknowledge the experience and worth of traditional medicine when we introduce western treatments for conditions such as diabetes. In many situations, traditional treatments contribute significantly.

There are times when partnership and collaboration are important to implement specific care. A good example is a case of infection, particularly foot infection. Amputation due to diabetes occurs at an alarming rate in many countries. For example, in Fiji, with a total population of only 750,000, at the hospital in Suva alone 39 diabetes-related amputations were performed in three months.

A main contributor is people's late presentation at a western-style medical clinic or hospital following an injury. They often use traditional medicine for a number of weeks and it is only when desperately ill that they seek medical advice. Unfortunately, in this situation, amputation is often lifesaving and the only option. It is not realistic to think that encouraging local people to seek western medical care swiftly will suffice when traditional medicine is entrenched in their culture and plays such an important and worthwhile role.

Therefore, it is necessary to collaborate with the traditional healers if local people are to get the best service. In countries such as the Republic of Kiribati, where traditional healers are registered, access and collaboration is easier.

Hopefully, by educating traditional healers to improve their skills, and by stressing the benefits of early antibiotic therapy for treatment of infection, the sick will present for western treatments earlier and the healers will increase their standing in the community.

This move has the potential to reduce these countries' devastating rates of amputations in people with diabetes.

Summary

Diabetes is a serious health issue found in almost all countries worldwide. The costs both in human and economic terms are enormous. Local and international diabetes organisations must work together to ensure that people with diabetes, wherever they are, receive an acceptable standard of diabetes care.

Chapter 35

The Impact of Diabetes

◆ By Dr Daniel McCarty & Professor Paul Zimmet ◆

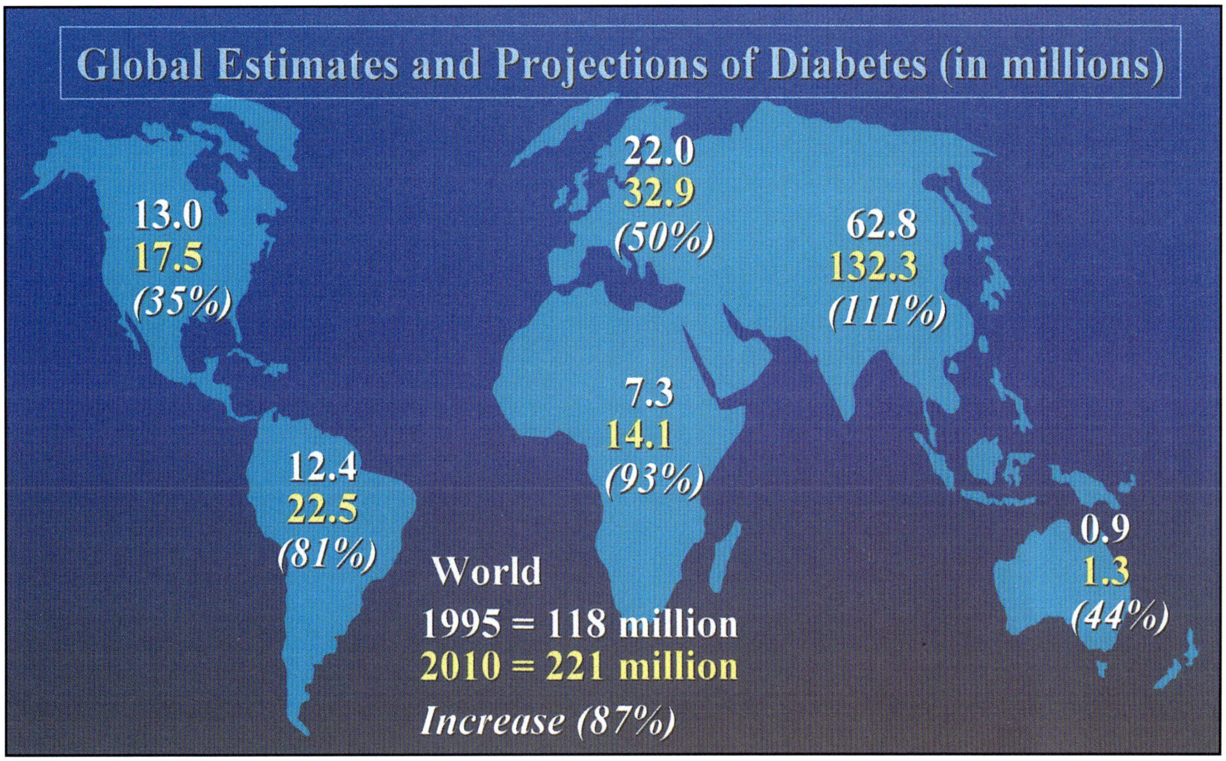

ALTHOUGH diabetes was very rare at the beginning of this century, it is now one of the most widespread and serious global health problems.

In Australia, studies suggest that the prevalence of type 1 and type 2 diabetes is increasing and recent findings indicate adult onset type 1 is more common than previously believed.

Diabetes is not only common, it is one of Australia's most challenging health problems, with impact across all sectors of the community, as indicated in Table 1 (page 125).

Why is type 2 diabetes becoming more common?

Paradoxically, for many countries like Australia, type 2 has evolved as a major health problem because we live longer.

During the past century, improved nutrition, better hygiene and the control of many infectious diseases have resulted in dramatically improved life expectancy. However, in so doing, these benefits have unmasked many age-related diseases such as type 2 diabetes, heart disease, hypertension (high blood pressure), strokes and many forms of cancer.

The term *epidemiologic transition* is used to describe the shift in disease patterns which occurred in developed countries in the past 50 years and which currently is occurring in many developing countries.

AT A GLANCE

- **An estimated 700,000 to 800,000 Australians have diabetes and numbers are increasing.**
- **About 25,000 Australians develop diabetes each year, with the total national cost of treatment exceeding $1 billion annually, or about $2,800 for every person with diabetes.**
- **Type 2 diabetes is by far the most frequent form of diabetes, representing about 80 per cent of all cases.**
- **Two major factors account for Australia's predicted rise in diabetes – we're getting older, putting more people at risk for type 2 diabetes; and the key diabetes risk factors – obesity and inactivity – are on the rise.**
- **Our main defence against diabetes in Australia is to reduce the risk factors associated with the disorder.**

This transition has changed type 2 diabetes from being a rare disease at the beginning of this century to its current position as a major global contributor to ill health.

In addition to shifting disease patterns, lifestyle change also greatly contributes to the upsurge in type 2 diabetes. This lifestyle phenomenon is well illustrated in Pacific and Indian Ocean island populations, and also in

Australian Aboriginal communities (see chapter 24 – Diabetes in Aboriginal People).

Rapid socio-economic development in the past 40 to 50 years has changed many peoples' way of life from traditional to modern. In virtually all populations, higher fat foods and decreased physical activity accompany the benefits of modernisation. These lifestyle changes plus increasing longevity account for the current dynamic increase in type 2 diabetes.

Ethnic differences in type 2 diabetes

Numerous reports from throughout the world continue to highlight the explosion of type 2 diabetes in relation to lifestyle change.

An example of a newly affected group in the Pacific region are the urbanised Wanigela people of the Koki settlement in Papua New Guinea. The Wanigela people now have one of the world's highest community rates of diabetes. However, diabetes is still a very rare disease among the Wanigela who live more traditional lifestyles in the country. The urban Wanigela probably experience more diabetes because they changed from a traditional diet (fresh vegetables, lower fat meats, and so on) to more modern foods (processed meals, canned meats, and so on) and they have greatly reduced their physical activity levels.

Studies in Mauritius, a multi-ethnic nation of Asian Indians, Chinese and Creoles in the Indian Ocean, also show the potential public health disaster from type 2 diabetes that could also affect other parts of the developing world.

Mauritius is a small country which has experienced rapid economic development.

Rates of diabetes among Mauritian Chinese, Indians and Creoles are equally high and significantly higher than rates found in Australia and Europe. The prevalence of diabetes among Mauritian Chinese and Indians has enormous public health implications for rapidly modernising countries, such as China and India. In fact, the epidemic may already be in full swing, with recent reports of prevalence as high as 5 per cent in the adult Beijing population .

Rapidly developing countries such as China and India inevitably will experience an epidemic of type 2 diabetes in the next few decades.

In addition to recent migrant groups, Australian Aboriginal people are also at very high risk for type 2 diabetes.

Why do some populations have such high rates of type 2 diabetes?

Australian Aboriginal people and other ethnic groups might be particularly prone to developing diabetes because for many thousands of years they have evolved and adapted to an environment which provided considerable seasonal variation in the availability of food.

Some researchers suggest that populations such as Australian Aboriginal people, may have developed a *thrifty genotype* or genetic helper which provided a survival advantage in times when food was scarce, but in present day conditions constitutes a disadvantage because there is continual access to high-energy, low-fibre, processed food, plus a decline in traditional physical activity levels.

How common is type 1 diabetes in Australia?

Type 1 diabetes remains one of the most common serious childhood diseases in the USA and Australia and recent studies suggest that it is increasing (Figure 2).

In 1997 about 4,000 Australians aged under 15 plus about 64,000 Australians aged over 15 were believed to have type 1 diabetes. Rates of type 1 diabetes in Australia are much the same as those in England and New Zealand, countries with very similar ethnic/genetic composition.

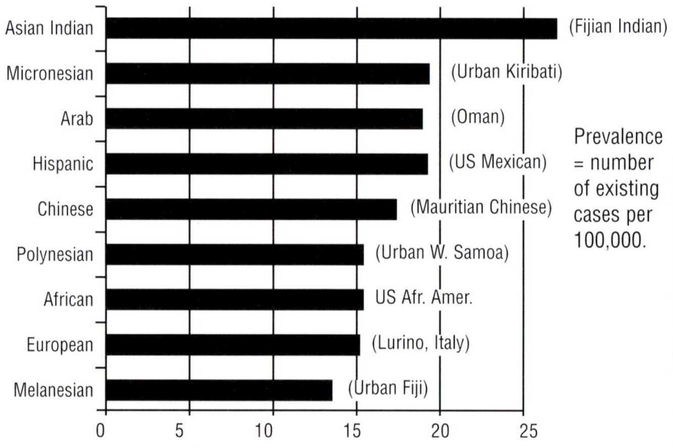

Figure 1. Highest reported rates of diabetes by ethnic group

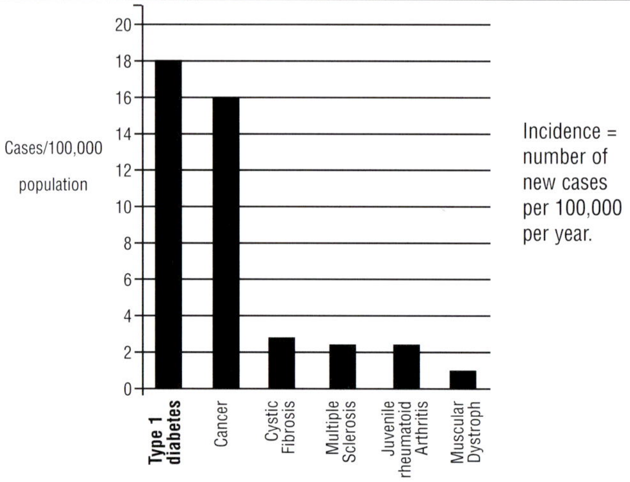

Figure 2. Incidence of type 1 diabetes compared with other chronic diseases in the US for children and young adults under 20. (From the American Diabetes Association, 1993).

How many Australians have diabetes?

To estimate the number of Australians with diabetes and forecast the future national burden of diabetes, we have plotted estimates of diabetes from the three largest Australian studies (see Figure 3).

It is estimated that there are 700,000 to 800,000 Australians with diabetes. Increasing trends in diabetes prevalence indicate that by 2010, Australians will experience a similar rate of diabetes to that of Caucasians in the USA between 1976 and 1980. Type 2 diabetes will be by far the most frequent form of diabetes, representing about 80 per cent of all cases. It is estimated that about 25,000 Australians develop diabetes each year, with the total national cost of treatment exceeding $1 billion annually, or about $2,800 for every person with diabetes.

Two major factors account for Australia's predicted rise in diabetes – underlying demographics and increase in known risk factors.

The age distribution of the Australian population is shifting to older age groups, putting more people at risk for type 2 diabetes. The rising prevalence of known risk factors such as obesity and inactivity will contribute to more type 2 diabetes in Australia.

Because we cannot influence the natural ageing of the Australian population, the only way to decrease the number of Australians with diabetes will be to reduce the risk factors associated with this disorder.

Table 1. The impact of diabetes in Australia

- In 1997 about 68,000 Australians had type 1 diabetes and 665,000 Australians had type 2 diabetes. Together, they represent 4 per cent of the total population.
- Diabetes is likely to affect 900,000 Australians by 2000 and 1.15 million Australians by 2010.
- Australian Aboriginal people suffer the 4th highest rates of type 2 diabetes in the world.
- Type 1 diabetes ranks as one of the most common serious childhood diseases in Australia. It is likely to have a higher incidence in young people under 20 than cancer, cystic fibrosis, multiple sclerosis, juvenile rheumatoid arthritis and muscular dystrophy.
- Compared with most countries in the world, Australia's rates of type 1 diabetes are very high.
- The incidence of gestational diabetes is increasing, particularly in ethnic populations.
- Risk factors for type 2 diabetes, such as obesity and physical inactivity, are increasing in Australia.
- Australian Aboriginal people and Torres Strait Islanders suffer exceptionally high rates of diabetes-related complications.
- The total cost of diabetes exceeds $1 billion annually (or about $2,800 per diagnosed case).

Diabetes in the future?

Although diabetes is likely to become more common in the future, we are not completely unprepared to meet the diabetes challenge in the next century. Of benefit, for example, are studies describing patterns and risk factors for diabetes.

Treatments have improved greatly in recent decades, as reflected by mortality studies which continue to demonstrate improved longevity for people with diabetes (see chapter 37 – Diabetes: Back to the Future).

The recently conducted Diabetes Control and Complications Trial in the USA confirmed that complications such as blindness can be reduced through careful glucose monitoring. Technologically advanced glucose monitoring devices are now available for this purpose.

Immunological techniques are being developed to identify high risk groups before the onset of type 1 diabetes and several primary prevention trials are under way for this type of diabetes.

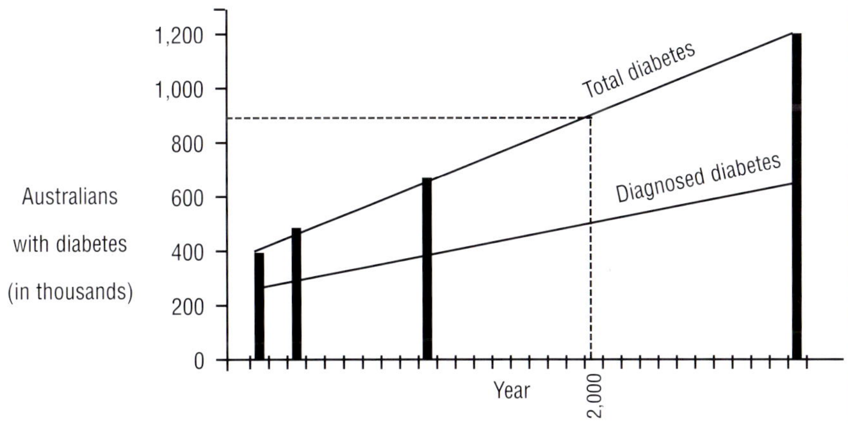

Figure 3. Estimated prevalence of diabetes in Australia 1980–2010. Diabetes has more than doubled.

The main behavioural, environmental and social determinants for type 2 diabetes have already been defined. These may provide the basis for intervention programs which emphasise healthy lifestyle practices such as exercise, good nutrition, maintenance of ideal body weight, smoking cessation and reduced alcohol consumption.

There is little doubt that diabetes will become even more common in the twenty-first century than it is today. However, if one considers how far we have come in our understanding of diabetes in the past few decades, our outlook should be very optimistic.

National Diabetes Strategy

◆ By Jeannette Baldwin ◆

THE National Diabetes Strategy (NDS) aims to reduce the personal and public impact of diabetes in Australia by proposing a core set of common goals, recommendations and practical implementation plans.

The strategy represents a major commitment by the Federal Government to combat the growing problem of diabetes in Australia.

AT A GLANCE

- **Diabetes is a chronic and costly disease that incurs an enormous personal and public health burden.**
- **An estimated 780,000 Australians have diabetes. Of these approximately 430,000 have diagnosed diabetes and another 350,000 have undiagnosed diabetes.**
- **The National Diabetes Strategy is about people who have diabetes, those who care for people with diabetes, and people who are at risk of developing diabetes.**
- **It is the blueprint for action to improve diabetes services in the next 10 years.**

Goals

- Prevent or delay development of type 1 and type 2 diabetes.
- Improve health-related quality of life and reduce complications and premature mortality in people with type 1 and type 2 diabetes.
- Achieve improved maternal and child outcomes for gestational diabetes and for women with pre-existing diabetes equivalent to those of non-diabetic pregnancies.
- Make progress towards a cure for type 1 diabetes.
- Advance knowledge and understanding about prevention, cure and care of diabetes through comprehensive research.
- Improve the capacity of the health system to deliver, manage and monitor services for preventing diabetes and care of people with it.

To achieve these goals a set of priority programs have been developed and recommended for immediate action. The programs aim to improve the quality and accessibility of diabetes care to reduce complications.

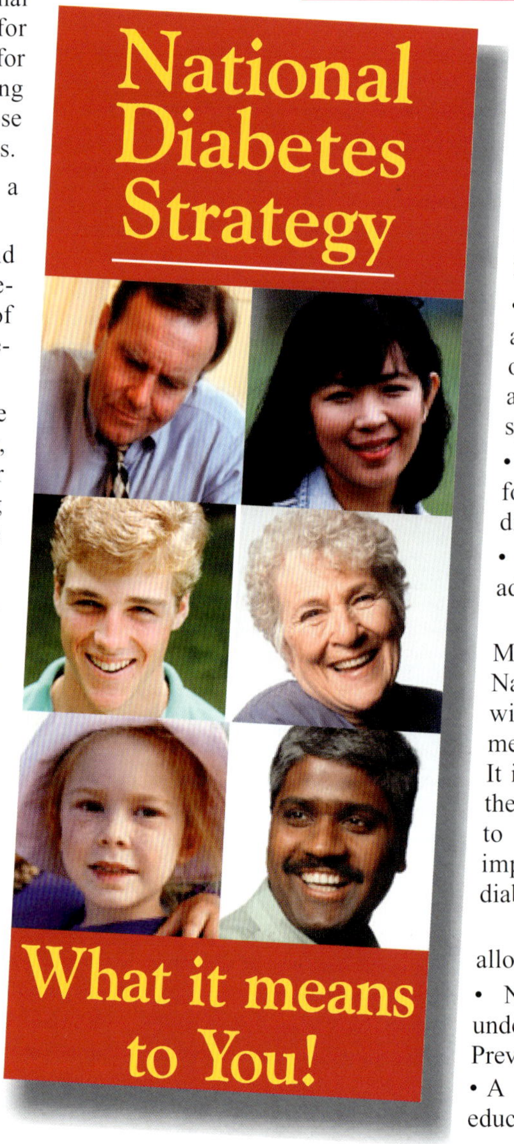

Priority Programs for Action

- Improving quality of diabetes care.
- Diabetes visual impairment prevention.
- Diabetes end stage renal disease prevention scheme.
- Improved diabetic foot disease management.
- Diabetic cardiovascular disease prevention.
- Systems for early detection of type 2 diabetes.

Other priority recommendations include:

- Optimising quality and accessibility of diabetes prevention of care for indigenous Australians and people from non-English-speaking backgrounds.
- Implementing national initiatives for detection and management of diabetes in pregnancy.
- Assessing needs of children and adolescents with diabetes.

In 1996 the Australian Health Ministers included diabetes as a 5th National Health Priority Area along with cancer, coronary heart disease, mental illness and accidental injuries. It is the purpose of the NDS to guide the additional funding now allocated to diabetes to initiate and support improvements to the outcomes of diabetes care and prevention.

Funding has already been allocated to a number of projects:

- NHMRC Retinopathy guidelines under the Diabetes Visual Impairment Prevention Program recommendation.
- A community awareness strategy to educate health professionals and the

community to the risks of type 2 diabetes to ensure earlier detection of the disease.

- A high-risk foot service for people with diabetes plus a network for diabetes foot care through training and the provision of telemedicine facilities in remote areas of Australia.

By providing an evidence-based framework, the strategy will guide the funding, planning, provision, organisation and monitoring of services for people with or at risk of type 1 diabetes, type 2 diabetes and gestational diabetes.

It is a thorough blueprint for action to improve and expand preventive, educational and research initiatives for diabetes during the next 10 years.

Chapter 37

Diabetes: Back to the Future

By Professor Leonard C. Harrison

A ROMAN physician, Aretaeus of Cappadocia (AD 30–90), was the first person we know of to ponder the cause of diabetes. Noting the symptom of frequent and copious urination, he assumed kidney weakness was the culprit.

It wasn't until the 17th century, at least in western civilisation, that this polyuria was associated with excretion of large amounts of glucose.

By the end of last century researchers realised that the pancreas was somehow involved in diabetes when tests showed dogs developed the condition after their pancreas was removed.

Yet in spite of its 5,000-year-old history and the ongoing research, diabetes is increasing.

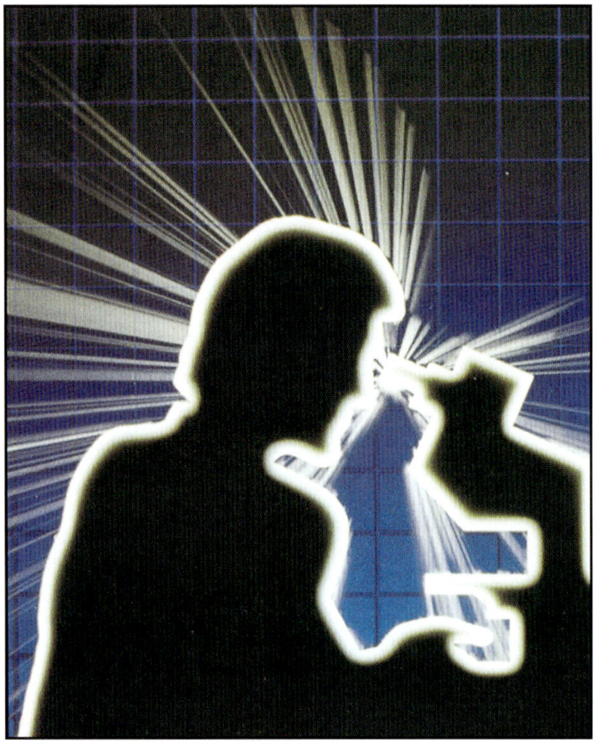

Discovery of insulin

Insulin, the hormone made by the beta cells in the islets of the pancreas, which regulates glucose in the body, was discovered by a team of four Canadian researchers in 1922.

They showed that extracts of dog pancreas could reverse diabetes.

They didn't know what insulin was or how it worked. However, since their discovery, four Nobel prizes have been awarded for research into insulin.

Insulin datelines

- 1922 – discovery of insulin
- 1953 – chemical sequence of insulin determined
- 1969 – physical structure of insulin seen via x-ray crystallography
- 1978 – gene for insulin cloned
- 1980s – genetically engineered pure human insulin first made available to patients.

AT A GLANCE

- **Thanks to research and new information, the outlook for people with diabetes has improved significantly in recent years.**
- **Most advances in the treatment of diabetes were made in the past 20 years, although the condition is one of the oldest recorded.**
- **Although there are treatment breakthroughs coming from biological and genetic engineering research, it makes more sense to prevent type 2 diabetes by education, behavioural and lifestyle changes than to hope for a miracle cure which many affected people couldn't afford anyway.**
- **Given the knowledge and techniques now available, plus the momentum of diabetes research internationally, we are at the threshold of a new era in which the outcome for people with diabetes will be dramatically improved by new forms of treatment.**

Insulin – a great discovery but not a cure

When insulin was first discovered, many thought it was a cure for diabetes. Although injected insulin prevented people with severe diabetes from wasting away and dying, the causes and complications of diabetes remained.

Younger people with the wasting type of diabetes no longer died; they survived to face longer term complications which shortened their lives.

It was decades before researchers realised the relationship of these complications to raised levels of blood glucose. Only recently, 70 years after insulin's discovery, did the Diabetes Control and Complications Trial definitively report that good control of blood glucose could prevent clinical complications.

Two major types of diabetes

For a time the discovery of insulin and its life-saving effect lulled us into a false sense of security.

Many older and frequently overweight people with diabetes didn't need insulin.

The lack of insulin, which distinguishes type 1 from type 2 diabetes, was not well appreciated until the late 1940s when an Australian biochemist, Joseph Bornstein, worked out a way to measure insulin in the blood.

He confirmed that there were two major types of diabetes: type 1 due to a lack of insulin and type 2 due to failure of the body to use glucose normally, even in the presence of insulin – *insulin resistance*.

A steep learning curve

While we look forward to the day when both types of diabetes can be prevented or cured, in the meantime, it helps to become an amateur diabetes researcher.

This is to comprehend the mechanics of the disorder and to learn what is and is not known so far.

Major breakthroughs, as reported in the newspapers, are rare. Progress usually occurs by small, gradual steps, with contributions from many researchers each adding pieces to the puzzle, while slowly a clearer picture emerges.

The pioneering discovery of insulin was preceded for 40 years by experiments with pancreatic extracts by other researchers in Europe and North America.

Almost everything we now know about diabetes was learned in the past 100 years; most of it in the past 20 years.

Many recent advances are spin-offs from the modern revolution in molecular biology – the ongoing study of our genetic material.

One way of getting a perspective on the progress in diabetes research over the past 20 years or so is to consider what we know now that we didn't know then. When we do this we come up with a long list (Table 1).

For example, we learned that beta cell destruction in type 1 diabetes is associated with a reaction by the body's immune system, in particular, white blood cells called T cells, against the beta cells which destroys them as if they were foreign. The ways in which T cells kill beta cells and the specific components of them that are recognised and targeted by the attacking T cells have been identified.

Table 1
Results of Diabetes Research 1975–1995

Basic	Treatment
Immune basis of type 1 diabetes	Highly purified animal insulins
Genes that predispose to type 1 diabetes	Genetically engineered human insulin
Primary genetic basis of type 2 diabetes	Strips and meters for self-monitoring
Viral and chemical trigger agents in type 1 diabetes	Insulin delivery devices, pens, pumps
Animal models of type 1 and type 2 diabetes	Effective treatments for hypertension
Cloning of genes for insulin, insulin receptor, glucose transporters etc.	Retinal photography and laser treatment
Glucose biochemistry and physiology	Dialysis/transplantation for kidney failure
Drugs to inhibit the effects of glucose	Combined kidney-pancreas transplantation
Drugs to enhance the effects of insulin	Long-term blood glucose monitoring with glycated haemoglobin (HbA1c)
Many new molecules involved in both type 1 and type 2 diabetes	Prevention of type 1 diabetes in animal models
	Trials for prevention of type 1 diabetes in humans

Genes have been discovered which predispose people to type 1 diabetes. We can now use blood tests to diagnose individuals in whom underlying beta cell inflammation and destruction is occurring, months to years before they develop symptoms and require insulin. This ability for early diagnosis before diabetes sets in is the beginning of preventive treatment intervention strategies.

Can we cure type 1 diabetes?

The only way we could cure type 1 diabetes would be by somehow restoring the ability to make insulin.

In 1911, more than a decade ahead of insulin's discovery, Dr John Ramsay attempted the first pancreas transplant at the Launceston General Hospital, Tasmania.

Transplantation of the whole or a segment of pancreas from human organ donor subjects is now technically feasible and effective in restoring insulin secretion. However, apart from the shortage of organ donor tissue, the major barrier to transplantation remains rejection by the body's immune system of tissue that is genetically different from its own. In order to prevent rejection and maintain survival of transplanted pancreas or the islet cells that make insulin, the recipients of the transplant must be given potent drugs to suppress their immune system. Unfortunately, these drugs can produce serious complications.

Until safe and specific treatments to prevent immune rejection are developed, transplantation of insulin-producing cells from human or animal pancreas is an option only for people with diabetes who require life-saving transplantation of another organ – usually the kidney for chronic kidney failure.

We can overcome the problem of tissue supply by using islet cells from animals. Foetal pig islet cells have been shown by researchers to reverse diabetes in mice and, following a preliminary trial in Sweden, offer the greatest hope.

Australian research into a cure of type 1 diabetes by overcoming the immunological barriers to transplanting foetal pig islet cells received a major boost thanks to a long-term program grant in 1995 from the Juvenile Diabetes Foundation International and National Institutes of Health, USA.

Other approaches to restoring beta-cell function include genetically engineering a person's own cells to make insulin and the development of insulin implant delivery devices linked to non-invasive blood glucose monitors.

Happily, many independent research groups and commercial ventures are competing to develop such techniques and cures.

Research in type 2 diabetes

The basis of type 2 diabetes has been an enigma for researchers and those seeking a cure. However, there is hope because modern approaches are beginning to identify genes that predispose to the condition. Also, several new molecules involved in insulin signalling to cells and in glucose metabolism have been discovered. One of the most recent and exciting molecules in this area is leptin, which is made by fat tissue and circulates to the brain to control energy balance. It was identified when researchers found a defect in the genes of obese mice that developed diabetes, and its discovery illustrates the power of modern genetic techniques.

Why not an oral cure?

It would be a major advance for people with both type 1 and type 2 diabetes if drugs that mimic insulin could be taken by mouth.

Researchers and pharmaceutical companies are working hard to discover such drugs and already have developed insulin-sensitising drugs called thiazolidinediones, which currently are being tested in humans.

On the threshold

Considering the pace of progress in diabetes research, future prospects look exciting (Table 2).

However, possibly a greater challenge than the discovery of new diagnostic and therapeutic tools will be their practical development and application.

Nowadays, there is often a long and expensive period of development, testing and approval before an important discovery can be translated into a human benefit. The social, political and economic factors that dictate accessibility to advances in health care will have a major impact, for example, on the epidemics of type 2 diabetes in developing societies of Africa, India, Asia and the South Pacific.

Table 2
Expected Benefits of Diabetes Research 1995–2015

Environmental agents, eg, viruses or chemical toxins, that trigger type 1 diabetes will be identified.	The artificial pancreas – a miniaturised insulin delivery pump connected to a non-invasive sensor for monitoring blood glucose – will be developed.
Specific and safe forms of therapy will prevent the development of type 1 diabetes.	Oral medications will be used to mimic the effects of insulin and to inhibit the effects of high glucose levels.
Specific and safe forms of therapy will block rejection of islet transplants and the recurrence of auto-immune diabetes in transplants.	Biochemical abnormalities in type 2 diabetes that are inherited and cause cells to be defective in their use of glucose will be discovered through genetic techniques.
Genetic engineering techniques will be used to transplant the insulin gene and its controlling mechanisms into a diabetic person's own cells, eg, skin cells.	

This emphasises the importance of preventing type 2 diabetes through education and behavioural and lifestyle changes.

The impact of high-fat, high-refined carbohydrate western fast foods and sedentary lifestyle on Australian Aboriginal people or on the coastal peoples of Papua New Guinea is a far more important consideration than the discovery of a drug for type 2 diabetes which they can't afford.

Evidence suggests that diabetes complications such as nephropathy and retinopathy are decreasing. These improvements are probably due to a combination of factors. They include better education; a shift away from less pure, long-acting insulins towards multiple daily doses of pure, short-acting insulins; better monitoring with home blood glucose testing strips and meters and by glycated haemoglobin; more effective control of high blood pressure with better drugs; and monitoring for complications and earlier intervention (for example, angiography and laser treatment for retinopathy).

Quick Read

1. **Living with someone with type 1 diabetes - page 1**

- Use whatever experiences you can glean from doctors, friends, your partner and literature.
- Build trust but not dependence.
- Know your personal limits and have a plan in place to hand over to others when it is needed.
- Know that no one can understand diabetes better than those who live with it every day.
- Above all, remember as a partner of a person with diabetes, you are the second most important person in the health care team.

2. **Living with diabetes - page 3**

- Maintain a positive attitude.
- Learn to manage your diabetes.
- Be diligent with care of your body.
- Thoroughly understand your eating plan.
- Ask questions of your health care team.
- Don't forget to enjoy life.

3. **Diabetes - what goes wrong? - page 5**

- Maintaining your blood glucose at a level just right for you is the essence of managing diabetes.
- Understand the mechanics of diabetes.

4. **Diabetes and Lifestyle - page 8**

- Don't get fat.
- Eat less fat.
- Eat complex carbohydrate.
- Spread your meals.
- Take 30.
- Take time out.
- Quit for life.

5. **Healthy Eating and Diabetes - page 10**

- Learn basic nutritional facts so you know which foods contain carbohydrates, proteins and fats.
- Know the energy values of foods so that wherever you are you can make wise meal choices.
- Ask your dietitian to help you review your nutrition needs and to explain aids such as the good-better-best and carbohydrate exchange systems which will assist in your diabetes control.
- Limit your fat and oil intake.
- Learn to differentiate between good and bad fats.
- Learn to correctly interpret the nutrition panels on food products.

6. **The Use of Tablets - page 14**

- Tablets are inappropriate for people with type 1 diabetes.
- Tablets are not a substitute for a meal plan.
- Over time, tablets may cease to be an effective treatment.
- Sensible eating may prolong the effectiveness of tablets for years.
- Regular glucose testing monitors the effectiveness of tablets.
- Any of the three families of tablets may cause side-effects.
- Illnesses can effect the effectiveness of tablets.

7. **Diabetes and Exercise - page 16**

- By taking appropriate precautions, most people with diabetes can exercise and play sport.
- Monitor yourself so you know what to do to avoid hypoglycaemia or hyperglycaemia.
- Blood glucose monitoring is vital to help you make appropriate adjustments to meal plans and medications, plus maintain blood glucose control during and after exercise.
- If you are middle-aged or older, have a thorough physical check-up, especially your feet, heart and eyes, before starting any exercise program.
- By taking a gradual and sensible approach, you can safely enjoy the benefits of regular physical activity even if you have some diabetes complications.

8. **Insulin and its Role - page 21**

- Five types of insulin are available and you and your doctor will decide which is right for you.
- Know your condition – have a good working knowledge of your diabetes.
- Know your insulin – remember its time of peak action and total duration.
- Test regularly – and monitor results.
- Record test results – and use your records to make informed decisions.
- Consider your diet – often a change of diet can be as useful as a change in insulin dosage.
- If in doubt, ask your doctor or diabetes nurse educator.

9. **Injections and Injectors - page 25**

- The daily injection process will become routine.
- Your doctor or diabetes nurse educator will teach you the correct injection and dose management techniques, while answering any of your treatment queries.
- A wide variety of injectors and injections are available, each designed for a particular purpose and individual's needs.
- Bruising, lumps and other responses to injections can be avoided if you have the know-how.

10. **Self-monitoring of Blood Glucose - page 31**

- Regular monitoring of blood glucose levels need not be a hassle and plays an active part in your ability to maintain a happy, enjoyable life.

- Keep asking questions about blood glucose testing and keep practising blood testing until you feel confident and comfortable about your technique.
- There are at least 10 good reasons why you should regularly monitor your blood glucose, including measuring the effectiveness of your treatment and preventing or delaying the onset of complications.
- Several factors – including equipment faults and human error – may influence the reliability of your test results.
- Record your results in a record book and take them to your diabetes adviser on each visit.

11. Testing Urine - page 36

- Urine testing helps your control over your diabetes management.
- Establish whether the urine threshold is normal before considering urine testing.
- Finding out your renal threshold lets you understand what the results mean.
- If you use insulin, measure your blood glucose, as urine testing won't provide enough information to determine any required changes in medication dosage.
- Urine tests – and other tests used in diabetes management – are not only your early warning system but a valuable management tool in diabetes control.

12. Hypoglycaemia and Hyperglycaemia - page 39

- This chapter describes the symptoms of low blood glucose and the symptoms of high blood glucose and explains how to treat each separate problem.
- Learn to recognise the symptoms of hypoglycaemia plus the simple treatment of eating sugar and teach those around you to do the same.
- Repeated prolonged attacks of severe hypoglycaemia may cause nervous system injury and brain damage and should be avoided at all costs.

13. Diabetes and Other Medications - page 43

- Make sure each doctor or pharmacist you consult knows you have diabetes and is aware of all the medications you use.
- Never take a new medication without determining if it may affect your diabetes and, if so, what precautions you should take.
- Be aware that problems are most likely to occur at times of dose change or when you stop and start medications. At these times, take extra care.

14. Sick Days - Feeling Unwell? - page 47

- Keep blood glucose test strips at home (and urine test strips for ketones if you are using insulin); check regularly that they have not passed the expiry date and that you know how to use them. If you're not sure how to use your blood and/or urine test strips correctly, ask a diabetes nurse educator, your doctor or a pharmacist.
- When you're ill, test your blood and urine more frequently than usual. Tests may have to be performed as often as every two hours if you are not improving quickly. Remember, you are looking for raised glucose levels in the blood and ketones in the urine. Ring your doctor if these remain high or increase over the course of several hours.
- Have a supply of quick-acting insulin available.
- Always continue injecting your insulin when you are ill, but seek advice from your doctor or diabetes nurse educator about dosage change.
- Have an adequate supply of suitable foods and fluids available and follow the general recommendations given in this chapter.
- Drink plenty of fluids; if you can't keep these down or have persistent vomiting or diarrhoea, seek immediate medical advice.
- Keep by the phone a list of contact numbers for your doctor, hospital and ambulance.
- Seek medical advice if you are ill and not getting better.
- If possible, have a friend or relative come and keep an eye on you.
- Persisting high blood glucose levels and/or ketones mean you need to talk to a doctor immediately.

15. Long Term Complications of Diabetes - page 51

How to reduce your chances of complications:

- Keep blood glucose levels between 4-8 mmol/L and lower than 11 mmol/L for most tests.
- Taking insulin injections more often may help control blood glucose – talk to your doctor.
- Do not smoke.
- Have regular physical exercise, keep your weight down to your healthy body weight, and keep your blood fats under control.
- If your blood pressure is high, have your doctor treat it.
- Have your blood pressure checked regularly plus occasional laboratory tests to check your blood fats, kidney function and average blood glucose control.
- Have your eyes checked regularly by a medical eye specialist (ophthalmologist) or by your diabetes specialist.
- Examine your feet regularly. From time to time have your doctor check them for blood vessel blockage, nerve damage, ulcers, ingrown toenails and tinea.

16. Diabetes and Eyes - page 56

- Educating people with diabetes, their doctors and the general public is important in the battle to prevent diabetic blindness – a battle we appear to be winning.
- Because diabetes can seriously and permanently affect vision, it is important to see your eye specialist regularly and well before you notice symptoms.
- Keep your diabetes well controlled.

17. Foot Care and Foot Wear - page 59

- The needs of every person with diabetes are individual. It is essential to visit a podiatrist or doctor for complete foot assessment.
- You can then be advised specifically on the necessary foot care. This assessment should be performed at least annually.
- Foot problems can be a serious complication of diabetes but, with early assessment, regular check-ups and proper care there is no reason why they cannot be overcome.
- You can have healthy feet with diabetes – it is up to you. Remember the old adage about feet: One pair must last a lifetime.

18. Diabetes and Oral Health - page 62

- Key factors are daily brushing and flossing, regular consultations with your dentist and eating the right foods.
- At the slightest suspicion of a gum, tooth, denture or mouth problem, see your dental professional.
- Eat nutritious snacks that don't contain sugars or acids.
- Drink plain water where possible.

19. Sexual Problems in Men - page 64

- Incidence of impotence increases with age and diabetes.
- Modern treatment is effective, relatively inexpensive and safe.
- About 70 per cent of impotence has a physical cause, the rest is psychological.
- The particular cause of the sexual problem determines the treatment.

20. Diabetes and Women's Health - page 66

- There is no evidence to suggest that women with diabetes encounter more sexual difficulties than other women.
- Women with diabetes often report cyclical change in their insulin requirements related to the menstrual cycle.
- High blood glucose levels can have a temporarily adverse effect on the sexual aspects of a woman's life.
- Diabetes increases the risks of thrush.
- Simple and effective treatments exist for most problems.

Diabetes and Pregnancy - page 68

- Women with diabetes have healthy pregnancies and healthy babies.
- Although there are potential problems, they can generally be averted by taking a disciplined and sensible approach to pregnancy supported by an experienced medical team.
- Pregnancy for a woman with diabetes is usually an enjoyable and rewarding experience.
- Seek advice from a dietitian to ensure food intake is adequate for you and the baby.
- Excellent diabetes control at the time of conception and during the first eight weeks of pregnancy minimises the risk of birth defects and miscarriage.
- Your baby should be monitored carefully in the last four to six weeks before delivery.
- Insulin requirements change throughout the pregnancy.

Diabetes, Menopause and Hormone Replacement Therapy (HRT) - page 72

- Menopause is a normal transition in every woman's life and some women experience no problems or symptoms during this average five-year phase.
- Women with diabetes who are approaching menopause and experience symptoms are advised to discuss the place of HRT with their doctors and health care professionals.
- HRT may be beneficial in reducing the risk of heart disease and osteoporosis.
- HRT has side effects which may be worse than the symptoms of menopause.
- It's not yet known whether HRT is as effective in women with diabetes as it is in women without diabetes.
- Post menopausal women with diabetes need to weigh up the possible effects of hormone treatment on glucose control and lipid metabolism.
- Expect your doctor to monitor your lipid profiles and blood glucose levels before and after you begin HRT.
- Menopause management differs with every woman.
- Each woman's particular wishes plus family medical history will be taken into account before menopause treatment decisions – if any – are made.
- You are entitled to a thorough explanation of the relative risks and benefits of all menopause treatments so that you can make an informed decision.

21. The School Child with Diabetes – page 76

- Alert all school staff that they have a child with diabetes in their care and offer appropriate information on diabetes management and how to deal with hypoglycaemia.
- Having a child with diabetes in class means added responsibility for the teacher(s).
- Expect the same standards of classroom behaviour from a child with diabetes as from any other child.
- Provide information to the school about the child's diabetes management needs.
- Offer school staff expert information on diabetes from professional organisations such as Diabetes Australia.
- Encourage communication between teachers, parents and the child with diabetes.
- There is a fine line between protecting the child and stifling natural potential.
- The child does not require certain special treatment but, at the same time, must not feel different from friends and classmates.

22. Diabetes and Teenagers – page 80

- Teenagers with diabetes may have particular needs but dislike being singled out for special treatment.
- Having diabetes need not compromise adolescent life.
- Young people with diabetes are often mature beyond their peers.
- This is a time for laying the groundwork for a healthy and confident adult life.
- Parents and their teenagers benefit from regular contact and discussions with competent doctors and diabetes health professionals.

23. Diabetes in the Elderly – page 82

- Early detection and control of diabetes may prevent or delay the onset of complications which otherwise might occur in older people.
- Major risk factors for developing diabetes are age, genetic predisposition, being overweight and reduced activity levels.
- The effects of diabetes in the aged differ from those in younger people.
- Ongoing diabetes education and regular monitoring will minimise the short and long-term impact of diabetes.

24. Diabetes in Aboriginal People – page 86

- It can be argued that humans are genetically programmed for a hunter-gatherer lifestyle.
- It makes sense to return to that lifestyle in our search for solutions to some current health programs.
- If successful, these solutions may have wider application than simply preventing and treating type 2 diabetes.
- Any aspect of a person's lifestyle which could worsen insulin resistance may act as a trigger to bring on diabetes.
- Diabetes is not only potentially reversible in Aborigines, but potentially preventable if people initiate major lifestyle changes.

25. Diabetes – A Problem in Any Language – page 89

- Certain migrant groups are more prone to type 2 diabetes.
- Australian residents are entitled to free health care through the public health service.
- Women from South East Asia, Africa, People's Republic of China, the Middle East and the Pacific Islands are more prone to develop gestational diabetes.
- For people with diabetes who are not confident in English, it is imperative that a professional interpreter is present during health care discussions.
- The Federal Government subsidises the cost of syringes and test strips. Contact Diabetes Australia to register for the subsidy.

26. How to Work with Your Health Care Team – page 93

- Maintain your ideal body weight.
- Be active every day.
- Set achievable goals.
- Take your medication correctly.
- Monitor your blood glucose levels regularly.
- Look after your feet.
- See your doctor regularly.
- Have annual checks with key specialists.
- Join Diabetes Australia to receive a variety of services to help you.

27. Rights and Responsibilities – page 96

- It is your responsibility to manage your diabetes and your right to access the resources you need.
- Among your rights is access to a professional health service and treatment plus confidentiality of your personal health care records.
- You are entitled to access to health information, support and supplies.
- Your other rights include a career of your choice, life and health insurance cover, appropriate job training and most civil licences and permits.
- Among your responsibilities is to declare your diabetes when applying for insurance, licences and permits.
- Failure to declare your diabetes to an employer may render you ineligible for workers' compensation.

28. Diabetes in General Practice – page 99

- Find a GP who is respectful and with whom you feel comfortable.
- Optimum diabetes care requires regularly scheduled GP consultations for adequate review and management.

- Look for a GP who is experienced in diabetes care and who has an organised approach.
- Use your GP as a health care resource to refer you on when you need specialist help.
- Don't be afraid to seek a second opinion.

29. Travelling with Diabetes - page 101

- Plan ahead by making lists.
- Carry a letter from your doctor saying you have diabetes and describing your medication requirements.
- Pack a traveller's survival kit which contains:
  - quick-acting carbohydrate (for example, glucose)
  - slow-acting carbohydrate snack (for example, dried fruits)
  - glucagon and syringes
  - quick-acting insulin (neutral, clear)
  - blood testing equipment
  - Medical Alert bracelet
  - basic first aid requirements
  - key contacts details at home and abroad
  - useful and relevant phrases in the language of your destination.

30. Diabetes and Discrimination - page 107

- It is illegal to use diabetes as a good reason not to employ a person unless there is good evidence that diabetes would prevent the person from adequately performing the genuine and reasonable requirements of the position.
- There are no specific discrimination laws relating to diabetes.
- Discrimination based on the condition is covered by the Human Rights and Equal Opportunity Commission Act 1986, the Disability Discrimination Act 1992 and others.
- Most problems relate to work or employment.
- Contact Diabetes Australia if you believe you have been discriminated against because of your diabetes.
- There is an official policy on driving and diabetes (phone 02 6289 1430 for information).

31. Insurance and Diabetes - page 110

- People with diabetes traditionally faced problems when seeking to take out insurance or obtain a driver's licence. However, improved life expectancy figures and consumer pressure are having an effect.
- Insurance policy prices are coming down due not only to improved health outcomes but to market competition and lobbying by Diabetes Australia.
- People with diabetes will benefit from adequate informed preparation before applying to an insurance company for cover.
- If you encounter any setbacks when seeking insurance, employment packages or specialised licences, contact your local Diabetes Australia office for advice.

32. Further Resources - page 113

- Each State and Territory has a Diabetes Australia office. Join for information, assistance, savings and advice.
- Reference literature and guidance on the latest and most up-to-date diabetes literature is available through Diabetes Australia.
- Information is also available from your health care team and, if they don't know the answers, they will refer you to others who do.

33. The Genetics of Diabetes - page 117

- Just because there is diabetes in the family does not mean that people genetically at risk will automatically contract diabetes.
- Genetic factors influence both types of diabetes, although each is a distinctly different clinical and genetic disorder.
- The majority of people with high risk antigens for type 1 diabetes never develop the condition.
- The overall chance of developing type 1 diabetes for a brother or sister of someone with the condition is 6 per cent, or about 1 in 20.
- Even though a person may have inherited a tendency to develop type 2 diabetes, food and exercise may postpone the onset of the condition or prevent it from developing.
- Relatives of people with type 2 diabetes are at risk of developing the condition.

34. Around the World with Diabetes - page 120

- Travelling in countries unfamiliar with type 1 diabetes presents special risks if you become ill or need surgery, as insulin must never be omitted.
- Lifestyle changes from strenuous rural existence to sedentary city life are linked to an ongoing and dramatic increase in type 2 diabetes.
- Because of countries' different approaches to health services, the International Diabetes Federation works at several levels to improve people's access to medication and care.
- Regardless of where they live, people with diabetes and their families face similar issues and problems, but the solutions need to be culturally specific.

35. The Impact of Diabetes - page 123

- An estimated 700,000 to 800,000 Australians have diabetes and numbers are increasing.
- About 25,000 Australians develop diabetes each year, with the total national cost of treatment exceeding $1 billion annually, or about $2,800 for every person with diabetes.
- Type 2 diabetes is by far the most frequent

form of diabetes, representing about 80 per cent of all cases.

- Two major factors account for Australia's predicted rise in diabetes – we're getting older, putting more people at risk of type 2 diabetes; and the key diabetes risk factors – obesity and inactivity – are on the rise.
- Our main defence against diabetes in Australia is to reduce the risk factors associated with the disorder.

36. National Diabetes Strategy - page 126

- Diabetes is a chronic and costly disease that incurs an enormous personal and public health burden.
- An estimated 780,000 Australians have diabetes. Of these approximately 430,000 have diagnosed diabetes and another 350,000 have undiagnosed diabetes.
- The National Diabetes Strategy is about people who have diabetes, those who care for people with diabetes, and people who are at risk of developing diabetes.
- It is the blueprint for action to improve diabetes services in the next 10 years.

37. Diabetes: Back to the Future - page 128

- Thanks to research and new information, the outlook for people with diabetes has improved significantly in recent years.
- Most advances in the treatment of diabetes were made in the past 20 years, although the condition is one of the oldest recorded.
- Although there are treatment breakthroughs coming from biological and genetic engineering research, it makes more sense to prevent type 2 diabetes by education, behavioural and lifestyle changes than to hope for a miracle cure which many affected people couldn't afford anyway.
- Given the knowledge and techniques now available, plus the momentum of diabetes research internationally, we are at the threshold of a new era in which the outcome for people with diabetes will be dramatically improved by new forms of treatment.

Acetone: See Ketones.

Adrenal: A gland of the endocrine system that produces essential hormones including adrenalin and cortisone.

Albumin: A water soluble protein present in the urine with kidney damage (albuminuria).

Alpha Cells: Cells in the pancreas that produce the hormone glucagon.

Angiography: A rapid series of pictures of blood vessels made after a dye has been injected.

Antibodies: Substances occurring naturally in the body that help fight infection.

Arteriosclerosis/ Atherosclerosis: Thickening,hardening and narrowing of the arteries.

Artery: A blood vessel that carries blood away from the heart.

Aspartame: A low calorie artificial sweetener.

Beta Cells: The insulin producing cells of the pancreas.

Callus: A hardened or thickened part of the skin caused by pressing or rubbing.

Calorie: A measure of the energy value of foods (now replaced by kilojoule). 1 calorie = 4.2 kilojoules.

Candida: A yeast like fungus infection often affecting the female genital area.

Capillary: Tiny blood vessels that connect the smallest arteries to the smallest veins.

Carbohydrate: Foods which contain sugars and starches.

Cardiovascular: Pertaining to the heart and blood vessels.

Cataract: An opacity in the lens of the eye.

Cell: The microscopic unit that forms the basis of all living things.

Cholesterol: A fatty substance produced by the human body and also found in animal tissue.

Claudication: Pain in the calf muscles occurring on exercise and disappearing with rest. Caused by decreased blood supply.

Coma: Loss of consciousness from any cause. In diabetes from very high or very low blood glucose levels.

Creatinine: A waste product normally removed by the kidneys.

Cyclamate: A low calorie artificial sweetener.

Cystitis: An inflammation of the urinary bladder.

Dehydrated: Loss of water or fluid from the body.

Dextrose: See glucose.

Dialysis: Artificial removal of waste products from the blood when the kidneys fail.

Diabetes: Disease in which the body cannot produce insulin or use insulin properly. Characterised by high blood glucose levels.

Digestion: Breaking down food in the stomach and intestines.

Electrocardiograph (ECG): The recording of the electrical activity of the heart.

Endocrine Glands: Glands that produce chemicals (hormones) which affect other body cells.

Enzyme: A substance that speeds up a chemical reaction.

Erectile dysfunction: See impotence.

Exchanges: Servings of food that contain the same food value. Also known as portions.

Fat Atrophy/ Hypertrophy:	Hollows (atrophy) or lumps (hypertrophy) that occur at sites of repeated insulin injection.
Fibre:	Food substances found in cereals, fruits and vegetables that are not digested but help the function of the intestines.
Fluorescein:	A harmless yellow coloured dye that is used to outline the vessels of the eye.
Fructosamine:	A glycated protein like glycated haemoglobin that measures glucose control over the preceding weeks.
Fructose:	A sugar found in fruits.
Gangrene:	Death of body tissue usually caused by lack of blood supply.
Gestational:	Referring to the period of pregnancy from conception to birth.
Glomerulus:	A tiny tuft of blood vessels that is part of the functional unit of the kidney.
Glucagon:	A hormone produced in the pancreas that increases blood glucose.
Glucose:	The form of sugar found in the human body.
Glucose Tolerance Test:	A diagnostic test for diabetes involving a drink of glucose and a series of blood glucose estimations.
Glycaemic index:	A system of ranking carbohydrate foods based on their blood glucose response compared to ingesting glucose.
Glycosuria:	The presence of glucose in the urine.
Haemoglobin:	The red coloured iron protein that carries oxygen in red cells.
Haemoglobin AM:	Alpha (glucagon producing) cells. See glycated haemoglobin.
HLA:	Human leucocyte antigens which are natural markers on white cells much the same as blood groups on red cells.
Hormone:	A chemical substance produced by endocrine glands which causes specific effects on other cells.
Hyperglycaemia:	Blood glucose higher than normal.
Hypertension:	High blood pressure.
Hypoglycaemia:	Blood glucose level lower than normal.
Impotence:	The inability in males to start, sustain or complete the act of sexual intercourse.
Insulin:	A hormone produced by the pancreas that lowers blood glucose.
Insulin Dependent Diabetes:	See Type 1 diabetes.
Insulin resistance:	When the body does not respond to insulin properly.
Intramuscular:	Administration of a medication through a needle into the muscles.
Intravenous:	Administration of a medication through a needle into a vein.
Islet Cell (of Langerhans):	Clusters of cells in the pancreas which include the beta (insulin producing) and alpha (glucagon producing) cells.
Juvenile Onset:	See Type 1 diabetes.
Keto-acidosis:	Uncontrolled blood glucose and ketone levels that cause dehydration, concentration of body fluids, build up of acids (acidosis) and coma.
Ketones:	Chemical substances from the breakdown of fat which can be dangerous in large amounts.
Ketones in the Urine (Ketonuria):	Warns of keto-acidosis.

Kilojoule:	A measurement of the energy of food which has replaced calorie (1 calorie = 4.2 kilojoules).
Lactic Acidosis:	A serious condition caused by the build up of lactic acid which is produced from glucose when there is not enough oxygen. Similar effects as ketoacidosis.
Lactose:	A sugar found in milk.
Laser (Light Amplification by Stimulated Emission of Radiation):	An intense narrow beam of light which can be used to heal damaged areas in the body (eg blood vessels in the eye).
Macrovascular:	Referring to the large blood vessels.
Maturity Onset Diabetes:	See Type 2 diabetes.
Metabolism:	The physical and chemical changes occurring in the body.
Microalbuminuria:	Leakage of small amounts of protein (albumin) into the urine. An early warning of kidney damage.
Microvascular:	Referring to the small blood vessels.
Millimole (mmol):	A measurement of the concentration of chemicals in the body.
Monilia:	See Candida.
Nephropathy:	Disease of the kidneys.
Neuropathy:	Disease of the nerves.
Non Insulin Dependent Diabetes:	See Type 2 diabetes.
Obesity:	The condition of severe overweight.
Oral Hypoglycaemic Agents:	Medications taken by mouth that stimulate the release or improve the action of insulin.
Pancreas:	A gland lying towards the back of the abdomen half way between the tummy button and line joining the nipples.
Photocoagulation:	Use of the laser to treat diabetic eye disease.
Plasma:	The liquid portion of blood.
Polyuria:	The passage of large amounts of urine.
Portions:	See exchanges.
Prandial:	Referring to meals eg pre-prandial: before meals; post-prandial: after meals.
Pruritus:	Itching.
Renal Threshold:	The blood glucose level above which glucose spills into the urine.
Retinopathy:	Damage to the retina of the eye.
Saccharin:	A low calorie artificial sweetener.
Somogyi Effect:	A rebound effect of low glucose followed by high blood glucose caused by too much insulin.
Sorbitol:	A sugar used to sweeten foods.
Subcutaneous:	Underneath the skin.
Sugars:	Simple carbohydrates which are sweet and occur widely in nature eg fructose, glucose, lactose, sucrose.
Sucrose:	A common widely available sugar from sugar cane or sugar beet.
Thrush:	See Candida.
Thyroid:	An endocrine gland in the base of the neck producing hormones controlling the body's metabolism.
Triglyceride:	A type of fat found in the blood and other parts of the body.

Type 1 Diabetes: Where little or no insulin is made, usually occurring under the age of 30 and requiring insulin injections for life. Also known as insulin dependent and juvenile onset diabetes.

Type 2 Diabetes: Insulin is present but doesn't work adequately. Usually occurs over the age of 30 and is controlled by diet and medication or diet and insulin. Also known as non insulin dependent and maturity onset diabetes.

Unit: The measurement of the dose of insulin.

Uraemia: Build up of poisons because of kidney failure.

Vein: A blood vessel that carries blood to the heart.

Abbreviations & Measures

Abbreviations

cc cubic centimetre

cm centimetre

g gram

kg kilogram

L litre

mg milligram

mmol = millimole
(eg. 5 mmol/L = 5 millimoles per litre)

Kj Kilojoule

Cal Calorie

lb pounds

Measures

1 level teaspoon = 5 ml

1 level tablespoom = 20 ml

1 cup = 250 ml

1 Kj = 1000 joules

1 Cal = 4.2 Kj

1 oz = 28.4 g

1000 g (1 kg) = 2.2 lbs

1 pint = 570 ml

1 fluid oz = 28.4 ml

1000 ml (1 litre) = 1.76 pints

Aboriginal people, and diabetes, 86-88, 124, 125, 135; lifestyle, 86-87; susceptibility to diabetes, 86
Acarbose, 14, 15, 18, 83
ACE inhibitors, 44, 52, 84
Acid blood, 37, 47, 78
Activity, 8; and hypoglycaemia, 39; physical, 16, 52
Actrapid, See Humulin R©, 28
Adalat™, 43, 46
Adolescence, 80
Adrenaline, 39, 45
Aerobic exercise, 19
Agon™, 46
Albumin, in urine, 52
Alcohol, 9, 12, 44, 52; and hypoglycaemia, 39; and medications, 45
Aldomet™, 46
Alford, Frank, 21-24
Allergy, to insulin, 30, 55
Allopurinol, 44
Allorin, 44
Ambulance insurance, 94
Ames Glucolet™, 35
Ames Glucostix, strips, 34
Amputation, 51, 53; See also Complications
Anaerobic exercise, 19
Angina, 46, 73
Angiogram, fluorescein, 57
Angiotensin converting enzyme inhibitors, see ACE inhibitors, 44
Antacids, 44-46
Antibiotics, 45; syrups, 43
Antidepressants, 44
Antifungal drugs, 44
Antigens, 117
Antihistamine syrups, 43, 46
Aspirin™, 44, 84
Atenolol, 45
Atromid-S™, 44
Atrophy, fatty, 24, 30, 54
Australian Diabetes Society, 71, 107, 112
Australian Paediatric Endocrine Group, 80
Autolet II - Austral Scientific™, 35
Automatic injectors, 28
Avomine™, 106
Ayers, Bernie, v, vii

Baby, large (macrosomic), 70, 71
Babysitting an infant or young child with diabetes, 114
Bactrim™, 45, 105
Baldwin, Jeannette, v, 126-127
Barfoot, Karen, v, 114-115
B-D Autolance™, 35
B-D Magni-Guide™, 28
B-D pen, 26, 27
Beta-blocker medications, 44, 45, 46, 84
Betacheck, strips, 34
Betaloc™, 45
Bladder infection, 53
Blindness, 56; See also Complications, Retinopathy
Blood fats, high, 54
Blood glucose, causes of high, 117; high, 40, 41, 54; low, 39, 40; monitoring, 31-35
Blood glucose control, 23, 24, 32, 38, 51, 83, 94, 97, 98, 111
Blood glucose levels, 17, 1821, 31, 32; factors influencing 32, 51
Blood glucose meters, 32-34
Blood glucose monitoring, 31, 41, 42, 60, 94, 96, 132; and illness, 48; during pregnancy, 69; during travel, 104; frequency of, 31; how to obtain blood for 34; in the elderly, 83; right to 96; schedules for, 31; testing techniques, 32; visual method 32, 104
Blood glucose test strips, types, 34
Blood pressure, high, 38, 46, 51, 52, 54, 58, 73, 84; low, 46; monitoring, 84, 94, 98
Blood vessels, blockage, 52; damage, to feet, 59, 60; factors affecting, 60
BM Advantage™, 33
BM Soft Touch™, 35
Boehringer Mannheim 20-800, strip, 34
Bornstein, Joseph, 129
Bowen, Kerry, v, 47-49
Brain, blockage of blood vessels, 52
Breast cancer, 74
Breast feeding, 71
Brown, Lynette, v, vii, 8, 9, 10-13
Bruising, 30
Brushing, tooth, 62
Busher injector, 28

Caesarean section, 70
Callus, 60
Campbell, Lesley, v, 66, 67
Camps, for school children, 79; for teenagers, 81; information sheet, 114
Cancer, breast, 74
Carbohydrates, 5, 10; and exercise, 17; complex, 8; digestion of and Acarbose, 15; effect on blood glucose, 11; exchange system, 13; extra when travelling, 102; metabolism of, 74
Carbohydrate spacing, 11
Cardiovascular disease, 16, 18,52, 73
Care of test strips, 32
Carer's groups, 2
Carter, John, v, 107, 110-112
Cartridge, for insulin pens, 26, 28
Cataract, 52, 56
Cerebrovascular disease, 52
Children, 76-79, 121; physical problems at school, 77; symptoms of hypoglycaemia in, 77; treatment of hypoglycaemia in, 77
Chisholm, Don, v, 16-19
Chlorporpamide, 15
Chlorpromide, 83
Chlorpropamide, 45
Cholesterol, 54, 55, 74, 97; HDL, 74; high, 54; LDL, 74
Clear insulin, 26, 83
Clinistix™ 37
Clofibrate, 44
Cloudy insulin, 22, 26, 27, 48, 83
Comfort Touch™ 35
Communication, importance of, 100
Community awareness, 126, 127
Complications of diabetes 51-55, 58, 59, 109, 131; and insurance, 110; and medications, 45, 46; and traditional medicine, 122; early screening for, 80; in the elderly, 83; long term, 133; minor, 54, 55; prevention of, 83, 84; risk factors for, 51, 54
Confidentiality, 96
Conquest magazine, 33, 113
Contraception, 66
Contraception, 66; barrier, 66; oral, 43, 66
Control, blood glucose, 6, 38, 58, 83, 94, 97, 98, 111; ideal 32
Control fluid, for blood glucose meters, 33
Corns, 60, 61
Coronary artery disease, 16, 18, 52, 73
Corticosteroids, 43
Cost of diabetes, 121, 125
Cough mixtures, 43, 46
Counselling, sexual, 65
Countdown magazine, 114
Couselling, genetic, 118
Creatinine, 98
Cromer, Thomas, v, 64, 65
Culture, 90
Cure for Type 1 diabetes, possibility of, 129
Customs, 90
Cystitis, 54

Dangerous activities, and diabetes, 9, 19, 112
Daonil, 15
Dehydration, 47, 49, 105
Delivery, of baby, 70
Dementia, 73
Dental health, and diabetes, 54, 62, 63
Dental Health Education Unit, South Australian Dental Service, 62, 63
Dental treatment, 63
Dentures, 63
Department of Health, travel advice, 105
Diabetes, among immigrants to Australia, 89; complications of, 51-55,131; discovery of types of, 128, 129; effects on vision, 56; gestational, 68, 71, 89, 119, 125; prevention of type 2, 87, 131; testing for, 71; treatment of, 71; in Australia, 124, 125; in the elderly, 82-85; symptoms in the elderly, 82; treatment in the elderly, 83; treatment in the future, 125
Diabetes Australia, 2, 25, 33, 79, 81, 91, 94, 96, 97, 109, 111, 113, 114; and discrimination, 107; policy on driving, 107
Diabetes Control and Complications Trial, 51, 80, 125, 128
Diabetes Education Service, Queen Elizabeth Hospital South Australia, v
Diabetes educators, 90, 114
Diabetes mellitus, definition of, 5
Diabex, 15
Diabinese, 15
Diaformin, 15
Diamicron, 15
Diarrhoea, 47, 49; and travelling, 105
Diastix™ 37
Diet, and tablets, 14
Dietitians, 90, 114
Dilantin™, 43, 44
Diment, Tony, v, 80, 81
Dining out, hints for, 12, 13
Diphenhydramine, 106
Disability Discrimination Act 1992, 107
Disclosing information, 108
Discrimination, 97, 107-109, 136
Disposal of sharps, 35
Distribution of diabetes in the world, 120
Diuretics, 43, 44, 84
Doctor, responsibilities of, 94; visiting regularly, 93, 94; when to call, 48
Documents, personal, 101, 102
Doxycycline, 105
Dramamine™ 106
Driver's licence, 97
Driving, and diabetes, 107, 112
Dry mouth, 63
Dunning, Trisha, v, vii, 21-24, 31-38
Dysfunction, erectile, 64, 65

Eating, healthy, 10-13, 132; in the elderly, 83
Education, access to, 89; nutrition, 13; sexual, 65
Effectiveness, of tablets, 14
Elderly people, definition, 82; diabetes in the, 82-85, 135
Electronic meters, 33
Eli Lilly, 27, 28
Emergency treatment, 48
Employment, and diabetes, 108
Epidemiologic transition, 123
Erectile dysfunction, 64, 65
Erection, physiology of, 64; vacuum-assisted, 65
Ethnicity, and diabetes, 89, 119; and Type 2 diabetes, 124
Euglucon, 15
Evans, Angela, v, 59-61
Examinations, and children with diabetes, 79; and older students with diabetes, 81
Exchange, carbohydrate, 13
Excursions, and school children, 79
Exercise, 8, 10, 16-19, 52, 87, 93, 132; and hypoglycaemia, 39; and school children, 79
Exercise and diabetes, 16-19
Eye damage, 52
Eyes, annual examination of, 95; damage to, 52; diabetes and, 56-58, 134; laser treatment, 58; monitoring, 84, 98; See also Retinopathy
Eyesight, aids for poor, 28

Family history, of diabetes, 51, 117
Fat, 11; body, 8; food, 8; reducing, 12
Fat atrophy, 24, 30, 54
Fat hypertrophy, 24, 30, 54
Fats, blood, 51; monitoring, 84
Fatty tissue, hollows in, 24, 30, 54; lumps in, 24, 30, 54
Feet, monitoring of, 95, 98; See Foot
Felodipine, 46
Fibre, dietary, 10, 87
Fingerprick devices, 34; automatic, 35
Flossing, dental, 62
Fluid, control, for blood glucose meters, 33
Fluid retention, 55
Fluids, 42, 48, 49, 63, 105
Fluorescein angiogram, 57
Food, for school children, 78, 79; selection, 11
Food labelling, 12
Foods, for sick days, 48, 49
Foot care, 3, 59-61, 93, 127, 134; damage to feet 53, 61; and exercise, 18, 19; monitoring, 59, 84; shape, 59, 60
Foot wear, 59-61, 134

Gangrene, 52
Gauge, needle, 25
General practice, and diabetes, 99, 100, 114, 135
Generic names, of medications, 43
Genetic engineering, 130
Genetics, and diabetes, 87, 88, 117-119, 136
Genotype, thrifty, 124
Gestational diabetes, 68, 71, 89, 119, 125; in Australian Aboriginals, 71; in ethnic groups, 71; testing for, 71; treatment of, 71
GI, 10, 11
Glcyaemic index, 10, 11
Glibenclamide, 15, 83
Gliclazide, 15, 83
Glimel, 15
Glipizide, 15, 83
Glucagon, 40, 41, 78, 105
Glucobay, 15
Glucometer™, 33
Glucophage, 15
Glucose, 5, 10; altered response to, 45; channels, 5, 6; and exercise, 16, 17; effects of, 51; in urine, 36; monitoring blood glucose, 31-35; testing urine for, 37
Glycated haemoglobin, 69, 94, 97
Glycogen, 41
Golden Guidelines, for lifestyle, 8, 9
Good-better-best, system of food selection, 11
GP, choosing, 99
GPs, and diabetes, 99, 100, 114
Gum, chewing, 63

Haemoglobin, glycated, 69, 94, 97
Harris, Gillian, v, 80, 81
Harrison, Leonard, v, 128-131

HbA1c, 69, 94, 97
HDL cholesterol, 74
Health care, right to, 90, 96
Health care team, 93-95, 135
Health insurance, 108
Health professionals, and teenagers, 80; in migrant communities, 90
Heart attack, 52, 73
Heart disease, 16, 18, 52, 73
Herbal medicines, 46, 74, 122
Heredity and diabetes, 117-119
History, family, 51, 117
History of insulin, 128
HLAs, 117, 118
Holmwood, Chris, v
Hormone Replacement Therapy, and diabetes, 72-74, 134
Horton, Joy, v, 1-2
HRT, 72-74, 134
Humalog™, 23, 83
Human Leucocyte Antigens, 117, 118
Human Rights and Equal Opportunity Commission Act 1986, 107
Humapen, 27
Humulin©, 23, 27, 48; NPH, 26, 28, 83, 106; R, 26, 28, 83, 106; UL, 83
Hunter-gatherer lifestyle, 86
Hyperglycaemia, 5, 6, 39-42, 63, 133; causes of, 40, 42; effect on blood, 40; effect on urine, 40; onset, 40; symptoms of, 40, 42; treatment, 40
Hypertrophy, fatty, 24, 30, 54
Hypoglycaemia, 2, 5, 6, 15, 39-42, 45, 51, 53, 68, 69, 83, 133; after exercise, 18; and tablets, 39; causes of, 39, 40; effect on blood, 40; effect on partner, 1; effect on urine, 40; in children, 39, 77-78; onset, 40; prevention of, 41; prevention of; recognition of, 18; symptoms of, 39, 40; treatment, 40, 41, 77-78; severe, 77, 78; when travelling, 105
Hypoglycaemic agents, oral, 14; See also Tablets
Hypoguard Supreme, strip, 34
Hypurin, 23

Identification, 101
IDF, 121
Illness, 23, 38, 47-49, 133; use of tablets during, 15; when travelling, 104; See also Sick days
Imodium™ 105
Impact of diabetes, 123-125, 136
Implants, penile, 65
Impotence, 46, 53, 64; definition of, 65; tests for, 65; treatment of, 65
In Control (book), 114
Independence, and teenagers, 81
Induction, of labour, 70
Infection, 53; foot, 60; gums, 62; mouth, 63; oral, 63; yeast, 66
Information, 3, 97; right to, 96; on overseas contacts, 113; on travel, 113
Infusion pump, 24
Injections, 25-30, 132; schedule, 3; site, choice of, 28, 29, 55, 95, 98; techniques 24, 29, 30
Injectors, 25-30, 132; automatic, 28; jet, 28; pens, 26, 27
Insulin, 21, 22, 23, 24, 25, 93, 132; mixed, 22, 23, 26, 28, 48; adjustment of dosage, 18, 23,24, 47, 51, 70, 103, 104; altered response to, 45; and illness, 23, 48; and infection, 23; and medications, 43, 44; and menstruation, 23; and travelling, 102; cartridges available, 28; clear, 26, 83;cloudy, 22, 26, 27, 48, 83; cost of, 121; during pregnancy, 69; history of, 128; immune reactions to, 24; intermediate-acting, 28, 48, 83; in the elderly, 83; isophane, 23, 83; lispro, 22, 28; long-acting, 22, 48; neutral, 22, 23; oedema, 55; packing, 102, 103; pens, 24-27; rapid onset short-acting, 22; reactions to, 24; response to, 17; resistance, 16, 30, 68, 129; sensitivity, 69; short-acting, 22, 28; soluble, 22, 23; storage of, 22; temperature of, 22; therapy, intensive, 51; timing of, and meals, 21; types of, 21-23; zinc suspension, 23; units, 22, 25, 103
Insurance, 97, 107, 110-112, 136; ambulance, 94; health, 108; information required, 110; life, 110, 113; travel, 101, 113
Intensive insulin therapy, 51
Intermediate acting insulin, 83
International Diabetes Federation, 121
International flights, food and drink on, 102
Interpreters, 90
Intracavernosal injection, 65
Intra-uterine contraceptive device, 66
Ischaemic heart disease, 52
Islet cells, 128; transplantation
Isophane, 23, 83
Isordil™, 46
Isosorbide, 46
Isotard, 23
Isotrate™, 46
Itinerary, need for detailed, 101
IUD, 66

JDFA, 114, 115
JDFI, 114
Jet injectors, 28
Jet lag, 104
Juvenile Diabetes Foundation Australia, 79, 81, 114, 115
Juvenile Diabetes Foundation International, 114, 130

Kaomagma, for diarrhoea in children, 105
Keogh, Ted, 64, 65
Keto-acidosis, 37, 47; in children, 78
Ketodiastix™ 37
Ketones, 47, 48; in urine, 36, 37
Ketonuria, 37
Kidneys, 36; and pregnancy, 69; annual examination of, 95; damage, 37, 52, 84; infection, 53, 54; monitoring, 84
Kidson, Warren, v, 51-55
Kids with Diabetes, video, 114
Kliogest™ 74

Labelling, food, 12
Labour, 70
Lancets, 35
Laser treatment, 58
Launceston General Hospital, Tasmania, 129
LDL cholesterol, 74
Leadership Needs Assessment Workshop, IDF, 121
Legs, blockage of blood vessels, 52
Length, of needle, 25
Letter from doctor, for travellers, 102
Libido, 64, 67
Licences and permits, 94, 97; for buses, taxis, articulated vehicles and dangerous goods vehicles, 112; for driving cars and motorcycles, 112
Life Insurance Federation of Australia, 111
Lifestyle, 88, 132; and diabetes, 8, 9; changes, 120, 123, 131; healthy, in the elderly, 83; healthy, 95

Lipids, 74, 84
Lipoprotein, high density, 97
Lispro insulin, 22, 23, 28
Liver, 17, 41
Lomotil™, 105
Long-acting insulin, 22
Look on the Bright Side, 114
Lopressor™, 45
Lowther, Bernadette, v, 89-91
Luggage, hand, 102
Lunch, for school children, 78, 79

Macrosomic baby, 70, 71
Macrovascular problems, 53
Maculopathy, 56, 58
Malaria, 105
Marathon running, 18
Marshall, Patricia, v, 10-13
Martin, Ian, 68-71
Mauritius, 124
McCarty, Daniel, v, 123-125
McElduff, Aidan, v, 107, 108, 109
McEwen, Ian, v, 3
McGill, Margaret, v, 120-122
Meal plan, 3, 13
Medical alert bracelet, 94
Medical assistance, 48
Medications, 93, 94, 133; and diabetes, 43-46; for diabetes in the elderly, 83; generic names, 43; herbal, 46; over the counter, 46; packing, 102; when travelling, 105; which affect blood glucose levels, 43, 44
MediSense Precision™ 33
Melizide, 15
Menopause, 67, 74; and diabetes, 72-74, 134; complications of, 72;
Menoprem 28™, 74
Mensch, Melba, v, 10-13, 47-49
Menstruation, 23, 66
Meridian™, 33
Metformin, 14, 15, 18, 44, 83
Methyldopa, 46
Metoprolol, 45
Microalbuminuria, 38, 98
Microvascular problems, 53
Migrant groups, and diabetes, 135
Mini Autolet™ 35
Minidiab, 15
Mitchell, Paul, v, 56-58
Mixed insulin, 22, 26, 28, 48
Mixtard, 22, 23, 28
Moffitt, Paul, v, vii, 101-106
Monilia, 66, 67
Monitoring, blood glucose, 31-35
Monoamine oxidase antidepressants, 44
Monotard™ 26, 27; See also Humulin
Motion sickness, 106
Mouthwash, 63
Murray, Shirley, v, 113, 114
Muscle cells, 5, 6, 17
Nails, toe, 60, 61
Nankervis, Alison, v, 68-71
Nathan, David, 96-98
National Diabetes Strategy, 126-127, 137
National Diabetic Services Scheme, 25, 91, 96, 108, 113
National Health Priority Area, diabetes as, 126
National Institutes of Health, USA, 130
Natural therapies, for menopause, 74
NDSS, 25, 91, 96, 108, 113
Necrobiosis lipoidica diabeticorum, 55
Needle, for insulin pens, 27; gauge, 25; length of, 25
Nephropathy, 37, 52, 84; and pregnancy, 69
Nerve damage, 46, 53; to feet, 59
Neuropathy, 46, 53; peripheral, 59
National Health and Medical Research Council (NHMRC), 105, 107, 112; booklet on HRT, 74; Retinopathy Guidelines, 58, 126
Nifedipine, 43, 46
Nitrate ointments, 46; patches, 46
Nitro-bid™ 46
Nitrodise™, 46
Non-English speaking background, diabetes and people of, 126
Non-steroidal anti-inflammatory medications, 44, 46
Noradrenaline, 45
Norfloxacin, 105
Noten™, 45
Novo Nordisk, 28
Novopen, 26, 27
Nutrition, for teenagers, 80; information, 12

O'Dea, Kerin, v, 86-88
O'Neal, David, v, 21-24
Obstetric management, 70
Oedema, insulin, 55
Oestrogen, 72
Ophthalmologist, examination by, 57, 95
Oral health, 54, 62, 63, 134
Oral hypoglycaemic agents, 14
Oral insulin, future possibility of, 130
Osteoporosis, 72, 73; risk factors for, 72
Over the counter medicines, 46
Overweight, 51, 54, 87, 98
Oxytetracycline, 44, 45

Pancreas, 5, 41, 128; transplantation, 129, 130
Papua New Guinea, 124
Paraesthesiae, 59
Parkin, Mary, v, 72-74
Penfill cartridge, 26, 28
Penile implants, 65
Pen injectors, 24, 25, 26
Penis, physiology of, 64
Peripheral vascular disease, 52, 73
Pfizer, 65
Phenothiazine, 43
Phenytoin, 43, 44
Phillips, Pat, v, vii, 5-6, 8, 9, 14, 15, 93-95
Physical activity, 8, 10, 16-19, 39, 52, 79, 87, 93, 132
Phytoestrogens, 74
Planning, for children's activities, 79; pregnancy, 69
Plates, dental, 63
Plendil™ 46
Podiatrist, 59, 95, 114
Polydipsia, 5, 6
Polyphagia, 5, 6
Polyuria, 5, 6
Popplewell, Phil, v, 82-85
Pre-ecalmpsia, in pregnancy, 70
Pregnancy, and diabetes, 68-71, 89, 119,134; and insulin, 22; and motion sickness treatments, 106; complications during, 69, 70; in women with pre-existing diabetes, 68-71; metabolic changes during, 68; planning, 69; renal threshold in, 36; testing urine for protein in, 37, 38; use of tablets during, 15
Premiums, insurance, 110, 111
Preventive treatment, 129
Progout, 44
Promothazine, 106
Prostaglandin E1, 65
Prostin™ 70
Protaphane, 23, 28, 83
Protein, in food, 10, 11; in urine, 36, 37, 38, 52
Provelle 28™, 74
Psychological problems, in children with diabetes, 79
Pump, infusion, 24
Pyelonephritis, 54
Pyramid, food, 11

Quick-acting insulin, 22, 28, 83
Quinine, 44, 45

Race, and diabetes, 89, 119, 124
Raine, June, 93-95
Ramsay, John, 129
Rapid onset short-acting insulin, 22
Rastinon, 15
Reaction, skin; to insulin, 30
Record keeping, blood glucose, 23, 95
Record keeping, urine test results, 38, 95
Reference material, for people with diabetes, 113
Reflectance meters, 33, 34
Reflolux S™, 33
Relationships, effect of diabetes on, 1, 67; with GP, 99; teenagers, 81
Relaxation, 8, 9, 80
Religion, 90
Renal threshold, 31, 36, 37
Research, 115, 137; current and future, 130; results of recent, 129
Resistance, insulin, 16, 30, 68, 129
Resources, for people with diabetes, 90, 113-115, 136
Responsibilities, 93, 94, 96-98, 135; diabetes and driving, 107; for diabetic control, 97, 98
Resprim™ 105
Restaurants, 12, 13
Retinopathy, 52, 56, 69; chance of, 56; examinations for, 57; exercise and, 19; laser treatment for, 58; proliferative, 56, 58; testing for, 57, 58; See also Eyes
Retinopathy Guidelines, NHMRC, 58, 126
Reversal of diabetes in Aboriginal people, 86, 87
Rights, and diabetes, 96-98, 108, 135; of people with diabetes, 96
Risk factors for complications, 51
Roads and Traffic Authority, 112
Royal Blind Society, 109
Running, 18, 108

Sainsbury, Joanne, vii
Saliva, artificial, 63
Salt, replacement of, 49
School, and diabetes, 76-79; information sheet, 114; school children, and diabetes, 135; staff, 76
Sea sickness, 106
Scuba diving, 97
Sensivity to insulin, during pregnancy, 69
Septrim™ 45, 105
Serjeantson, Susan, v, 117-119
Sex life, women's, 67
Sexual problems, in men, 64, 65, 134
Sharps containers, 35
Shenfield, Gillian, v, 43-46
Shopping, 12
Short-acting insulin, 22
Sick days, 23, 38, 47-49, 133; when travelling, 104
Side effects, of tablets, 14
Sildenafil, 65
Silink, Martin, v, 76-79
Site for injection, choice of, 28, 29
Skin, redness or sores, 55; reactions, to insulin, 30
Smoking, 9, 45, 51, 54
South Australian Dental Service, Dental Health Education Unit, 62, 63
Specialist care, 97, 100, 114
Sport, 16; and school children, 79; See also Exercise
Starch, 10; See also Carbohydrate
Sterilisation, 66
Stocks, Alan, v, 25-30
Storage, of cartridges, 27; of insulin, 22, 102, 103
Stress, 8, 9, 80; and hyperglycaemia, 42
Strips, for blood glucose testing, 34
Stroke, 73
Subsidy, for products to manage diabetes, 25, 91, 96, 108, 113
Sugar, 10; See also Glucose
Sulphonamide, 44
Sulphonylureas, 14, 17, 18, 44, 45, 83
Superannuation, 111
Supplies, access to, 96
Support, access to, 96; groups, 81
Swelling, ankles, 55; face, 55
Syringes, 24, 25

Tablets, 14, 15, 93, 94, 132; adjustment of dose, 18; and breast feeding, 71; and hypoglycaemia, 39; and other medications, 43, 44; during pregnancy, 69; effect of, 14; for diabetes in the elderly, 83; side effects of, 14
Taft, Pincus, 14, 15
Teacher, added responsibility of, 76
Teenagers, and diabetes, 80-81, 135
Tenormin™ 45
Testape™, 37
Testing techniques, blood glucose, 32
Test strips, blood glucose, 34; care of, 32
Tetracycline, 105
The Only Remedy is a Cure, 115
Thomson, Glenys, 118
Threshold, renal, 31, 36, 37
Thrifty genotype, 124
Thrombosis, risk of, 66
Thrush, 66
TIA, 52
Time zones, and insulin injections, 103
Tobacco, 9, 45, 51, 54
Toenails, 60, 61
Tolbutamide, 15, 45
Traditional lifestyle, of Australian Aboriginal people, 86, 87
Traditional medicine, 122
Tradition, 90
Tranquilisers, 43
Transiderm Nitro™, 46
Transient ischaemic attack, 52, 73
Transplantation, islet cell, 130; pancreas, 129, 130
Travacalm™ 106
Travel, preparation for, 101-106, 120, 136 ; direction of flight and insulin, 104; documents for, 102, 104; jet lag, 104; traveller's survival kit, 101
Treatment, dental, 63
Treatment of hyperglycaemia, 40, 41
Treatment of hypoglycaemia, 40, 41
Triathlons, 18
Triglycerides, 74, 97
Twins, and diabetes, 117, 119
Type 1 diabetes, 82, 129; and hyperglycaemia, 42; and illness, 47; genetics of, 117- 119; rate of in Australia, 124
Type 2 diabetes, 16, 17, 82, 129; and hyperglycaemia, 42; and illness, 47; causes of, 125; ethnic differences in, 124; genetics of, 117-119; increasing rate of, 120, 123; in the elderly, 83; lifestyle disease, 8; prevention of, 87, 88, 131; research in, 130

Ultrasound examinations, 70
Ultratard™ 23, 26
Underwriting rules, insurance, 111
Unistick™, 35
Units, insulin, 22, 25, 103
Unsworth, Maureen, v, 93-95, 96-98
Update newsletter, 114
Urinary protein, 98; substances tested for, 36; testing, 36-38, 104, 133
Vaccinations, for the elderly, 84

Vacuum-assisted erection, 65
Vaginal infection, 53
van Netten, Dianne, 10-13
Vascular disease, 52; peripheral, 73
Vasodilation, 65
Viagra, 46, 65
Virus, as trigger for diabetes, 117
Vision, effects of diabetes on, 56
Visual testing, blood glucose, 32, 104; reasons for inaccuracy, 34; strips available, 34
Vomiting, 42, 47, 48, 49

'Walk for the Cure', 115
Wanigela people, 124
Warfarin, 44
Weight, 8, 10, 51, 87, 93, 94, 98; ideal, 84; loss, 11
Welborn, Timothy, v, 39-42
Western Pacific Region, of IDF, 121
Westmead Children's Hospital, Feeding Guide, 49
Withdrawing insulin, 25, 26, 29
Women's health, 134; diabetes and, 66, 67
Work, 97, 108

Xanthelasma, 55
Xanthoma, 55
Xerostomia, 63

Yeast infection, 66
Your Friend Has Diabetes, 114

Zimmett, Paul, v, 123-125
Zyloprim, 44